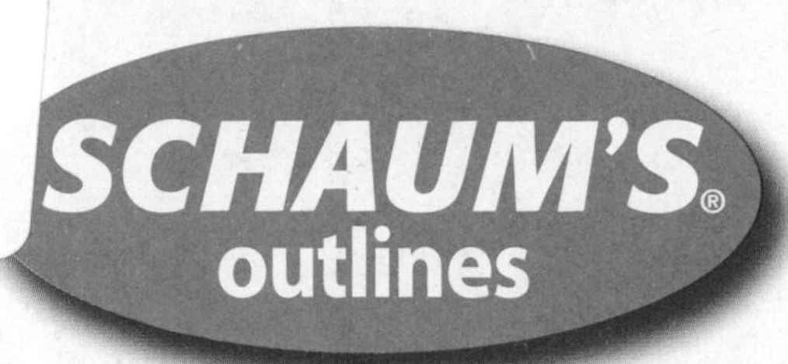

Critical Care Nursing

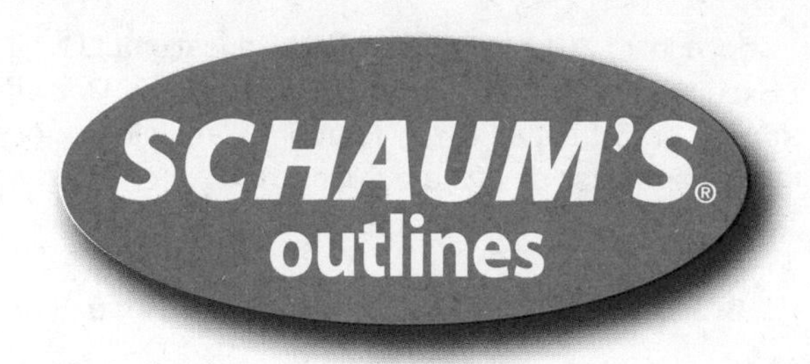

Critical Care Nursing

James Keogh, RN

Schaum's Outline Series

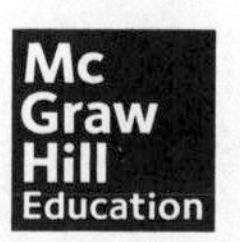

New York Chicago San Francisco Lisbon London Madrid
Mexico City Milan New Delhi San Juan Seoul
Singapore Sydney Toronto

1 2 3 4 5 6 7 8 9 10 QVR/QVR 2 0 1 9 8 7 6 5 4 3

ISBN 978-0-07-178992-9
MHID 0-07-178992-8

e-ISBN 978-0-07-178993-6
e-MHID 0-07-178993-6

Library of Congress Control Number: 2012948444

This book is printed on acid-free paper.

James Keogh, RN-BC, BSN, MBA, is a registered nurse and has written *Schaum's Outline of Pharmacology, Schaum's Outline of Nursing Laboratory and Diagnostic Tests, Schaum's Outline of Medical-Surgical Nursing*, and *Schaum's Outline of Medical Charting* and co-authored *Schaum's Outline of ECG Interpretation*. His books can be found in leading university libraries including Yale University School of Medicine, University of Pennsylvania Biomedical Library, Columbia University, Brown University, University of Medicine and Dentistry of New Jersey, Cambridge University, and Oxford University. He is a former member of the faculty of Columbia University and a member of the faculty of New York University.

This book is dedicated to Anne, Sandy, Joanne, Amber-Leigh Christine, Shawn, Eric, and Amy, without whose help and support this book couldn't have been written.

Contents

CHAPTER 1 **Critical Care Basics** 1

1.1 Definitions 1.2 Physiological Compensation 1.3 Measuring Patient Risk Factors 1.4 Critical Care Thinking 1.5 Analyzing Findings 1.6 Critical Care Stressors 1.7 Critical Care and the Family 1.8 Documentation 1.9 Ethical Challenges of Critical Care 1.10 Cost of Critical Care 1.11 Critical Care Standards 1.12 Critical Care Legal Issues

CHAPTER 2 **Multisystem Critical Care** 21

2.1 Definitions 2.2 Cellular Function 2.3 Digestion 2.4 Cells and Glucose 2.5 Oxygen, Carbon Dioxide, and Blood 2.6 Cardiovascular System 2.7 Blood 2.8 Immune System 2.9 Kidneys 2.10 Fluids and Electrolytes 2.11 Acid-Base 2.12 Endocrine System 2.13 Neurologic System

CHAPTER 3 **Cardiovascular Critical Care** 43

3.1 Definitions 3.2 Critical Care Cardiovascular Assessment 3.3 Critical Care Chest Pain Assessment 3.4 Cardiac Tests 3.5 Cardiac Medication 3.6 Aortic Aneurysm 3.7 Angina (Angina Pectoris) 3.8 Myocardial Infarction (MI) 3.9 Cardiac Tamponade 3.10 Cardiogenic Shock 3.11 Endocarditis 3.12 Congestive Heart Failure (CHF) 3.13 Hypertension and Hypertensive Crisis 3.14 Hypovolemic Shock 3.15 Myocarditis 3.16 Pericarditis 3.17 Pulmonary Edema 3.18 Thrombophlebitis 3.19 Atrial Fibrillation 3.20 Asystole 3.21 Ventricular Fibrillation 3.22 Ventricular Tachycardia 3.23 Cardiac Arrest 3.24 Fibrinolytic Therapy 3.25 Acute Stroke 3.26 Acute Coronary Syndrome 3.27 Cardiac Contusion 3.28 Coronary Artery Bypass Graft (CABG) 3.29 Valve Surgery 3.30 Vascular Surgery 3.31 Vascular Assist Device 3.32 Balloon Catheterization 3.33 Synchronized Cardioversion 3.34 Pacemaker

CHAPTER 4 **Respiratory Critical Care** 117

4.1 Definitions 4.2 Respiratory Tests 4.3 Respiratory Medication 4.4 Acute Respiratory Distress Syndrome (ARDS) 4.5 Asthma 4.6 Atelectasis 4.7 Bronchiectasis 4.8 Bronchitis 4.9 Cor Pulmonale

4.10 Emphysema 4.11 Pleural Effusion 4.12 Pneumonia
4.13 Pneumothorax 4.14 Respiratory Acidosis 4.15 Tuberculosis
4.16 Acute Respiratory Failure 4.17 Pulmonary Embolism
4.18 Respiratory Arrest 4.19 Respiratory Procedures

CHAPTER 5 **Gastrointestinal Critical Care** 163

5.1 Definitions 5.2 Gastrointestinal Tests 5.3 Gastrointestinal Medications
5.4 Appendicitis 5.6 Cirrhosis of the Liver 5.7 Crohn's Disease
5.8 Diverticulitis 5.9 Gastroenteritis 5.10 Gastroesophageal Reflux
Disease (GERD) 5.11 Gastrointestinal Bleeding 5.12 Gastritis
5.13 Hepatitis 5.14 Hiatal Hernia (Diaphragmatic Hernia)
5.15 Intestinal Obstruction and Paralytic Ileus 5.16 Pancreatitis
5.17 Peritonitis 5.18 Peptic Ulcer Disease (PUD) 5.19 Ulcerative
Colitis 5.20 Abdominal Trauma 5.21 Gastrointestinal Procedures

CHAPTER 6 **Renal Critical Care** 208

6.1 Definitions 6.2 Renal Tests 6.3 Urinary Medication 6.4 Acute
Glomerulonephritis 6.5 Kidney Trauma 6.6 Kidney stones (Renal
Calculi) 6.7 Pyelonephritis 6.8 Renal Failure 6.9 Urinary Tract
Infection 6.10 Bladder Cancer 6.11 Kidney Cancer 6.12 Acute
Tubular Necrosis 6.13 Renal Procedures

CHAPTER 7 **Endocrine Critical Care** 239

7.1 Definitions 7.2 Endocrine Tests 7.3 Endocrine Medication
7.4 Hypothyroidism (Myxedema) 7.5 Hyperthyroidism (Graves' Disease)
7.6 Addison's Disease 7.7 Syndrome of Inappropriate Antidiuretic
Hormone Secretion (SIADH) 7.8 Cushing's Syndrome 7.9 Diabetes
Insipidus 7.10 Primary Aldosteronism (Conn's Syndrome)
7.11 Pheochromocytoma 7.12 Hyperparathyroidism
7.13 Diabetes Mellitus 7.14 Metabolic Syndrome
(Syndrome X/Dysmetabolic Syndrome)

CHAPTER 8 **Environmental Critical Care** 267

8.1 Definitions 8.2 Environmental Tests and Procedures
8.3 Environmental Medication 8.4 Hyperthermia 8.5 Hypothermia
8.6 Burns 8.7 Poisoning

CHAPTER 9 **Neurologic Critical Care** 287

9.1 Definitions 9.2 Neurologic Tests and Procedures 9.3 Neurologic
Medication 9.4 Cerebral Hemorrhage 9.5 Bell's Palsy 9.6 Brain Abscess
9.7 Brain Tumor 9.8 Cerebral Aneurysm 9.9 Encephalitis 9.10 Guillain-Barré
Syndrome 9.11 Meningitis 9.12 Spinal Cord Injury 9.13 Cerebrovascular
Accident (CVA) 9.14 Seizure Disorder 9.15 Concussion 9.16 Contusion
9.17 Subdural Hematoma 9.18 Diffuse Axonal Injury 9.19 Skull Fracture
9.20 Intracerebral Hematoma 9.21 Subarachnoid Hemorrhage

CHAPTER 10 Hematologic and Immune Critical Care 325

10.1 Definitions **10.2** Hematologic and Immune Tests **10.3** Hematologic and Immune Medication **10.4** Anemia **10.5** Aplastic Anemia (Pancytopenia) **10.6** Iron Deficiency Anemia **10.7** Pernicious Anemia **10.8** Disseminated Intravascular Coagulation (DIC) **10.9** Hemophilia **10.10** Leukemia **10.11** Multiple Myeloma **10.12** Polycythemia Vera **10.13** Sickle Cell Anemia **10.14** Deep Vein Thrombosis **10.15** Idiopathic Thrombocytopenic Purpura (ITP) **10.16** Acquired Immunodeficiency Syndrome (AIDS) **10.17** Anaphylaxis **10.18** Kaposi's sarcoma (KS) **10.19** Lymphoma **10.20** Scleroderma **10.21** Septic shock

INDEX 375

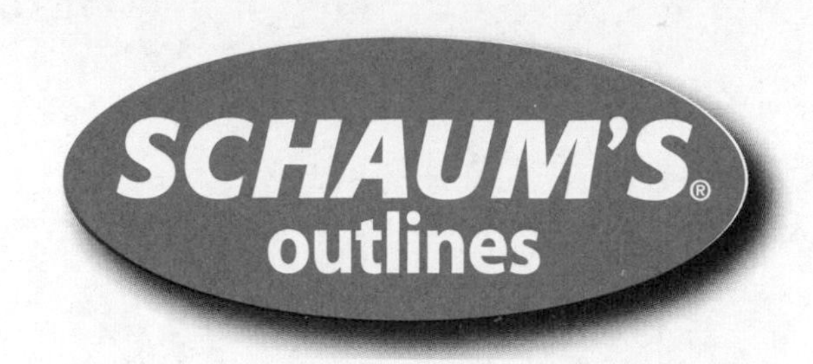

Critical Care Nursing

Critical Care Basics

1.1 Definitions

A critical care patient:

- Is at high risk for or has a life-threatening illness.
- Is unstable.
- Requires intense and constant care in a critical care unit (CCU).
- Has massive disruption of physiology that requires medical intervention to maintain the physiology until normal physiology is restored.

Differences between critical care and emergency medicine:

- Critical care:
  - Focuses on stabilizing an unstable patient who is in a critical stage.
  - A diagnosis is required to initiate care.
  - The environment is controlled.
  - Care can continue for months.
- Emergency medicine:
  - Focuses on stabilizing an unstable patient who is in a crisis stage.
  - A diagnosis is not required to initiate care.
  - The environment is less controlled.
  - Care continues for less than 24 hours.
- CCU:
  - High patient-to-nurse ratio (2:1).
  - Invasive monitoring equipment (e.g., intracranial pressure monitoring) is used to monitor the patient continually.
  - Mechanical devices (e.g., continuous dialysis, mechanical ventilation) used to sustain life.

1.2 Physiological Compensation

- Physiological compensation is the reaction to change by systems within the body. For example, the fight-or-flight response occurs in some stressful situations. Heart and respiratory rates increase and some blood vessels contract, whereas other blood vessels dilate to increase the availability of oxygenated blood as a way to compensate for fighting or running. When blood glucose levels reach 200 mg/dl, the kidneys excrete more water to flush glucose from the blood. Physiological reserve is the body's ability to compensate for change. The lower the physiological reserve, the less likely that the body can compensate to change, leading to the potential of life-threatening illness.
- The physiological reserve decreases with aging and disorders of one or more systems within the body.
  - Aging: Decreased physiological reserve of the liver in the elderly may result in reduced metabolism of some medications, leading to the risk of ineffective therapeutic effect of the medication and the risk of an overdose of the medication.
  - Disorders of systems: Decreased physiological reserve of the immune system may lead to immunodeficiency, increasing the risk of infection that the immune system is unable to fight.
- A goal of the CCU staff is to provide therapeutic support to the patient when the patient's physiological reserves are decreased. The combination of therapeutic support and the available physiological reserves may enable the body to compensate physiologically for the change.

1.2.1 Measuring the physiological reserve

- Physiological reserve is measured by indicators that are based on the performance of a specific system.
  - Cardiac system: A physiological reserve can be measured as the difference between the patient's resting heart rate and the heart rate at which ischemia angina occurs during a stress electrocardiography or echocardiography.
  - Pulmonary system: A physiological reserve can be measured as partial pressure of end-tidal CO_2 ($PaCO_2$) in arterial blood gas. A rise in CO_2 indicates a low pulmonary system physiological reserve.
  - Renal system: A physiological reserve can be measured as glomerular filtration rate using the 24-hour creatinine clearance test, where a value less than 20 ml/minute indicates decreased renal system physiological reserve.
  - Hematopoietic (blood production) system: Physiological reserves can be measured as serum hemoglobin and platelet count. Decreased physiological reserves for hemoglobin are below 7g/l and below 50,000 for platelet count.
- Measuring the physiological reserves of other systems is difficult, and efforts to do so can produced misleading results.

1.2.2 Multiorgan dysfunction syndrome

- Multiorgan dysfunction syndrome is when the physiological reserves of an organ cannot compensate for a change. This leads to a cascade effect that taxes the physiological reserves of other organs, which depletes those organs' physiological reserves, resulting in multiorgan dysfunction.
- For example, respiratory distress leads to a rise in CO_2 in arterial blood gas, resulting in increased heart rate to provide oxygenated blood to organs throughout the body. When cardiac reserves are

depleted, the heart rate slows. Organs, including the heart, no longer receive oxygen, leading to multiorgan dysfunction.

- A goal of the CCU is to enlist a preemptive strategy that uses therapeutic interventions to assist an organ to compensate before the physiological reserve is depleted, thereby postponing or preventing multiorgan dysfunction syndrome from occurring.

1.3 Measuring Patient Risk Factors

- There are many methods used by some CCUs to assess the patient's risk of mortality based on the patient's current presentation and history.
  - Acute Physiology and Chronic Health Evaluation (APACHE): This is a computer system developed by William A. Knaus at George Washington, University Hospital in Washington, D.C., that uses a database of more than 18,000 medical records to predict a patient's risk of dying in a hospital. The projection by APACHE is 95% accurate.
  - Simplified Acute Physiology Score (SAPS): This system predicts mortality of patients in CCUs according to the severity of disease. The SAPS score is a value between 0 and 163 that is converted to a mortality prediction of between 0% and 100%. The mortality prediction is a statistical projection. The SAPS score is calculated using 12 physiological measurements after the first 24 hours in the intensive care unit.
  - Mortality Probability Model (MPM): This is a system that predicts mortality of a patient in the intensive care unit by 15 factors that include cardiac function, liver function, renal function, and age. MPM is used within 1 hour of admission to the CCU.
  - Multiple organ failure (MOF): This is an assessment of a patient's mortality based on the number of organs that have exhausted their physiological reserves.
  - Sequential Organ failure Assessment Score (SOFA): This is a system that monitors the patient's status while in the CCU. The total SOFA score is based on the score for six physiological functions: respiratory, cardiovascular, hepatic, coagulation, renal, and neurologic. A higher score for each physiological function indicates a decline in physiological reserves.

1.4 Critical Care Thinking

- Critical care thinking is an approach to problem solving that focuses on the entire patient rather than the patient's current diagnosis. The patient is admitted to the CCU because of current or potential lack of physiological reserves of multiple organs to compensate for the current diagnosis.
- The initial goal when the patient is admitted to the CCU is to assess each of the patient's organs and systems to identify a list of problems or potential problems. A problem is any abnormal physiology.
- The secondary goal is to reverse all abnormal physiology by identifying and treating the underlying cause of the abnormal physiology. For example, a high serum potassium level is an abnormal physiology caused by malfunctioning kidneys. Intravenous (IV) administration of glucose and insulin can lower serum potassium levels; however, kidney dialysis may be necessary to address the underlying cause of the problem, which is kidney failure in this example.
- Each assessment seeks to answer the question, Why should the patient be treated in the CCU?

- The list of problems or potential problems is dynamic. Some problems resolve while new problems are presented as a result of cascading organ and system failure. Therefore, every organ and system must be evaluated in each assessment to develop a whole picture of the patient's status.
- Revise the list of problems or potential problems after each assessment is completed.
- Revise treatment for each problem or potential problem as necessary.
- Ask the question, Is the situation futile? Collectively, the patient's organs and systems have limited physiological reserves. Treatment in the CCU provides additional physiological reserves until the patient's organs and systems can compensate for the physiological imbalance. However, there is a time when the patient's organs and systems will never be able to compensate for the physiological imbalance. Life support provided by the critical care unit maintains the patient's life. Removing life support results in death. Therefore, the situation is futile.

1.4.1 Critical care assessment

- The critical care assessment begins with the patient's history. Typically, the patient's history has been documented by the sending unit (i.e., emergency department, medical surgical unit) prior to the patient's arrival to the CCU. The patient may be unable to provide a history because of his or her condition.
- Trust but verify all documented information about the patient. The patient is transferred to the CCU because the sending unit is unable to treat the patient. The CCU staff must reassess the patient.
- Develop a baseline of the patient's health related to the patient's age.
  - Identify current and past medical problems and chronic medical conditions. Be sure to identify conditions that may have resulted from work or environmental exposure to toxins.
  - Identify the presenting problem that caused the patient to be admitted to the hospital. The presenting problem may be different from the current problem that caused the patient to be admitted to the CCU.
- Develop a timeline of events.
  - Chief complaint that brought the patient to the hospital.
  - Complications that caused the patient to be admitted to the CCU.
  - Potential problems that may likely occur if interventions are not initiated.
- Objective assessment of the patient's physiological reserves.
- Develop a problem list. Each problem must have a treatment and desired outcome that is measured objectively by physiological targets.

1.4.2 Physical assessment

- Begin the physical assessment by introducing yourself to the patient, and explain that you are going to assess the patient. Do this even if the parent is unresponsive because the patient may be able to hear and understand you.
- Take a minute to review the output of monitors that are connected to the patient. These readings provide insight into the current status of the patient. Typically, they include a cardiac monitor, blood pressure, respiratory monitor, ventilator settings, infusion pumps, and drainage from the patient's body.

- Perform a head-to-toe assessment. Be sure to roll the patient to assess the patient's back and assess the skin and skin breakdown.
- Determine the patient's level of consciousness using the GCS (see 1.4.3 Glasgow Coma Scale).
- Head:
  - Eyes open. Pupils equal and reacting to light.
  - Mouth free from trauma.
  - Patent airway.
  - All tubes are patent.
- Chest:
  - Heart sounds.
  - Respiration.
  - Chest expansion.
  - Lungs.
  - Drainage tubes are patent.
- Arms and hands:
  - Skin.
  - Range of motion (ROM).
  - Patent IV lines.
- Abdomen:
  - Bowel sounds present.
  - Bowel movement.
  - Urinary output.
  - Drainage tubes are patent.
  - Femoral line patent.
- Legs and feet:
  - Skin.
  - ROM.
- Note normal and abnormal results.

1.4.3 Glasgow Coma Scale

- GCS assesses the conscious state of the patient.
- GCS was developed at the University of Glasgow's Institute of Neurological Sciences. There are three tests performed to assess the patient using GCS. These are:
  - Eye responses.
  - Verbal responses.
  - Motor responses.
- Each test results in a score (Table 1.1). The sum of these scores is used to assess the conscious state of the patient.

TABLE 1.1 Glasgow Coma Scale

	1	2	3	4	5	6
Eyes	Does not open eyes	Opens eyes in response to painful stimuli	Opens eyes in response to voice	Opens eyes spontaneously	N/A	N/A
Verbal	Makes no sounds	Incomprehensible sounds	Utters inappropriate words	Confused, disoriented	Oriented, converses, normally	N/A
Motor	Makes no movements	Extension to painful stimuli (decerebrate response)	Abnormal flexion to painful stimuli (decorticate response)	Flexion/withdrawal to painful stimuli	Localizes painful stimuli	Obeys commands

1.5 Analyzing Findings

- Primarily focus on physiological reserves of critical systems. A physiological reserve is a dynamic value within a range from normal to critical, similar to a fuel gauge. Each critical system has a unique range.
  - Respiratory system: The physiological reserve of the respiratory system can be measured by the arterial oxygenation value. The lower the value, the less oxygen is available to organs.

TABLE 1.2 Arterial Oxygenation Range

PaO_2/FiO2 (mmHg) Arterial Oxygenation	Range
<400	Normal
<300	
<200	Critical mechanical ventilation used
<100	

  - Neurologic system: The neurologic system reserve is measured by the GCS value (see 1.4.3 Glasgow Coma Scale). The lower the value, the lower the reserve.

TABLE 1.3 Glasgow Coma Scale Physiological Reserve Measurements

Glasgow Coma Scale	Range
13–14	Normal
10–12	
6–9	Critical
<6	

- Cardiovascular system: The physiological reserve of the cardiovascular system is measured by the mean arterial pressure (MAP). MAP is the average arterial pressure during a cardiac cycle. Abnormal values indicate a risk that organs will not be perfused with blood.

TABLE 1.4 Cardiovascular System Physiological Reserve Measurements

Mean Arterial Pressure (MAP)	Range
> or =70 mmHg	Normal
< 50 mmHg	Critical

- Liver: The physiological reserve of the liver is measured by total bilirubin in serum. Bilirubin is the byproduct of hemoglobin in red blood cells. The liver removes bilirubin from blood. The higher the value, the less the liver is removing bilirubin.

TABLE 1.5 Liver Physiological Reserve Measurements

Bilirubin (mg/dl)	Range
1.2–1.9	Normal
2.0–5.9	
6.0–11.9	
>12	Critical

- Coagulation: The physiological reserve of coagulation is measured by the amount of platelets in blood. Platelets coagulate blood when a blood vessel ruptures. The lower the value, the fewer platelets are available to coagulate blood.

TABLE 1.6 Coagulation Physiological Reserve Measurements

Platelets ($\times 10^3$/mcl)	Range
<150	Normal
<100	
<50	Critical
<20	

- Renal: The physiological reserve of kidneys is measured by the amount of creatinine in blood. Creatinine is a byproduct created when muscle is metabolized. Kidneys filter creatinine, which is excreted in urine. The higher the value, the greater decrease in kidney function.

TABLE 1.7 Renal Physiological Reserve Measurements

Creatinine (mg/dl)	Range
1.2–1.91	Normal
2.0–3.4	
3.5–4.9	Critical
>5.0	

1.5.1 Critical factors

- The focus of a critical care assessment progresses to the patient's critical factors. Determine whether the factor is normal or abnormal. If abnormal, then identify the underlying cause of why the factor is abnormal. The treatment plan developed by the patient's healthcare team should include interventions that return the factor to within acceptable limits.
- Neurologic
  - GCS
  - Ramsay Sedation Score
  - Sedation Agitation Scale (SAS)
- Respiratory
  - Respiratory rate.
  - Partial pressure of arterial O_2 (PaO_2).
  - Partial pressure of end-tidal CO_2 ($PaCO_2$).
- Cardiovascular
  - Heart rate.
  - Blood pressure.
  - MAP to measure end-organ perfusion.
  - Urinary output to measure end-organ perfusion.
  - Anemia.
    - Hematocrit (Hct) low.
    - Hemoglobin (Hgb) low.
    - Total iron-binding capacity low.
    - Iron low.
    - Ferritin low.
    - Red blood cells (RBCs) low.
  - Risk for bleeding
    - Platelet count $<$37,000.
    - Partial thromboplastin time (PTT) high.
    - Prothrombin time (PT) high.
    - International normalized ratio (INR) high.
- Nutrition
  - Malnutrition
    - Prealbumin: decreased.
    - Albumin: decreased.
- Gastrointestinal
  - Bowel sounds.
  - Bowel movement.
  - Passing flatus.
- Fluid balance
  - Dehydration
    - Blood:
      - Hct high.

      - Hgb high.
      - RBC high.
      - Albumin high.
    - Urine specific gravity: high.
  - Overhydration
    - Blood:
      - Hct low.
      - Hgb low.
      - RBC low.
      - Albumin low.
    - Urine specific gravity: low.
- Pancreas
  - Amylase high.
  - Lipase high.
- Liver function
  - Albumin low.
  - Alanine aminotransferase (ALT) high.
  - Aspartate aminotransferase (AST) high.
  - Total bilirubin high.
  - Direct bilirubin high.
- Renal function
  - Urine output less than 1 ml/kg/hr.
  - Creatinine high.
  - Blood urea nitrogen (BUN) high.
- Endocrine
  - Blood glucose.
- Immune system
  - CD4 low.
  - White blood cell count (WBC) <2000.
  - Erythrocyte sedimentation rate (ESR) high.
  - Neutrophils high.
  - Eosinpohils high.
  - Lymphocytes high.

1.6 Critical Care Stressors

- The CCU is stressful for the patient because of stressors that are common to a CCU. Stressors can exacerbate the patient's condition and deplete physiological reserves. Common stressors are:
  - The fear of death: Admitting a patient to the CCU implies to everyone, including the patient, that the patient's medical condition is unstable.

  - The fear of permanent disability: The patient has grounds to be concerned that life as the patient knows it has changed and that the patient will not be able to return to a fully functional life. Regardless of whether this is or is not the prognosis, the thought of permanent disability stresses the patient.
  - Discomfort: In many situations, the patient is in bed with tubes such as an IV, Foley catheter, and nasogastric (NG) tube inserted into the patient's body, all of which can cause discomfort and pain.
  - Loss of autonomy: The patient has little or no autonomy other than to refuse treatment. This may be the first time in the patient's life when the patient has loss of independence.
  - Lack of privacy: The patient is under constant observation by the healthcare team, who are strangers to the patient.
  - Loss of dignity: The patient lies in the bed naked except for a poorly fitted gown and a sheet. The patient is likely unable to urinate or have a bowel movement privately.
  - Sleep disruption: The circadian rhythm and rapid eye movement (REM) sleep is disrupted by medication, treatment, and the distraction of the critical care unit.
  - Boredom: The patient lies in bed 24 hours a day for weeks broken only by brief, timed visits from a few relatives.
  - Separation: The patient is likely to experience separation anxiety from family and friends. All contact with those other than the healthcare team is carefully controlled by the healthcare team.
  - Lack of coping skills: Stressors are managed by using coping skills, such as walking, as a distraction. The critical care patient's coping skills usually cannot be implemented in a CCU; therefore, the patient has little ability to cope with critical care unit stressors.
  - Frustration: The patient can easily become frustrated by lack of autonomy, lack of coping skills, and lack of immediate resolution of the patient's disorder.
- The critical care nurse must realize that the patient has a feeling of powerlessness that leads to hopelessness. Stressors and the lack of coping may hinder the restoration of physiological reserves.
- The nurse cannot eliminate all stressors related to the CCU. However, the nurse can take steps to reduce the level of stress for the patient.
  - Acknowledge: Tell the patient that you realize the stress he or she is experiencing. Identify each stressor. This validates the patient's feelings.
  - Educate the patient: The appropriate member of the healthcare team needs to explain to the patient the patient's diagnosis and prognosis. Address the patient's concerns about death and permanent disability.
  - Provide the patient with milestones: A milestone is an outcome that is easily recognized and understood by the patient. A milestone gives the patient some autonomy in that the patient will know that the treatment is progressing without being told so by the healthcare team.
  - Discomfort: Focus on making the patient comfortable even when the patient does not complain.
  - Communication: Always talk to the patient and develop a way for the patient to communicate with you if the patient is unable to talk. Assume that the patient is able to hear your conversation, especially when you and other healthcare team members are talking at bedside. If possible, include the patient in your conversation.
  - Minimum disruption: Within the limitations of the treatment plan, organize interventions on a predictable schedule. This minimizes disrupting the patient and provides order for the patient's day.
  - Interact with the patient: Within the limitations of the treatment plan and the patient's condition, spend a few caring moments with the patient during which you explore the patient's feelings and, if appropriate, nontreatment-related small talk. These moments help the patient feel like a person rather than a patient.

1.7 Critical Care and the Family

- Although the patient is the primary concern of the critical care nurse, the patient's family is also a focus of the nurse. Family members experience new stressors when a loved one is admitted to the CCU. And as with the patient, family members may lack coping skills to handle those stressors.
- The critical care nurse must receive written consent from the patient to discuss the patient's medical condition and treatment with family members.
- Identify the patient's family members and their relationship to the patient.
- Ask the family to designate a family liaison. A family liaison is a family member who will facilitate communication between the healthcare team and the family. The healthcare team contacts the family liaison, and the family liaison disseminates the information to the family. Furthermore, the family liaison may facilitate family members' visits with the patient.
- Family members have some of the same stressors as the patient. These include the following:
  - The fear of death: Family members realize that the patient is unstable but probably are concerned that the patient may die.
  - The fear of permanent disability: The patient may play a key role in the family, such as providing financial resources or supportive resources (e.g., child care). Permanent or temporary disability may have a serious impact on other family members.
  - Separation: The family is likely to experience separation anxiety from the patient. One or two family members may visit with the patient for 15 minutes and then leave. The lack of the patient's presence is felt at home.
  - Lack of coping skills: Family members may be unable to cope with the patient's condition and other stressors related to the patient's stay in the CCU.
  - Frustration: The family can easily become frustrated with minimum visits, lack of immediate improvement in the patient's condition, lack of response by the patient, and issues at home related to the patient being admitted to the CCU (e.g., financial, child care, transportation).
- The nurse can assess how family members are coping with stressors by reaching out to the family whenever possible. The goal is to establish mutual trust.
  - Acknowledge: Validate family members' concerns by identifying each stressor.
  - Active listening: Take time to listen to family members. Give family members your undivided attention.
  - Explore feelings: Help family members process feelings by assisting family members to think rationally.
  - Educate the family: The appropriate member of the healthcare team needs to explain to the patient's family the patient's diagnosis, treatment plan, and prognosis. Address the family's concerns about death and permanent disability.
  - Provide the patient and family with milestones: A milestone is an outcome that is easily recognized and understood by family members.
  - Communication: Keep open a line of communication between the healthcare team and the family. Be honest and direct. If you promise to call the family liaison, then be sure to call. If you arrange for the family liaison to call you at a particular time, then be available to take the call. Tell family members:
    - Facts known and unknown about the patient's health.
    - Treatment plan.
    - Interventions.
    - Outcomes of interventions.

- Set expectations: Family members do not know what to expect when the patient becomes unstable and is admitted to the CCU. The healthcare team needs to set the family expectations immediately and reset expectations during the course of treatment. Family members need to know:
  - Will the patient recover?
  - Will the patient regain all functionality (e.g., return to work, care for children)?
  - When will we know whether the patient is improving?
  - What is wrong with the patient?
  - How much is treatment going to cost the patient/family?
- Explain unit rules: Although some family members may be familiar with visiting patients in the hospital, many family members are unfamiliar with the unique rules of the CCU. Take time to explain the rules and the rationale behind the rules.

- Give family members time to adapt to the fact that the patient is in an unstable condition by helping family members work through the stages of adaptation. Stages of adaptation are:
  - Disbelief: The family does not believe that the patient can be so ill.
  - Developing awareness: The family learns about the diagnosis, treatment, and prognosis and how the patient's unstable condition impacts the family.
  - Reorganization: The family accepts that the patient is unstable and then plans to change.
  - Resolution: The family learns from others who have been in a similar situation about what changes are needed.
  - Identifying change: The family decides what needs to change and implements the change.

1.8 Documentation

- Background: Documentation should begin with a brief description of the patient's medical history and the events leading to admission to the CCU.
- Current problems: Next should be a list of current problems. A current problem is an abnormal condition that requires an intervention to resolve.
- Review of systems: The status of each system is then documented based on the results of the patient assessments. Both normal and abnormal findings should be documented. This enables the healthcare team to track the patient's progression while in the CCU.
- Impression: The impression is an opinion about the patient's status based on interpretation of the patient's history, events leading to admission to the CCU, current problem list, and the status of the patient's systems.
- Plan: Documentation concludes with the treatment plan. The treatment plan focuses on current problems. A current problem may be the result of cascading organ failure that needs treatment until the underlying condition resolves. For example, the patient may have low respiratory reserves. The treatment plan may call for the patient to be placed on a mechanical ventilator while the underlying cause of the respiratory problem is being treated.

1.9 Ethical Challenges of Critical Care

- Ethics is a moral philosophy of choosing right from wrong based on a standard. For example, the nurse who stays with a patient who is in crisis makes an ethical choice based on a moral and nursing standard.

- Ethical dilemma is a conflict between two ethical standards, each justifying opposing actions. For example, a scarce organ becomes available for transplant. Should it be given to a 70-year-old patient or a 24-year-old patient? The ethical principle of justice states that all patients are treated as equals. However, the 24-year-old patient will have a longer natural life span than the 70-year-old patient and therefore would be more deserving of the scarce organ.
- A frequent ethical challenge in critical care is the conflict between the cost of critical care and medical futility. Medical futility occurs when the patient's physiological reserves are depleted and it is believed that they are unable to be restored.
- Medical technology is used in the CCU to supplement the patient's depleting physiological reserves of one or more organ or system. As the underlying cause resolves, the patient's physiological reserves are naturally restored and the supplementary physiological reserves provided by medical technology are removed.
- Common ethical challenges are:
  - What should happen if the patient's physiological reserves are not naturally restored? The patient remains alive because of the supplemental support of medical technology.
  - Who determines whether maintaining the patient on life support is medically futile?
  - Maintaining the patient on life support is costly to the healthcare facility and to the patient and patient's family. The cost is justified if the patient's physiology is restored. Is the cost justified if life support is medically futile?
  - Further complicating the ethical dilemma is the limited availability of critical care resources. The patient whose condition is medically futile is using critical care resources that can be used for a patient whose physiological reserves can be naturally restored with the assistance of critical care medical technology.

1.9.1 Ethical principles

- Autonomy: Autonomy is when the patient makes decisions about his or her healthcare. The critical care nurse must provide the patient with objective and complete information about the diagnosis, all treatment options, and medical probability of all outcomes. The critical care nurse must accept the patient's decision about treatment.
- Beneficence: Beneficence is the requirement that the nurse promote the well-being of the patient by preventing harm to the patient. That is, the nurse must do something that prevents the patient from being harmed. A common conflict occurs when the patient refuses treatment (autonomy) and by doing so the patient's condition worsens (the patient is harmed).
- Nonmaleficence: Nonmaleficence is for the nurse to do no harm. That is, the nurse must not do anything that will harm the patient. There can be conflict between nonmaleficence and beneficence as illustrated by giving an intramuscular injection. Administering the injection does harm to the patient (contrary to nonmaleficence); however, the medication that is injected prevents the patient from being harmed further by the disorder (beneficence).
- Veracity: Veracity requires that the nurse be truthful to the patient. Conflict between veracity and beneficence can arise when the desired treatment (beneficence) results in material discomfort to the patient. In order to obtain consent (autonomy) for the procedure, the nurse minimizes the discomfort when explaining the treatment to the patient (contrary to veracity).
- Fidelity: Fidelity is faithfulness to the patient. The nurse is expected to maintain a trusting relationship with the patient. Fidelity often conflicts with beneficence. For example, the patient may reveal pertinent information to the nurse and ask the nurse not to share the information with the healthcare team. Fidelity conflicts may be avoided by applying veracity, that is, telling the patient what is and is not feasible. In the previous example, the nurse may have told the patient that

the information may be shared with the healthcare team in order to provide the patient with the best possible care.

- Justice: Justice requires the nurse to treat all patients equally. Conflicts with justice frequently occur in critical care nursing when resources are limited and must be allocated to a patient population. Some patients will have access to the resource and others will have no access, although these patients have the same diagnosis and require the same treatment.

1.9.2 Handling an ethical dilemma

- A framework should be used to assist the healthcare team in resolving an ethical dilemma based on critical care nursing standards and ethical principles. Here is a commonly used decision framework:
    - Identify the problem: Evaluate evidence-based data to assess the patient's diagnosis and prognosis.
    - Define the ethical problem: An ethical problem arises from conflicts in applying ethical principles and nursing standards.
    - Gather information: Expand data collection to include nonmedical data such as the patient's economic status, ethnicity, religion, and support network to develop a holistic picture of the patient.
    - Identify the decision maker: Identify the person on the healthcare team who is responsible for making the ethical decision. The nurse must be aware that resolution of an ethical dilemma may not reside with the nurse. In situations such as treatment, the practitioner makes the ethical decision. In other situations, such as the right to refuse treatment, the patient decides and the nurse respects patient autonomy and then notifies the practitioner. And in other situations, such as allocation of scarce resources, the facility's ethics committee may decide the issue.
    - Review the basis for the ethical dilemma: Clearly identify the principles that are in conflict.
    - Identify options: Before focusing on a course of action, identify and explore all alternatives that may resolve the ethical dilemma.
    - Make the decision: Select the best alternative and then enact that alternative.
    - Assess the outcome: Determine whether the decision resolves the ethical conflict. If not, then use the framework to reassess the ethical dilemma.

1.10 Cost of Critical Care

- The expense of critical care is considerably higher than other care units because of increased use of technology, expensive medications, and a relatively small staff-to-patient ratio. For example, a medical-surgical unit may have a 1:8 nurse-to-patient ratio. Typically, a CCU has a 1:2 nurse-to-patient ratio.
- The healthcare team is confronted by competing interests. There is a general philosophy in society that an all-out effort must be made to sustain everyone, regardless of medical futility. However, the rising cost of healthcare has hospital administrators and medical economics proposing cost effectiveness in medical treatment.
- The healthcare team is guided by an evidence-based approach to provide cost-effective treatment. An evidence-based approach states that treatment decisions are based on documented evidence that a specific treatment will produce a desired outcome to restore the patient's physiological reserves.

1.11 Critical Care Standards

- The American Association of Critical Care Nurses (AACN) established standards for critical care nursing. Standards are organized into the nursing process. These are:
  - Assessment: The nurse collects healthcare data about the patient.
  - Diagnosis: The nurse determines a diagnosis by analyzing patient healthcare data.
  - Outcome: The nurse determines the patient outcome.
  - Planning: The nurse develops interventions to achieve the outcome.
  - Implementation: The nurse develops a care plan to implement interventions.
  - Evaluation: The nurse assesses the patient to determine whether the interventions achieve the outcome.
- The AACN defines the responsibilities of a critical care nurse as:
  - Support the patient in making an informed decision about the patient's medical care.
  - Advocate for the patient to receive care.
  - Respect the patient's beliefs.
  - Educate the patient about healthcare and treatments.
  - Support the patient's healthcare decision.
  - Monitor the quality of care of the patient.
  - Be a liaison between the patient/patient's family and the healthcare team.
- The AACN defines the standards of practice of a critical care nurse as:
  - Quality of care: The nurse systematically evaluates nursing practices.
  - Individual practice evaluation: The nurse reviews regulations, laws, and standards of practice.
  - Education: The nurse maintains knowledge and competency in critical care nursing.
  - Collegiality: The nurse helps to develop a collegial relationship with others on the healthcare team.
  - Ethics: The nurse cares for the patient in an ethical manner.
  - Collaboration: The nurse collaborates with members of the healthcare team when caring for the patient.
  - Research: The nurse will use and develop evidence-based interventions.
  - Resource utilization: The nurse will be cognitive of cost, effectiveness, and safety when planning interventions.

1.12 Critical Care Legal Issues

- A critical care nurse must provide care within the standards of care. Failing to do so may expose the nurse to litigation-based factors law, which are:
  - Negligence: Negligence is failing to act. In critical care, negligence is failure to act as a prudent nurse with similar education and work experience would do under similar circumstances. There must have been an obligation to act. In negligence, the failure to act resulted in injury to the patient and that injury would not have occurred if the nurse had acted appropriately.
  - Malpractice: Malpractice is professional misconduct by the nurse because the nurse has a special standing as a licensed nurse.

- Duty: Duty is obligation to care for a patient based on the nurse-patient relationship. The nurse-patient relationship begins when the nurse renders care to the patient. Duty may occur even if the nurse is not assigned to the patient. For example, a nurse who walks into a patient's room and sees reddening of an IV site has the duty to act even if the nurse is not assigned to the patient.
- Breach: A breach is a failure to act based on the standard of care. Here are commonly breached standards:
  - Failure to adhere to self-determination: The nurse must act in accordance with the patient's wishes.
  - Failure to diagnose: The nursing diagnoses must be appropriate and evidence based. Legal action may occur if the patient is treated for inappropriate diagnoses.
  - Failure to take appropriate action: The nurse must take appropriate action. For example, a heparin lock must be removed when the nurse notices a reddening of an IV site. Failure to act can lead to injury to the patient.
  - Failure to document: The nurse must document findings, interventions, and patient response. Failure to document properly can lead to intervention by others on the healthcare team that may cause injury to the patient. For example, failure to document medication administration may lead to double dosing the patient.
  - Failure to maintain patient privacy: Patient information is disseminated on a need-to-know basis. Releasing patient information inappropriately is a breach of the standard of care.
  - Failure to be the patient's advocate: The nurse is obligated to act on the patient's behalf, including questioning treatment orders. For example, a resident ordered nitroglycerin for an asymptomatic patient without reviewing the patient's current treatment. The patient was ambulatory and had received his maintenance dose of blood pressure medication 30 minutes before the resident issued the order. The nurse politely brought this issue to the resident, who refused to change the nitroglycerin order. The nurse called the attending physician, who ordered the nitroglycerin to be held until the attending assessed the patient. Nitroglycerin administered shortly after administration of blood pressure medication would have caused a dramatic drop in the patient's blood pressure.
- Wrongful death: Survivors of the patient or the patient's estate can bring action against the nurse if the nurse's action or inaction led to the patient's death.
- Defamation: Defamation occurs when the nurse says (slander) or writes (libel) something that is false that injures the patient's reputation.
- Loss of consortium: Loss of consortium occurs when the patient's relationship with one or more family members suffers because of the negligence of the nurse. Emotional distress is an example of loss of consortium, which is difficult to prove.
- Damages: Damages is a monetary amount imposed by the courts to compensate the patient who has been injured by a nurse who had the duty to act and breached that duty.

Solved Problems

1.1 What is a critical care patient?

A critical care patient:

- Is at high risk for or has a life-threatening illness.
- Is unstable.
- Requires intense and constant care in a CCU.

- Has massive disruption of physiology that requires medical intervention to maintain the physiology until the physiology is restored.

1.2 What is a key difference between critical care and emergency medicine?

Emergency medicine does not require a diagnosis to initiate care, whereas critical care requires a diagnosis to initiate care.

1.3 What is physiological compensation?

Physiological compensation is the reaction to change by systems within the body.

1.4 What is a physiological reserve?

Physiological reserve is the body's ability to compensate to change. The lower the physiological reserve, the less likely that the body can compensate to change, leading to the potential of life-threatening illness.

1.5 What can affect physiological reserve?

- Aging: Decreased physiological reserve of the liver in the elderly may result in reduced metabolism of some medications, leading to the risk of ineffective therapeutic effect of the medication and the risk of an overdose of the medication.
- Disorders of systems: Decreased physiological reserve of the immune system may lead to immunodeficiency, increasing the risk of infection because the immune system is unable to fight.

1.6 What is the goal of the CCU staff?

A goal of the CCU staff is to provide therapeutic support to the patient when the patient's physiological reserves are decreased. The combination of therapeutic support and the available physiological reserves may enable the body to physiologically compensate for the change.

1.7 How is a physiological reserve measured?

Physiological reserve is measured by indicators based on the performance of a specific system.

1.8 What is multiorgan dysfunction syndrome?

Multiorgan dysfunction syndrome is when the physiological reserves of an organ cannot compensate for a change, leading to a cascade effect that taxes the physiological reserves of other organs. This effect depletes those organs' physiological reserves and results in multiorgan dysfunction.

1.9 When should therapeutic interventions be enlisted?

A goal of the CCU is to enlist a preemptive strategy that uses therapeutic interventions to assist an organ to compensate before the physiological reserve is depleted, thereby postponing or preventing multiorgan dysfunction syndrome from occurring.

1.10 What is the initial goal when the patient is admitted to the critical care unit?

The initial goal when the patient is admitted to the critical care unit is to assess each of the patient's organs and systems to identify a list of problems or potential problems. A problem is any abnormal physiology.

1.11 What is the secondary goal when the patient is admitted to the CCU?

The secondary goal is to reverse all abnormal physiology by identifying and treating the underlying cause of the abnormal physiology. For example, a high serum potassium level is an abnormal physiology caused by malfunctioning kidneys. Glucose and insulin administered by IV can lower serum potassium levels; however, kidney dialysis may be necessary to address the underlying cause of the problem, which is kidney failure in this example.

1.12 To what does the term *medically futile* refer to?

Collectively, the patient's organs and systems have limited physiological reserves. Treatment in the CCU provides additional physiological reserves until the patient's organs and systems can compensate for the physiological imbalance. However, there is a time when the patient's organs and systems will never be able to compensate for the physiological imbalance. Life support provided by the CCU maintains the patient's life. Removing life support results in death. Therefore, the situation is futile.

1.13 What is a critical care problem list?

A problem list is a list of depleted physiological reserves. Each problem must have a treatment and desired outcome that is measured objectively by physiological targets.

1.14 What is a critical care stressor?

A critical care stressor is a factor of being in the critical unit that exacerbates the patient's condition.

1.15 What are common critical care stressors?

- The fear of the death.
- The fear of permanent disability.
- Discomfort.
- Loss of autonomy.
- Lack of privacy.
- Loss of dignity.
- Sleep disruption.
- Boredom.
- Separation.
- Lack of coping skills.
- Frustration.

1.16 Why is it important for the critical care nurse to reduce the level of stress for the critical care patient?

Stressors and the lack of coping may hinder the restoration of physiological reserves.

1.17 What are common ways the critical care nurse can reduce stress for the patient?

- Acknowledge: Tell the patient that you realize the stress he or she is experiencing.
- Identify each stressor. This validates the patient's feelings.
- Educate the patient: The appropriate member of the healthcare team needs to explain to the patient the patient's diagnosis and prognosis. Address the patient's concerns about death and permanent disability.

- Provide the patient with milestones: A milestone is an outcome that is easily recognized and understood by the patient. A milestone gives the patient some autonomy in that the patient will know that the treatment is progressing without being told so by the healthcare team.
- Discomfort: Focus on making the patient comfortable even when the patient does not complain.
- Communication: Always talk to the patient and develop a way for the patient to communicate with you if the patient is unable to talk. Assume that the patient is able to hear your conversation, especially when you and other healthcare team members are talking at bedside. If possible, include the patient in your conversation.
- Minimum disruption: Within the limitations of the treatment plan, organize interventions on a predictable schedule. This minimizes disrupting the patient and provides order for the patient's day.
- Interact with the patient: Within the limitations of the treatment plan and the patient's condition, spend a few caring moments with the patient during which you explore the patient's feelings and, if appropriate, nontreatment-related small talk. These moments help the patient feel like a person rather than a patient.

1.18 How can the critical care nurse help the critical care patient work through the stages of adaptation?

- Give family members time to adapt to the fact that the patient is in an unstable condition by helping family members work through the stages of adaptation. Stages of adaptation are:
    - Disbelief: The family does not believe that the patient can be so ill.
    - Developing awareness: The family learns about the diagnosis, treatment, and prognosis and how the patient's unstable condition impacts the family.
    - Reorganization: The family accepts that the patient is unstable and then plans to change.
    - Resolution: The family learns from others who have been in a similar situation about what changes are needed.
    - Identifying change: The family decides what needs to change and implements the change.

1.19 What is an ethical dilemma?

Ethical dilemma is a conflict between two ethical standards with each justifying opposing actions.

1.20 What is a common ethical challenge in critical care?

A frequent ethical challenge in critical care is the conflict between the cost of critical care and medical futility. Medical futility occurs when the patient's physiological reserves are depleted and are unable to be restored.

1.21 What is autonomy?

Autonomy involves the patient making decisions about his or her own health care. The critical care nurse must provide the patient with objective and complete information about the diagnosis, all treatment options, and medical probability of all outcomes. The critical care nurse must accept the patient's decision about treatment.

1.22 What framework can be used to handle an ethical dilemma?

- A framework should be used to assist the healthcare team resolve an ethical dilemma based on critical care nursing standards and ethical principles. Here is a commonly used decision framework:
    - Identify the problem: Evaluate evidence-based data to assess the patient's diagnosis and prognosis.

- Define the ethical problem: An ethical problem arises from conflicts in applying ethical principles and nursing standards.
- Gather information: Expand data collection to include nonmedical data, such as the patient's economic status, ethnicity, religion, and support network to develop a holistic picture of the patient.
- Identify the decision maker: Identify the person on the healthcare team who is responsible for making the ethical decision. The nurse must be aware that resolution of an ethical dilemma may not reside with the nurse. In situations such as treatment, the practitioner makes the ethical decision. In other situations, such as the right to refuse treatment, the patient decides and the nurse respects patient autonomy and then notifies the practitioner. And in other situations, such as allocation of scarce resources, the facility's ethics committee may decide the issue.
- Review the basis for the ethical dilemma: Clearly identify the principles that are in conflict.
- Identify options: Before focusing on a course of action, identify and explore all alternatives that may resolve the ethical dilemma.
- Make the decision: Select the best alternative and then enact that alternative.
- Assess the outcome: Determine whether the decision resolves the ethical conflict. If not, then use the framework to reassess the ethical dilemma.

1.23 What are critical care standards?

The AACN established standards for critical care nursing. Standards are organized into the nursing process. These are:

- Assessment: The nurse collects healthcare data about the patient.
- Diagnosis: The nurse determines a diagnosis by analyzing patient healthcare data.
- Outcome: The nurse determines the patient's outcome.
- Planning: The nurse develops interventions to achieve the outcome.
- Implementation: The nurse develops a care plan to implement interventions.
- Evaluation: The nurse assesses the patient to determine whether the interventions achieve the outcome.

1.24 What is the legal concept of duty?

Duty is obligation to care for a patient based on the nurse-patient relationship. The nurse-patient relationship begins when the nurse renders care to the patient. Duty may occur even if the nurse is not assigned to the patient. For example, a nurse who walks into a patient's room and sees reddening of an IV site has the duty to act even if the nurse is not assigned to the patient.

1.25 What is the focus of a critical care assessment progresses?

The focus of a critical care assessment progresses to critical factors of the patient. Determine if the factor is normal or abnormal. If abnormal, then identify the underlying cause of why the factor is abnormal. The treatment plan developed by the patient's healthcare team should include interventions that return the factor to within acceptable limits.

Multisystem Critical Care

2.1 Definitions

- Multisystem critical care focuses on all systems in the patient's body. Each system has a physiological activity and physiological reserve. Decreased physiological reserve of one system may have a cascading effect on other systems in the body as the other systems attempt to compensate for the disorder.
- The critical care healthcare team anticipates cascading system failure and provides technological assistance (e.g., medication, mechanical/electronic devices) to increase physiological reserves until the underlying disorder stabilizes.
- This chapter focuses on understanding key elements of normal physiology and the impact a physiological disorder has on other systems, providing a foundation to anticipate cascading system failure.
- Monitoring the body's systems continually in the critical care unit enables the healthcare team to learn quickly when compensation occurs or when a physiological reserve is stressed.

2.2 Cellular Function

- A cell is the basic building block of the body. Each cell has a specific physiological activity and is grouped together with similar cells to form tissues and organs.
- Physiological activities occur within cells. The hypothalamus gland controls the rate at which these activities occur.
  - A low level of thyroid hormone in blood triggers the hypothalamus to release thyroid-releasing hormone (TRH).
  - TRH triggers the anterior pituitary gland to release thyroid-stimulating hormone (TSH).
  - TSH triggers the thyroid to release triiodothyronine (T3) and thyroxine (T4) into blood.
  - T4 moves into the cell and is converted to T3. The more T4 and T3 in a cell, the higher the physiological activity of the cell.
- To carry out physiological activities, cells require nutrients:
  - Glucose: Glucose is the energy source of cells.
  - Oxygen.

- Enzymes: An enzyme is a protein that increases the rate of a chemical reaction inside the cell.
- Electrolytes: An electrolyte is an element that acquires a positive or negative charge when dissolved in water.
- Inside cells
  - Potassium.
  - Magnesium.
  - Phosphorus.
  - Calcium (cells of bone and teeth).
  - Chloride.
  - Sodium.
- Outside cells
  - Sodium.

- A critical care patient's diet must be adjusted to compensate for the patient's condition. Although the patient is immobile, the patient may require increased carbohydrates, protein, fat, and other nutrients to support the body's effort to compensate for failing systems.
- Waste byproducts of physiological activity of the cell are removed from the cell.
- Blood transports nutrients to cells and removes waste byproducts from cells.
- Most cells have a life span, after which, the cell dies (apoptosis). The cell membrane ruptures, releasing the contents of the cell in the blood. The length of a cell's life depends on the nature of the cell.
- Cell growth
  - Thiamin (Vitamin B1): Thiamin is a coenzyme needed for cellular metabolism.
  - Carbohydrates, lipids, and protein can be broken down by cells (catabolism) and used for energy.
  - Amino acids can be combined by cells into protein (anabolism).

2.3 Digestion

- Many nutrients required by cells are contained in food. The digestion process breaks down ingested food so nutrients can be absorbed into the blood and transported to cells.
- Three key nutrients that are absorbed during digestion are:
  - Carbohydrates: A compound composed of sugar (glucose).
  - Fats: A compound used for cell membranes, to insulate organs from shock, and to help to stabilize body temperature.
  - Protein: A compound that is broken down into essential amino acids. An amino acid is a chemical that is necessary for cells to conduct physiological activities.
- Digestion begins with mechanical and chemical digestion in the mouth, where teeth break food into small pieces. Saliva moistens the food and produces amylase (an enzyme) that starts breaking down carbohydrates. Saliva also kills some bacteria.
- Mechanical/chemical digestion in the mouth converts food into soft pliable material called bolus. Voluntary movement moves the bolus from the oral cavity to the pharynx. The epiglottis closes, preventing the bolus from entering the larynx and respiratory system and enables the bolus to enter the esophagus.

- Involuntary muscles along the esophagus move the bolus using a peristaltic wave through the lower esophageal sphincter into the stomach. The lower esophageal sphincter is a ring of muscles at the end of the esophagus that acts like a valve between the esophagus and the stomach. The lower esophageal sphincter prevents stomach contents from returning to the esophagus.
- The bolus enters the top part of the stomach (cardia), which is a holding area. Smooth muscles in the stomach move the bolus to the body of the stomach and then to the lower stomach (antrum). The stomach secretes digestive juices:
  - Pepsin is a digestive enzyme that breaks down protein in the bolus. Pepsin is needed only when a bolus is in the stomach. The stomach secretes pepsinogen, which is a chemical that is converted into pepsin by hydrochloric acid. When the bolus enters the stomach, the stomach secretes gastrin. Gastrin causes gastric motility (turning) and causes the stomach to secrete hydrochloric acid, which transforms pepsinogen into pepsin to digest protein.
- Digestion in the stomach causes the bolus to be transformed into a semifluid mass called chyme. Chyme moves from the stomach through the pyloric sphincter into the small intestine. The pyloric sphincter is a ring of muscles at the end of the stomach that acts like a valve between the stomach and the small intestine.
- The small intestine is where nutrients from the chyme are absorbed. The small intestine is divided into:
  - Duodenum: The duodenum is where chyme is further digested by digestive juices from the gallbladder and the pancreas. The bile duct from the gallbladder connects to the sphincter of Oddi in the duodenum. Bile enters the duodenum to break down fat in the chyme.
    - The pancreatic duct from the pancreas connects to the sphincter of Oddi in the duodenum. Digestive enzymes from the pancreas enter the duodenum.
      - Amylase breaks down carbohydrates into glucose.
      - Lipase breaks down fat into fatty acids and glycerol.
      - Trypsin breaks down protein into amino acids.
  - Jejunum: Muscles in the small intestine move digested chyme from the duodenum to the jejunum. The jejunum absorbs glucose, amino acids (building blocks of protein), vitamins, and minerals into the blood.
  - Ileum: Absorbs fatty acids, glycerol, fat-soluble vitamins, and remaining nutrients.
- Muscles in the small intestine move chyme through the ileocecal valve into the cecum, which is the beginning of the large intestine. The cecum is the beginning of the large intestine, commonly referred to as the site of the appendix.
- The large intestine is divided into:
  - Ascending colon.
  - Transverse colon.
  - Descending colon.
  - Sigmoid colon.
- As the chyme moves through the large intestine, water and materials are reabsorbed. Bacteria in the large intestine further digest chyme to produce vitamin K and other nutrients. Undigested chyme is called fecal material and is formed into a stool.
- Stool is moved from the sigmoid colon to the rectum, where stool is stored. When fecal material reaches a specific volume, barrel receptor nerves in the rectum signal the urge to defecate. The anus is an opening to the rectum. The urge to defecate causes the anal sphincter to open, releasing fecal material.

2.3.1 Digestion and the Liver

- Nutrients absorbed by the small intestine are carried to the liver by portal blood veins. The liver processes (metabolizes) nutrients and stores fat and glucose.
- The liver secretes bile into the gallbladder, where bile is held until it is released into the duodenum. Bile contains bile acid, which is used to assist in the absorption of fats and fat-soluble vitamins (vitamins A, D, E, and K).
- The liver detoxifies alcohol, medication, and toxins, transforming them into chemicals that are safe to eliminate through urine and feces.
- The liver makes protein, such as albumin and clotting factors. Albumin assists in maintaining the volume of blood by causing fluid to remain in blood vessels. The liver also processes and stores carbohydrates (glucose).
- The liver can regenerate rapidly.

2.4 Cells and Glucose

- Cells use blood glucose as an energy source. When the small intestines breaks down carbohydrates into glucose, levels of glucose in the blood rise, triggering beta cells in the pancreas to secrete insulin into the blood.
- Insulin causes cells to carry blood glucose across the cell membrane and into the cell, where glucose is used to energize the cell's physiological activity. Potassium is also transported into the cells during this process.
- Excess blood glucose is stored as glycogen in the liver, muscle, and fatty tissue. When blood glucose levels sufficiently decline, alpha cells in the pancreas secrete glucagon. Glucagon is a hormone that causes glycogen in the liver to be converted to glucose through glycogenolysis. As glycogen in the liver is depleted, fatty tissue and eventually muscle are converted to glucose.

2.5 Oxygen, Carbon Dioxide, and Blood

- Air inspired through the nose and mouth is warmed and filtered. Air travels through the pharynx, larynx, and trachea before entering the left or right bronchi, and then into the bronchioles. Bronchioles contain alveoli, which are small sacs that contain small blood vessels.
- Oxygen attaches to hemoglobin in red blood cells (RBCs, or erythrocytes) in the alveoli, causing carbon dioxide to be released from hemoglobin and to move into the bronchioles through the respiratory system and exhaled.
- RBCs travel through arteries of the cardiovascular system, distributing oxygen to cells throughout the body. Oxygen is released from hemoglobin and moves into a cell. Carbon dioxide, a byproduct of cell metabolism, moves from the cell and attaches to hemoglobin. RBCs return through veins of the cardiovascular system, returning to the alveoli where carbon dioxide and oxygen are exchanged.

2.6 Cardiovascular System

- The cardiovascular system distributes RBCs (i.e., oxygen, carbon dioxide), white blood cells (WBCs), nutrients, and other elements in blood throughout the body, making it available to cells, which is called profusion.

- Profusion of cells depends on cardiac output. Contraction of the heart pushes blood through arteries. Movement of patients (e.g., walking) assists the return flow of blood through veins back to the heart.
- The amount of blood ejected from the left ventricle of the heart in 1 minute is called cardiac output. Cardiac output needs to be 4 to 8 L/min to adequately perfuse cells throughout the body.
- Cardiac output depends on three activities:
  - Preload: Preload is the amount of blood returning to the right side of the heart from the veins.
  - Afterload: Afterload is the arterial pressure in the body. The heart is pushing blood against pressure in the aorta and arteries. The higher the afterload resistance, the harder the heart has to push to eject blood.
  - Contractility: Contractility is the capability of the heart to contract the ventricles.

2.6.1 Maintaining cardiac output

- The cardiovascular system distributes RBCs (i.e., oxygen, carbon dioxide), WBCs, nutrients, and other elements in blood throughout the body, making it available to cells, which is called profusion.
- At rest normal cardiac activity is:
  - Cardiac output: 5.6 L/min for men and 4.9 L/min for women.
  - Heart rate: Between 60 and 100 beats per minute.
  - Blood pressure is between 90/60 mmHg to 120/80 mmHg.
- The cardiovascular system uses four mechanisms to compensate for physiological deficiencies of other systems that result in abnormally high or low blood volume.
  - Central nervous system: A decrease in carbon dioxide in the blood is detected by nerves in the atria, aorta, and carotid sinuses. The sympathetic nervous system stimulates the adrenal gland to secrete epinephrine and norepinephrine into the blood. Epinephrine increases contractions of the heart, resulting in increased cardiac output. Epinephrine and norepinephrine cause vasoconstriction, resulting in increased blood pressure. When the cardiac rate is high, the parasympathetic nervous system causes decreased cardiac contractions, leading to vasodilation.
  - Kidneys: The kidneys detect decreased perfusion and secrete renin into the blood. The liver detects renin in the blood and releases angiotensinogen into the blood. Angiotensinogen converts renin into angiotensin I. The angiotensin-converting enzyme (ACE) in the lungs converts angiotensin I into angiotensin II, which is a vasoconstrictor that results in increased blood pressure. Increased angiotensin in blood causes the adrenal gland to secrete aldosterone. Aldosterone causes the kidney to absorb more sodium and water, leading to an increase in blood volume and blood pressure. When blood volume is high, less renin is secreted by the kidneys, leading to decreased vasoconstriction and a decrease in the absorption of sodium and water. This results in decreased blood pressure.
  - Hypothalamus: Nerves in the hypothalamus detect when there is a concentration of blood, which occurs as a result of low blood volume. The hypothalamus triggers the pituitary gland to secrete antidiuretic hormone (ADH) into the blood. ADH causes the kidneys to retain water, resulting in increased blood pressure. As the volume of blood increases, ADH is no longer secreted and the kidneys no longer retain excess water.
  - Cardiac muscles: As cardiac muscles expand, cardiac cells release B-type natriuretic peptide (BNP) into the blood, causing the kidneys to absorb less water and create more urine (diuresis), resulting in vasodilation. However, decreased blood volume results in less expansion of cardiac muscles and a decrease in the release of BNP, resulting in less water absorption by the kidneys leading to an increase in water retention and increase blood pressure.

2.6.2 The working heart

- Cardiac contractions are controlled by the cardiac conduction system.
  - Sinoatrial (SA) node: The cardiac cycle begins with an impulse from the SA node located in the upper right wall of the right atrium. It causes contraction of the atrium.
  - Atrioventricular (AV) node: Next, the AV node, located in the lower interatrial septum, sends an impulse to the bundle of His (AV bundle), which transmits the impulse to the ventricles through the left and right bundle branches.
  - The Purkinje fibers: The Purkinje fibers contact the impulse from the interventricular septum through the apex to the ventricles.
- Blood is pumped through four chambers of the heart.
  - Right atrium: The right atrium receives venous blood from the superior vena cava, inferior vena cava, and the coronary sinus. This blood is saturated with 70% oxygen and 30% carbon dioxide.
  - Tricuspid value: The tricuspid value separates the right atrium from the right ventricle and controls the flow of venous blood from the right atrium to the right ventricle.
  - Right ventricle: Blood in the right ventricle is pumped through the pulmonic valve into the pulmonary artery, where the blood travels to the lungs for exchange of carbon dioxide for oxygen.
  - Left atrium: The left atrium receives oxygenated blood from the pulmonary vein and then passes the blood through the mitral valve into the left ventricle.
  - Left ventricle: The left ventricle pumps blood through the aortic valve and into the aorta and then enters the systematic circulation.
- Coronary circulation is blood supplied to cardiac tissues.
  - Coronary arteries: Blood from the aorta enters the ascending aorta and then moves into the right and left coronary arteries, where blood is supplied to cardiac tissues.
  - Coronary veins: Coronary veins take deoxygenated blood to the coronary sinus, which leads into the right atrium.
- Collateral circulation consists of blood vessels in the heart other than the coronary arteries that dilate whenever one or more coronary artery is blocked, thereby providing oxygenated blood flow to the heart.

2.7 Blood

- Blood transports elements to cells throughout the body. An adult has about 5 L of blood, 3 L of which is plasma. These elements are:
  - WBCs (leukocytes): Combat infection.
  - RBCs (erythrocytes): Carry oxygen and carbon dioxide and define blood type.
  - Plasma: Fluid portion of blood.
  - Platelets (thrombocytes): Clot blood.
  - Nutrients: Elements required for cell activity.
  - Electrolytes: Elements that conduct an electrical impulse.
  - Hormones: Chemical messengers.
  - Protein: Elements required for the structure, function, and regulation of cells.
  - Waste: A byproduct of cellular activity.

2.7.1 Red blood cells

- When oxygen levels in the blood are low, the kidneys secrete the erythropoietin hormone. The erythropoietin hormone causes stem cells in the bone marrow to make more RBCs.
- Bone marrow releases immature RBCs called reticulocytes. Once mature, the RBC is called an erythrocyte. An erythrocyte has hemoglobin containing heme, which is a protein used by oxygen and carbon dioxide to adhere to the RBCs. The RBC transports oxygen to cells and removes carbon dioxide from cells.
- Bone marrow requires vitamin B12, foliate, folic acid, and iron form an RBC. Iron is a material contained in hemoglobin, and it gives RBC its color. Iron binds to oxygen.
- The normal range for RBC count for a man is 4.7 million cells/mcL to 6.1 million cells/mcL. Women is 4.2 million cells/mcL to 5.4 million cells/mcL.
- The life of an RBC is 120 days, after which the RBC is removed in the liver and spleen. The liver converts hemoglobin of dead RBC into bilirubin, which is excreted as bile, in feces (brown color), and in urine (yellow color of urine).

2.7.2 White blood cells

- WBCs (leukocytes) are part of the immune system and they combat infection. There is normally about 4500 to 10,000 white blood cells/mcL. The life span of a WBC can be from a few hours to months, depending on its type.
- There are six types of WBCs. These are:
  - Neutrophils: Fifty-eight percent (58%) of WBCs are neutrophils. Neutrophils ingest bacteria (phagocytosis). Neutrophils are also referred to as PMNs, polys, or segs.
  - Bands: Three percent (3%) of WBCs are bands. Bands are immature neutrophils.
  - Eosinophils: Two percent (2%) of WBCs are eosinophils. Eosinophils kill parasites and become active in an allergic reaction.
  - Basophils: One percent (1%) of WBCs are basophils. Basophils release histamine during an allergic reaction, resulting in increased permeability of the capillaries. Basophils also release heparin to prevent blood clotting, enabling WBCs to reach bacteria.
  - Monocytes: Four percent (4%) of WBCs are monocytes. Monocytes are in the blood for about 20 hours, transform into macrophages, and move into tissues, where they live for years. Macrophages remove old and damaged cells and destroy bacteria.
  - Lymphocytes: Lymphocytes are WBCs directed by the immune system to defend the body against invading microorganisms. There are two types of lymphocytes. These are:
    - B lymphocytes (B cells): B lymphocytes are created and mature in bone marrow and are activated by T cells. B lymphocytes are transformed into plasma cells when either activated helper T cells or an invading microorganism is present. B lymphocytes produce antibodies (in plasma) that can recognize bacteria and viruses that have invaded the body and destroy specific bacteria and viruses (antigens). These antibodies are called immunoglobulins or gamma globulins. There are five types of immunoglobulins: IgG, IgM, IgE, IgA, and IgD. Each binds to an antigen, causing the antigen to clump and break open. B lymphocytes activate the complement system. The complement system consists of enzymes that cause neutrophils and macrophages to go to and kill the antigen.

- T lymphocytes (T cells): T lymphocytes are created in bone marrow and mature in the thymus gland. There are several types of T lymphocytes, of which the more common are:
  - Helper T cells: Helper T cells have a protein on the cell member called CD4 and are used to direct the immune system by releasing cytokines. Cytokines transform B cells into plasma cells that form antibodies. Cytokine also causes the production of cytotoxic T cells and suppressor T cells.
  - Cytotoxic T cells: Cytotoxic T cells secrete chemicals that kill invading microorganisms.
  - Suppressor T cells: Suppressor T cells turn off the immune response once the invading microorganism is destroyed and prevent the immune response from destroying normal cells.
  - Memory T cells: Memory T cells remain, looking for the invading microorganism should it return.

2.7.3 Platelets

- Platelets (thrombocytes) develop from megakaryocytes that are formed in bone marrow. Thrombin causes megakaryoctes to break up into fragments called platelets. Fibrinogen causes platelets to attract other platelets to form a platelet plug (thrombus) that prevents blood from leaking through broken blood vessels. A fibrin mesh called a clot forms. Platelets also stimulate blood vessel repair and help to begin the coagulation process.
- Clotting factors are proteins used in the coagulation cascade (coagulation process) to prevent bleeding from broken blood vessels. The liver uses vitamin K to produce coagulation factors. Vitamin K is made available by dietary sources and produced by normal intestinal flora.
- Thromboplastin is a plasma protein that converts prothrombin to thrombin. Two common blood tests measure prothrombin time (PT) and activated partial thromboplastin time (aPTT). Both tests measure blood coagulation and are used together to evaluate all coagulation factors. The international normalized ratio (INR) is another coagulation test that compares the time it takes blood to clot in a patient to the average time for blood to clot.

2.7.4 Plasma

- Plasma is straw-colored fluid in blood consisting of 90% water. It carries RBCs and WBCs and nutrients to cells throughout the body and waste from cells to the kidneys and lungs, where the waste is excreted from the body.
- Contractions of the heart push plasma through blood vessels, creating blood pressure (hydrostatic pressure). Protein in plasmas causes oncotic pressure, which keeps plasma within blood vessels and transports nutrients, carbohydrates (glucose), lipids (cholesterol), vitamins, medication, and hormones throughout the body. The main proteins in plasma are:
  - Albumin: Albumin causes plasma to remain within blood vessels.
  - Globulins (immunoglobulins): Globulins are antibodies that attack microorganisms that invade the body (see 2.7.2 White blood cells).
  - Fibrinogen: Fibrinogen is used to create blood clots (see 2.7.2 White blood cells).
- Electrolytes are also contained in plasma (see 2.10 Fluids and Electrolytes) and transported throughout the body.
- Serum is the fluid that remains after blood cells and clotting factors are removed. Serum is tested in many blood tests.

2.7.5 Blood type and Rh blood group

- Blood is classified by blood type as A, B, AB, and O, based on the antigens (agglutinogens) on the surface of the RBCs. Blood type forms during infancy but is not present at birth. There are two agglutinogens, A and B. RBCs can have one antigen (A or B), both antigens (AB), or neither antigen (O).

- Plasma has antibodies that are the opposite of the blood type. An antibody attacks an antigen.
  - Type A blood (A antigen) has B antibodies in the plasma. Administering type B blood to a patient who has type A blood causes an antibody reaction to the transfusion.
  - Type B blood (B antigen) has A antibodies in plasma. Administering type A blood to a patient who has type B blood causes an antibody reaction to the transfusion.
  - Type AB blood has no A or B antibodies in plasma. Therefore, no antibody reaction occurs when transfusing type A or B blood.
  - Type O blood (no antigen) has A antibodies and B antibodies in plasma. Administering any other blood type than type O blood to a patient who has type O blood causes an antibody reaction to the transfusion.
- A patient with blood type AB can receive blood of any blood type (universal recipient).
- A donor with blood type O can donate blood to any patient (universal donor).
- Blood is also grouped by Rh antigens that are located on RBCs. The most common Rh antigen is the D antigen. Rh antigens develop at birth. The blood is considered Rh+ if the D antigen is present and Rh– if the D antigen is not present.
  - A patient with Rh+ blood can receive Rh+ and Rh– blood.
  - A patient with Rh– blood can receive only Rh– blood.
  - When there is no time to test the blood type and Rh group, administer blood type O Rh–.

2.8 Immune System

- The immune system protects the body from microorganisms (bacteria, viruses, toxins, and parasites) by attacking these microorganisms before they can impede physiological activity of the cells within the body. Microorganisms include:
  - Bacteria: Single-cell organisms that are able to reproduce and frequently release toxins that interrupt the physiological activity of cells.
  - Virus: A fragment of DNA in a protective shell that attaches to a cell and injects its DNA into the cell, in a sense taking over the cell. As the cell ruptures, the viral DNA attacks other cells.
  - Toxin: A substance that is poisonous to cells. The substance might be man-made or produced by a cell.
  - Parasite: An organism that lives on or in another organism.
- The immune system creates a barrier that prevents the microorganism from entering the body or cell and has specialized cells (see 2.7.2 White blood cells) to attack and kill the microorganism. In addition, the immune system destroys the body's imperfect cells (i.e., cancer).
- The immune system consists of:
  - Skin: The skin provides a barrier between microorganisms and cells within the body. The epidermis contains antibacterial substances that kill many microorganisms. Saliva, tears, and mucus contain enzymes that kill bacteria.
  - Thymus: The thymus is a gland where T cells mature (see 2.7.2 White blood cells).
  - Spleen: The spleen is a blood filter where foreign cells and mature RBCs are removed from the blood.

- Lymph system: The lymph system consists of lymph vessels, lymph nodes, and lymph. Lymph is blood plasma that receives nutrients and water from blood and carries nutrients and water to cells. Lymph surrounds cells. Protein and waste from cells enter the lymph. Lymph vessels drain and filter these byproducts of physiological activity of cells and remove bacteria. Lymph is collected in lymph nodes. Lymph nodes filter lymph. The filtered lymph is then returned into blood. The lymph nodes swell with bacteria and antibodies when the body has a bacterial infection. The swelling subsides as the antibodies destroy the bacteria.
- Bone marrow: Bone marrow produces WBCs, some of which are transformed into antibodies that attack microorganisms (see 2.7.2 White blood cells).
- Complement system: The complement system consists of protein produced by the liver that freely floats in blood. It is activated by antibodies. These proteins cause invading cells to rupture (lysing) and signal the phagocytes to remove cell parts.
- Hormones: Hormones are chemical messengers that signal. Immune system hormones are called lymphokines.
  - Corticosteroids: Corticosteroids are hormones that suppress the immune system.
  - Tymosin: Tymosin is a hormone that causes production of WBCs.
  - Interleukin: Interleukin is a hormone produced by macrophages once the macrophage destroys the invading cell. Interleukin causes the hypothalamus to increase body temperature to a degree that kills bacteria.
  - Tumor necrosis factor (TNF): TNF is a hormone produced by macrophages that causes tumor cells to be killed and helps create new blood vessels.
  - Interferon: Interferon is a hormone produced by many cells when a virus is detected. Interferon causes cells to produce a protein that prevents the virus from replicating in other cells.

2.8.1 Inflammation vs. infection

- Inflammation is a response to cell damage caused by injury or a microorganism. Inflammation is different from an infection. An infection is the invasion of a microorganism into the body that causes an inflammation response. However, the inflammation response can also occur in reaction to cell damage caused by injury, not by a microorganism.
- The inflammation response begins with damage to cells. The pattern recognition receptors (PRRs) at the injury site cause blood vessels at the site to dilate (vasodilation), resulting in increased blood flow to the site. PRRs also release bradykinin, which stimulates nerves at the site, causing the patient to focus on the injury.
- Increased blood flow causes the site to become warm, swollen, and redden (red blood cells are closer to the surface of the skin). Blood vessels also become more permeable, enabling plasma and white blood cells to enter the injured tissue. WBCs remove damaged cells. Plasma contains nutrients that promote new cell growth at the site. As damaged cells are removed and new cells grow, PRRs decrease and eventually stops the inflammation response at the site, resulting in contraction of blood vessels to their normal size (no swelling), and stopping the release of bradykinin (no pain).
- There are two categories of inflammation:
  - Acute inflammation: Acute inflammation occurs in response to an injury or invasion by a microorganism. Once damaged cells are removed and replaced by new cells, the inflammation process stops.
  - Chronic inflammation: Chronic inflammation is persistent inflammation caused by continued injury (e.g., osteoarthritis) or a malfunction to the immune system resulting in the inflammation response not being shut off once new cells replace damaged cells.

- Infection occurs as a result of the invasion of a microorganism. The presence of the microorganism causes the immune response, which includes the inflammation response.
- Infection occurs when the chain of infection is in place:
  - Etiologic agent: There is a microorganism.
  - Reservoir: There is a place where the microorganism can grow (i.e., the body).
  - Portal of exit: There is a method of leaving the reservoir (airborne [sneeze, cough], contact [touch], ingestion).
  - Transmission: The microorganism moves to the patient.
  - Portal of entry: The microorganism enters the patient (i.e., through the nose, mouth, eyes, or break in the skin).
  - Susceptible host: Barriers to infection are compromised. The patient's immune system (i.e., antibodies, WBCs) is unable to quickly kill the microorganism.

2.9 Kidneys

- Kidneys receive 20% of the blood pumped by the heart through the renal artery, where waste (urea, ammonia, toxins, and drugs) and excess fluid are removed and passed through the ureters as urine and into the bladder. The urinary bladder holds about 350 ml of urine. The renal vein returns filtered blood. When urine volume reaches 25% of the bladder's volume (87 ml), barrel receptors signal the brain to urinate. Muscles in the urethra relax and urine is released. A goal of the kidney is to maintain a constant composition of blood.
- The nephron is the fundamental unit in the kidney. The nephron contains glomerulus, which is a filter that retains proteins and cells in blood and extracts excess fluid and waste into a tubule. Fluid that passes into the tubule contains nutrients (electrolytes) that are returned to the blood if needed by the body.
- The kidneys also release:
  - Erythropoietin (EPO): The EPO hormone stimulates bone marrow to form RBCs.
  - Renin: Renin regulates blood pressure.
  - Calcitirol: Calcitirol is the active form of vitamin D that is necessary to maintain calcium in bone.
- Renal function is measured by the glomerular filtration rate (GFR). The GFR is the percentage of renal function; 60% renal function would be asymptomatic; 25% renal function will result in serious physiological effects, and 15% or less renal function requires dialysis or kidney transplant.
- Blood urea nitrogen (BUN) is another test that measures glomerular filtration. Excess protein in the blood is converted to urea and excreted by the kidneys. Blood should contain between 7 mg/dl to 20 mg/dl of urea. An amount higher than 20 mg/dl might indicate decreased glomerular filtration. However, a value higher than 20 mg/dl can also indicate dehydration.
- Renal disorders occur when nephrons lose filtering capacity. Acute renal failure results from poisoning or injury. Chronic renal failure occurs slowly from diseases such as renal disease, diabetes, and high blood pressure. High blood glucose levels acts like a poison to the nephrons. High blood pressure damages glomeruli, resulting in loss of filtering capacity.

2.10 Fluids and Electrolytes

- Fluids are approximately 60% of body weight. Ninety percent (90%) of fluids come from water in foods and ingestion of fluid. Ten percent (10%) is from the byproduct of metabolic oxidation. Daily requirements of fluids for a normal adult are 2500 ml.

- Fluids are in two locations within the body:
  - Intracellular (ICF): Inside the cell.
  - Extracellular (ECF): Outside the cell.
    - Intravascular fluid (plasma): In blood vessels (3 L).
    - Interstitial fluid (lymphatic): Between cells (9 L).
- Fluid is normally lost through:
  - Skin (sweat) (500 ml/day).
  - Urine (800 to 1500 ml/day).
  - Feces.
  - Lungs.
- Electrolytes are elements that can conduct an electrical impulse required for physiological activities within the cell when dissolved in water. Electrolytes are partly nutrients that are the end product of metabolized food. They are located inside and outside cells. Unbalanced electrolytes may be life threatening. Electrolyte levels must be balanced or the patient will become symptomatic as the result of too many or too few electrical impulses.
- Hormones maintain electrolyte levels:
  - Insulin: Insulin moves potassium from blood into the cell.
  - Calcitonin: Calcitonin moves calcium from blood into bone.
  - Parathyroid hormone (PTH): PTH moves calcium from bone into blood.
- The kidneys also control the amount of electrolytes in blood by selective filtering of electrolytes. A high level of an electrolyte in blood causes the kidneys to excrete some of that electrolyte. A low level of an electrolyte in blood causes the kidneys to retain that electrolyte.
- Electrolytes that are found mostly inside cells are:
  - Potassium.
  - Magnesium.
  - Phosphorus.
  - Calcium.
  - Chloride.
- The electrolyte found mostly outside of cells is sodium.
- Inverse relationships with electrolytes that cause an unbalance of electrolytes:
  - Potassium and sodium: Retention of sodium results in excretion of potassium. Retention of potassium results in excretion of sodium.
  - Calcium and phosphorus: Retention of calcium results in excretion of phosphorus. Retention of phosphorus results in excretion of calcium.
  - Magnesium and chloride: Retention of magnesium results in excretion of chloride. Retention of chloride results in excretion of magnesium.

2.10.1 Tests: Fluids and electrolytes

- Fluids:
  - Urine specific gravity: 1.002 to 1.030.
    - High: Dehydration.
    - Low: Too much fluid.

- Hemoglobin (Hgb): 13.2 to 16.2 g/dl (male); 12.0 to 15.2 g/dl (female).
  - High: Dehydration.
- Hematocrit (Hct): 40% to 52% (male); 37% to 46% (female).
  - High: Dehydration.
- Blood urea nitrogen (BUN): 7 to 250 mg/dl.
  - High: Dehydration, decreased kidney function.
- Creatinine (Cre): 0.5 to 1.4 mg/dl.
  - High: decreased kidney function.

- Electrolytes:
  - Calcium (serum): 8.9 to 10.4 mg/dl.
  - Chloride (serum): 98 to 110 mEq/L.
  - Potassium (serum): 3.6 to 5.0 mEq/L.
  - Sodium (serum): 137 to 145 mEq/L.

2.10.2 Treatment: Fluids and electrolytes

- Fluids volume excess (FVE):
  - Restrict sodium intake.
  - Treat the underlying cause.
  - Administer:
    - Loop diuretics
      - Furosemide (Lasix): Risk for hypokalemia.
    - Potassium-sparing diuretics
      - Spironolactone (Aldactone): Risk for hyperkalemia.
- Fluids volume deficit (FVD):
  - Increase fluid:
    - Orally.
    - Intraveously (IV).
  - Treat the underlying cause.
- Low sodium levels
  - Restrict fluid intake.
  - Administer: Normal saline IV.
- High sodium levels
  - Slowly replace fluids.
- Low potassium levels
  - Administer: Potassium chloride in 5% dextrose solution (D5W).
- High potassium levels
  - Dialysis.
  - Administer:
    - Kayexalate.
    - Insulin.
    - Glucose.

- Low calcium
  - Administer: Calcium chloride.
- High calcium
  - Administer: Furosemide (Lasix).
- Low magnesium
  - Administer:
    - Magnesium gluconate.
    - Magnesium oxide.
- High magnesium
  - Dialysis
  - Administer: Calcium gluconate.
- Low phosphorous
  - Administer: Potassium phosphate.
- High phosphorous
  - Dialysis.
- Low chloride
  - Treat underlying cause.
- High chloride
  - Treat underlying cause.

2.10.3 Critical thinking: Fluids and electrolytes

- Fluids:
  - Intake and output must be monitored to ensure that the patient is not dehydrating. Critical care patients can dehydrate quickly. Fluid intake and output should be approximately the same volume.
  - Increased fluid loss:
    - Causes:
      - Fever.
      - Rapid breathing.
      - Surgical drainage.
      - Suction.
      - Fistulas.
      - Sweating (diaphoresis).
      - Burns, because skin no longer holds fluid
      - Hemorrhage.
      - Vomiting.
      - Diarrhea.
  - Signs:
    - Tenting of skin.
    - Low or no urination.

    - Decreased visible veins in hands and neck.
    - Decreased blood pressure.
    - Weak, rapid pulse.
    - Dry mucous membranes.
    - Weight loss.
    - Cool extremities.
    - Increased urine specific gravity.
    - Increased thirst.
- A patient on a high ventilator setting will need increased fluids because fluid is lost through rapid breathing.
- A patient with less body fat (e.g., elderly, women) retains less fluid.
- Make sure there is sufficient fluid to maintain perfusion of organs. Insufficient fluid may result in vascular collapse, resulting in no blood flowing to organs, which leads to organ death.
- A critical care patient usually receives most if not all fluids IV because the patient may have limited or no ability to ingest food and water.
- Monitor urine output to be sure that the patient does not become overhydrated (fluid overload) because fluids are usually supplied through IV.
- The pituitary gland stores ADH, which causes water retention in the vascular space.
- The hypothalamus controls the thirst response, which occurs when fluid volume is decreased. A critical care patient's thirst response may be impaired.
- Small intestine disorders may affect absorption of fluid from ingested food. Ninety percent (90%) of fluid from ingested food is absorbed by the small intestine.
- Plasma protein (albumin) holds fluid in the vascular space. A decrease in plasma protein from liver disease (not making enough), malnourishment (decreased protein intake), or severe burns may cause fluid to move to interstitial space from the vascular space.
- Isotonic dehydration occurs when there is a fluid volume deficit, where equal amounts of fluid and sodium are lost. The sodium serum value remains unchanged. Signs are:
  - Fluid volume excess occurs with too much fluid,
    - Caused by:
      - Albumin infusion.
      - Excessive IV normal saline or lactated ringers.
      - Renal failure.
      - Increased aldosterone.
      - Increased steroid administration.
      - Increased ADH.
      - Blood product infusion.
    - Signs are:
      - High blood pressure.
      - Edema.
      - Weight gain.
      - Bounding pulse.
      - Tachycardia.
      - Jugular vein distension.

    - Fluid in lungs.
    - Productive cough.
    - Increased urination.
- Fluid backs up when there is decreased cardiac output, leading to pulmonary edema (fluid in the lungs).
- Electrolytes:
  - Monitor electrolyte balance. Electrolytes can become unbalanced by:
    - Vomiting.
    - Diarrhea.
    - Nasogastric suctioning.
    - Drainage.
    - Diuretics.
    - Anorexia.
    - Poor nutrition.
    - Tumors.
    - Chemotherapy.
    - Trauma, especially crushing injuries.
  - Unbalanced electrolytes must be balanced.
  - Potassium:
    - Serum potassium levels can decrease, leading to arrhythmias when administering insulin IV. Insulin pulls glucose and potassium into cells from the vascular space.
    - Too much or too little potassium and magnesium can result in arrhythmias, respiratory arrest, and seizures.
    - Impaired kidney function may result in increased potassium levels.
  - Calcium:
    - Excessive levels of the parathyroid hormone (PTH) can cause serum calcium levels to increase and calcium levels in bone to decrease.
    - Excessive calcitonin can cause serum calcium levels to decrease and calcium levels in bone to increase.
  - Sodium:
    - Rapid changes in sodium can result in serious complications, leading to seizures and brain damage.
    - Low blood volume causes the kidneys to retain sodium and water in the vascular space.
    - Administering diuretics may decrease sodium.
    - Hypernatremia: Too much sodium is caused by a decrease in water or increase in sodium intake.
    - Sodium is found in food and medication, including IV fluids; it can lead to hypernatremia.
    - Hyponatremia: Too little sodium is caused by an increase in water intake or a decrease in sodium.
    - Adrenal glands secrete aldosterone. Aldosterone causes sodium and water to be retained and potassium to be excreted. Malfunction of the adrenal glands or administering aldosterone will affect electrolyte balance.
    - Dehydration occurs when sodium is retained and fluid is lost.

2.11 Acid-Base

- The pH scale is used to measure the level of hydrogen ion in fluid. The pH scale has a range from 0 to 14. A pH value of 7 is neutral. A pH value less than 7 means there is a high level of hydrogen ions (acidity). A pH value more than 7 means there is a low level of hydrogen ions (alkalinity). Fluid in the body must remain at a pH value between 7.35 and 7.45; otherwise, nutrients in the fluid lose functionality.
- Acid-base balance is measured by the pH level of blood and the amount of carbon dioxide (CO_2) and bicarbonate (HCO_3) in blood. The lungs and kidneys regulate blood pH. The respiration rate determines the amount of CO_2 (acid) in blood. The concentration of urine by the kidneys determines the amount of HCO_3 (base) in the blood.
- An acid-base imbalance occurs when too much or too little CO_2 and/or HCO_3 is retained in blood.
- Acidosis: Acidosis occurs when blood pH falls below 7.35. This means that there is too much CO_2 in the blood. Acidosis occurs when the lungs are not removing enough CO_2 or the kidneys are not retaining sufficient HCO_3.
- Alkalosis: Alkalosis occurs when blood pH rises above 7.45. This means there is too much HCO_3 in the blood. Alkalosis occurs when the lungs are removing too much CO_2 or the kidneys are retaining too much HCO_3.
- If the underlying cause of the acid-base imbalance is inappropriate respiration, then the acid-base imbalance is referred to as respiratory acidosis or respiratory alkalosis.
- If the underlying cause of the acid-base imbalance is dysfunctional kidneys, then the acid-base imbalance is referred to as metabolic acidosis or metabolic alkalosis.
- A blood gas test is used to measure the pH of blood and the amount of CO_2 and HCO_3 in blood. Table 2.1 shows the possible results of a blood gas test.

TABLE 2.1 Blood Gas Test Results

Disorder	pH	Carbon Dioxide	Bicarbonate
Respiratory acidosis	<7.4	High	Low
Respiratory alkalosis	>7.4	Low	High
Metabolic acidosis	<7.4	High	Low
Metabolic alkalosis	>7.4	Low	High

- The body compensates for an acid-base imbalance by altering respiratory and kidney function over a time period. Table 2.2 shows the possible results of a blood gas test after the body compensates for the acid-base imbalance.

TABLE 2.2 Blood Gas Test Results after Compensation

Disorder	pH	Carbon Dioxide	Bicarbonate
Respiratory acidosis	<7.4	High	High
Respiratory alkalosis	>7.4	Low	Low
Metabolic acidosis	<7.4	High	High
Metabolic alkalosis	>7.4	Low	Low

2.12 Endocrine System

- The endocrine system consists of glands that secrete hormones into blood. Hormones are chemical messengers that signal specific actions by parts of the body.
- Hormones are controlled by the pituitary gland and a feedback system. The feedback system detects the level of hormone in blood and then adjusts the level by causing more or less hormone to be released by a gland in the endocrine system.
- Glands of the endocrine system are:
  - Adrenal glands: Adrenal glands are above each kidney and produce more than 30 steroid hormones. The outer layer (cortex) secretes cortisone. Cortisone reduces the inflammation process. The inner layer (medulla) secretes epinephrine and norepinephrine. Both hormones increase the heart rate, release more glucose into the blood, constrict blood vessels, and dilate bronchioles.
  - Pancreas: The pancreas is located behind the stomach and secretes insulin and glucagon. Insulin moves glucose from the blood into cells when the blood glucose level is high. Glucagon stimulates the liver to release glucose when the blood glucose level is low.
  - Pituitary gland: The pituitary gland, located at the base of the brain, controls other glands.
    - The anterior lobe secretes:
      - Somatotropin: A growth hormone that encourages cell reproduction.
      - Thyrotropic hormone: A TSH that stimulates the thyroid gland to secrete hormones.
      - Adrenocorticotropic hormone (ACTH): A hormone that stimulates the cortex of the adrenal gland to secrete cortisone.
      - Follicle-stimulating hormone (FSH) and luteinizing hormone (LH): Hormones that stimulate testes in males and ovaries in females.
      - Prolactin: Stimulates the mammary glands to secrete milk.
    - The posterior lobe secretes:
      - Oxytocin: Stimulates smooth muscles (important in childbirth).
      - Vasopressin: Stimulates the kidneys to increase blood pressure.
  - Testes are contained in the scrotum and secrete testosterone, which causes secondary male sex characteristics.
  - Ovaries are located in the pelvis and secrete:
    - Estrogen and progesterone: Stimulate ovulation and cause secondary female sex characteristics.
  - The thyroid gland, located in the front of the neck, secretes hormones that control metabolism throughout the body.
  - Parathyroid glands, located in the back of the thyroid gland, secrete parathyroid hormone, which controls the level of calcium in blood.
  - Three mechanisms are used to release hormones into the blood. These are:
    - Neural mechanism: The sympathetic nervous system stimulates the adrenal gland (sympathetic-adrenal response) to secrete acetylcholine, resulting in the secretion of epinephrine. Epinephrine causes the fight-flight response.
    - Hormonal mechanism: A hormone from one gland is secreted to stimulate another gland to secrete a hormone.
    - Humoral mechanism: A high or low concentration of a hormone or other substance causes a gland to secrete more or fewer hormones.

2.13 Neurologic System

- The network of neurons (nerve cells) transmits impulses throughout the body. Neurons are covered by a fatty substance called myelin, which insulates the neuron. The end of a neuron (synaptic terminal) contains tiny sacs that contain a neurotransmitter. A neurotransmitter is a chemical that transmits impulses to another neuron when stimulated by an electrical impulse.
- The nervous system has two major divisions:
  - Central nervous system: The central nervous system consists of the brain and spinal cord, which are protected by bone, tissue, and cerebrospinal fluid.
  - Peripheral nervous system: The peripheral nervous system receives impulses from the central nervous system and carries the impulses to the designated site in the body. The peripheral nervous system consists of cranial nerves (nerves directly connected to the brain) and spinal nerves (nerves from the spinal cord). The peripheral nervous system has two divisions:
    - Somatic nervous system: Nerves that control voluntary muscles.
    - Autonomic nervous system: Nerves that control involuntary body functions.
- The brain is divided into:
  - Cerebellum: Located at the back of the skull, the cerebellum controls movement, posture, and balance.
  - Thalamus: Located inside the brain, the thalamus receives impulses from the body and relays the impulses to the appropriate part of the brain. The thalamus is involved in body temperature, pain, and touch.
  - Hypothalamus: Located around the thalamus, the hypothalamus controls involuntary movement, such as circulating blood and cardiac contractions.
  - Pituitary gland: Attached to the hypothalamus, the pituitary gland controls many hormones in the body.
  - Cerebral cortex: The cerebral cortex covers the inner part of the brain and is divided into two areas called cerebral hemispheres. Each hemisphere regulates voluntary action.
  - Corpus callosum: The corpus callosum connects the cerebral hemispheres.
  - Medulla: Located at the base of the brain, the medulla is where the hemispheres cross, resulting in a hemisphere controlling the opposite side of the body.
  - Cerebrospinal fluid: Cerebrospinal fluid is a clear fluid that surrounds the spinal cord and the brain. Cerebrospinal fluid is produced by blood vessels called the choroid plexus located in ventricles in the brain. Ventricles are chambers. Five ounces of cerebrospinal fluid circulates around the spinal cord and brain.

Solved Problems

2.1 What causes a multisystem critical condition?
Multisystem critical care focuses on all systems in the patient's body. Each system has a physiological activity and physiological reserve. Decreased physiological reserve of one system may have a cascading effect on other systems in the body as the other systems attempt to compensate for the disorder.

2.2 How should the critical care team manage a multisystem critical condition?
The critical care healthcare team anticipates cascading system failure and provides technological

assistance (e.g., medication, mechanical/electronic devices) to increase physiological reserves until the underlying disorder stabilizes.

2.3 What controls the rate of physiological activities within cells?
The hypothalamus gland.

2.4 Why must the diet of a critical care patient be adjusted?
A critical care patient's diet must be adjusted to compensate for the patient's condition. Although the patient is immobile, the patient may require an increase in carbohydrates, protein, fat, and other nutrients to support the body's effort to compensate for failing systems.

2.5 Why is it important that the critically ill patient have sufficient thiamin?
Thiamin is a coenzyme needed for cellular metabolism.

2.6 Why might a patient with liver disease have an increased risk of bleeding?
Vitamin K is required to produce clotting factors. A diseased liver may not be able to absorb vitamin K.

2.7 What is the role of glucagon?
When blood glucose levels decline, alpha cells in the pancreas secrete glucagon. Glucagon is a hormone that causes glycogen in the liver to be converted to glucose through glycogenolysis.

2.8 What occurs when glycogen in the liver is depleted?
As glycogen in the liver is depleted, fatty tissue and eventually muscle are converted to glucose.

2.9 What can cause an insufficient amount of oxygen to reach cells?
An insufficient quality of red blood cells.

2.10 What action returns blood flow to the heart?
Movement of the patient (i.e., walking) assists the return flow of blood through veins back to the heart.

2.11 What results in a high afterload?
The higher the afterload resistance, the harder the heart has to push to eject blood.

2.12 What are the four mechanisms the cardiovascular system uses to compensate for physiological deficiencies of other systems that result in abnormally high or low blood volume?

- Central nervous system: A decrease in carbon dioxide in blood is detected by nerves in the atria, aorta, and carotid sinuses. The sympathetic nervous system stimulates the adrenal gland to secrete epinephrine and norepinephrine into the blood. Epinephrine increases contractions of the heart, resulting in increased cardiac output. Epinephrine and norepinephrine cause vasoconstriction, resulting in increased blood pressure. When cardiac rate is high, the parasympathetic nervous system causes decreased cardiac contractions, leading to vasodilation.
- Kidneys: Kidneys detect decreased perfusion and secrete renin into the blood. The liver detects renin in the blood and releases angiotensinogen into the blood. Angiotensinogen converts renin into angiotensin I. The angiotensin-converting enzyme (ACE) in the lungs converts angiotensin I into angiotensin II, which is vasoconstrictor that leads to increased blood pressure. Increased angiotensin in blood causes the adrenal gland to secrete aldosterone. Aldosterone causes the kidney to absorb more sodium and water, leading to an increase in blood volume and blood pressure.

When blood volume is high, less renin is secreted by the kidneys, leading to decreased vasoconstriction and a decrease in the absorption of sodium and water. This results in decreased blood pressure.

- Hypothalamus: Nerves in the hypothalamus detect when there is a concentration of blood, which occurs as a result of low blood volume. The hypothalamus triggers the pituitary gland to secrete antidiuretic hormone (ADH) into the blood. ADH causes the kidneys to retain water, resulting in increased blood pressure. As the volume of blood increases, ADH is no longer secreted and the kidneys no longer retain excess water.
- Cardiac muscles: As cardiac muscles expand, cardiac cells release B-type natriuretic peptide (BNP) into the blood, causing the kidneys to absorb less water and create more urine (diuresis), resulting in vasodilation. However, decreased blood volume results in less expansion of cardiac muscles and a decrease in the release of BNP. This results in less water absorption by the kidneys, leading to increased water retention and increased blood pressure.

2.13 Why would a patient who has liver disease be at risk for bleeding?
Clotting factors are proteins used in the coagulation cascade (coagulation process) that prevent bleeding from broken blood vessels. The liver uses vitamin K to produce coagulation factors. Vitamin K is made available by dietary sources and produced by normal intestinal flora.

2.14 How do the kidneys influence blood pressure?
The kidneys detect decreased perfusion and secrete renin into the blood. The liver detects renin in the blood and releases angiotensinogen into the blood. Angiotensinogen converts renin into angiotensin I. The angiotensin-converting enzyme (ACE) in the lungs converts angiotensin I into angiotensin II, which is vasoconstrictor that leads to increased blood pressure. Increased angiotensin in blood causes the adrenal gland to secrete aldosterone. Aldosterone causes the kidney to absorb more sodium and water, leading to an increase in blood volume and blood pressure. When blood volume is high, there is less renin secreted by the kidneys, leading to decreased vasoconstriction and a decrease in the absorption of sodium and water. This results in a decrease in blood pressure.

2.15 How do cardiac muscles influence blood pressure?
As cardiac muscles expand, cardiac cells release B-type natriuretic peptide (BNP) into the blood, causing the kidneys to absorb less water and create more urine (diuresis), resulting in vasodilation. However, decreased blood volume results in less expansion of cardiac muscles and a decrease in the release of BNP, resulting in less water absorption by the kidneys. This leads to increased water retention and increased blood pressure.

2.16 How do basophils prevent blood clotting?
Basophils release heparin to prevent blood clotting.

2.17 What are the types and roles of T cells?

- Helper T cells: Helper T cells have a protein on the cell member called CD4, which is used to direct the immune system by releasing cytokines. Cytokine transforms B cells into plasma cells that form antibodies. Cytokine also causes the production of cytotoxic T cells and suppressor T cells.
- Cytotoxic T cells: Cytotoxic T cells secrete chemicals that kill invading microorganisms.
- Suppressor T cells: Suppressor T cells turn off the immune response once the invading microorganism is destroyed and prevents the immune response from destroying normal cells.
- Memory T cells: Memory T cells remain, looking for the invading microorganism should it return.

2.18 What is the role of fibrinogen?
Platelets (thrombocytes) develop from megakaryocytes that are formed in bone marrow. Thrombin causes megakaryoctes to break into fragments called platelets. Fibrinogen causes platelets to attract other platelets, which form a platelet plug (thrombus) that prevents blood from leaking through broken blood vessels. A fibrin mesh called a clot forms. Platelets also stimulate blood vessel repair and help begin the coagulation process.

2.19 What is the role of albumin?
Albumin causes plasma to remain within blood vessels.

2.20 What is the difference between inflammation and infection?
Inflammation is a response to cell damage caused by injury or by a microorganism. Inflammation is different from an infection. An infection is the invasion of a microorganism into the body that causes an inflammation response. However, the inflammation response can also occur in reaction to cell damage caused by injury, not by a microorganism.

2.21 What is the function of pattern recognition receptors?
The inflammation response begins with damage to cells. The pattern recognition receptors (PRRs) at the injury site cause blood vessels at the site to dilate (vasodilation), resulting in increased blood flow to the site. PRRs also release bradykinin, which stimulates nerves at the site, causing the patient to focus on the injury.

2.22 What is the difference between acute and chronic inflammation?

- Acute inflammation: Acute inflammation occurs in response to an injury or invasion by a microorganism. Once damaged cells are removed and replaced by new cells, the inflammation process stops.
- Chronic inflammation: Chronic inflammation is persistent inflammation caused by continuing injury (e.g., osteoarthritis) or a malfunction of the immune system. This results in the inflammation response not being shut off once new cells replace damaged cells.

2.23 What is the chain of infection?

- Etiologic agent: There is a microorganism.
- Reservoir: A place where the microorganism can grow (i.e., the body).
- Portal of exit: A method of leaving the reservoir (airborne [sneeze, cough], contact [touch], ingestion).
- Transmission: The microorganism moves to the patient.
- Portal of entry: The microorganism enters the patient (i.e., through the nose, mouth, eyes, or break in the skin).
- Susceptible host: Barriers to infection are compromised. The patient's immune system (i.e., antibodies, WBCs) is unable to kill the microorganism quickly.

2.24 What is the function of EPO in the kidneys?
EPO is released by the kidneys and stimulates bone marrow to form in RBCs.

2.25 What is the function of histamines?
Histamines increase the permeability of capillaries, enabling blood to flow to repair injured tissues.

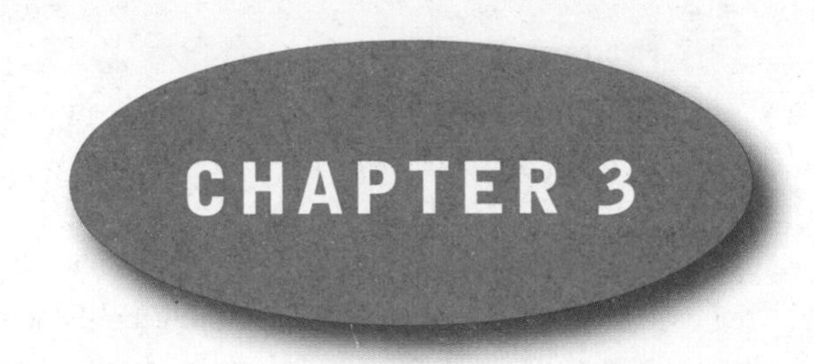

Cardiovascular Critical Care

3.1 Definitions

- Cardiovascular critical care is necessary when cardiovascular reserves are insufficient to sustain circulation. When this happens, the patient becomes unstable, requiring mechanical and/or pharmaceutical treatment to supplement cardiovascular reserves.
- The cardiovascular system distributes oxygen and nutrients to cells throughout the body and removes carbon dioxide and metabolic waste from cells to organs that facilitate removal of waste from the body. The cardiovascular system also transports hormones throughout the body.
- Decreased cardiovascular reserves may result in a cascading failure of systems throughout the body.
- The goal of cardiovascular critical care is to assist the patient's cardiovascular system and maintain sufficient circulation and blood pressure to perfuse organs.
- A patient may be admitted to the critical care unit for a condition other than a cardiac condition. However, a cascading failure of systems other than the cardiovascular system may result in cardiovascular instability. Therefore, always carefully monitor the cardiovascular system for abnormalities.

3.1.1 Cardiovascular blood flow

- Blood flow to and from the heart:
  - Deoxygenated blood returns to the right atrium of the heart from the inferior and superior vena cava.
  - Deoxygenated blood flows from the right atrium to the right ventricle when the right atrium contracts.
  - Deoxygenated blood in the right ventricle flows through the pulmonary arteries into the lungs when the right ventricle contracts.
  - Carbon dioxide, which is attached to the hemoglobin in red blood cells, is replaced by oxygen.
  - Oxygenated blood returns from the lungs to the left atrium through four pulmonary veins.
  - Oxygenated blood flows into the left ventricle when the left atrium contracts.
  - Oxygenated blood flows from the left ventricle through the aorta to the arterial system, providing oxygenated blood to cells throughout the body.

- Heart valves:
  - A heart valve enables blood to flow in one direction by preventing the backflow of blood by the pressure of blood in the chamber (passive pressure).
  - The atrioventricular valves (AV):
    - Tricuspid valve: The valve between the right atrium and the right ventricle.
    - Mitral valve: The valve between the left atrium and the right ventricle.
  - Semilunar valves:
    - Pulmonic valve: The valve between the right ventricle and the pulmonary artery.
    - Aortic valve: The valve between the left ventricle and the aorta.
- Blood supply to the heart:
  - Oxygenated blood is carried by coronary arteries to cardiac cells.
  - Coronary arteries are connected to the aorta through the coronary ostium opening, which is located above the aortic valve.
  - The coronary ostium opens when the left ventricle is filling with blood, resulting in blood flow to the coronary arteries.
  - The right coronary artery supplies blood to:
    - Bundle of His.
    - AV node.
    - SA node.
    - Right atrium.
    - Right ventricle.
    - A segment of the left ventricle.
  - The left coronary artery supplies blood to:
    - Left atrium.
    - Anterior wall of the left ventricle.
    - Right bundle branch.
    - Right ventricle.
    - Interventricular septum.
    - Left anterior fasciculus.
  - Circumflex artery supplies blood to:
    - Lateral wall of the left ventricle.
    - Later wall to the left atrium.
    - SA node in 50% of patients.
    - Posterior left ventricle.
- Deoxygenated blood is carried by cardiac veins from cardiac cells to the coronary sinus.
- Deoxygenated blood is carried by the coronary sinus to the right atrium.

3.1.2 Cardiac cycle

- Systole:
  - Ventricles contract.
    - Pressure in the right ventricle forces the pulmonary valve to open, enabling deoxygenated blood to flow into the pulmonary artery.

        - Pressure in the left ventricle forces the aortic valve to open, enabling oxygenated blood to flow throughout the body.
        - Atriums relax and fill with blood.
- Diastole:
    - Ventricles relax and fill with blood.
        - Thirty percent (30%) of blood enters the ventricles through atrium contraction.
        - Seventy percent (70%) of the blood enters the ventricles through gravity.
    - Atriums contract (atrial kick), forcing blood into the ventricles.
- Cardiac output:
    - Cardiac output is the volume of blood ejected by the heart in 1 minute and is calculated as:

      cardiac output = heart rate × stroke volume
- Stroke volume:
    - Stroke volume is the volume of blood ejected by the heart during each cardiac contraction.
    - Factors influencing stroke volume are:
        - Preload:
            - Preload is the stretching ability of cardiac fibers.
            - The higher the ability to stretch, the higher the force of the cardiac contraction.
        - Afterload:
            - Afterload is the pressure that the left ventricle must generate to overcome resistance in the arterial system.
            - The higher the afterload, the higher workload on the heart to eject blood.
        - Contractility:
            - Contractility is the ability of the heart to contract and it is influenced by the preload.
            - The greater the contractility, the higher the force of the cardiac contraction.

3.1.3 Cardiac impulses

- The SA node generates the impulse that stimulates the atrium to contract.
- The AV node sends an impulse to the atrioventricular bundle (bundle of His) causing the ventricles to contract.

3.2 Critical Care Cardiovascular Assessment

- A cardiovascular assessment begins by asking the patient about cardiovascular complaints:
    - Is the patient alert and oriented?
    - Does the patient:
        - Experience chest pain?
        - Have difficulty breathing when lying down?
        - Experience palpitations?
        - Feel that his heart beats irregularly?

- Feel tried?
- Experience cramping in the legs?
- Have leg pain?
- Have swelling in the legs?
- Feel dizzy?
- Experience nausea?
- Experience sweating?
- Frequently urinate?

- Inspect the patient:
  - Position the patient on his or her back with the head of the bed raised 30 degrees or 45 degrees.
  - Expose areas of the body as needed during the inspection.
  - Skin color (view mucous membranes in dark-skinned patients):
    - Shiny: May indicate diminished arterial blood flow.
    - Cynanosis (bluish): May indicate diminished cardiac output.
    - Pallor: May indicate diminished tissue perfusion.
  - Body hair:
    - No body hair: May indicate diminished arterial blood flow.
  - Edema (arms/legs): May indicate:
    - Venous insufficiency: Veins are unable to return blood to the heart.
    - Left side heart failure: Insufficient output by the left ventricle.
    - Thrombophlebitis: Inflammation of a vein caused by a blood clot.
    - Varicosities: Valves in veins deep in the leg malfunction, resulting in pooling of blood. This leads to increased venous pressure that causes surface veins to enlarge.
    - Carotid artery: The carotid artery should not be pounding or have a weak pulse, and the pulse should remain unchanged when the patient changes position.
    - Internal jugular vein: The internal jugular vein's pulsating should change when the patient changes position. Jugular vein distention may indicate increased central venous pressure (CVP).
- Palpate the patient:
  - Skin:
    - Cool: May indicate diminished tissue perfusion.
  - Capillary refill: Capillary refill should be less than 3 seconds.
  - Pulse: Compare the same pulse on each side of the body.
    - Weak pulse: Weak pulse may indicate decreased cardiac output or arterial atherosclerosis, resulting in increased peripheral vascular resistance.
    - Bounding pulse: Bounding pulse may indicate hypertension or increased cardiac output related to hyperthyroidism, anemia, aneurism, or exercising.
    - Epigastric pulsation: Epigastric pulsation may indicate aortic aneurysm.
    - Grading pulses:
      - 0 = Absent
      - 1 = Weak
      - 2 = Normal

- 3 = Increased
- 4 = Bounding

- Pedal pulse:
  - Absent: May indicate diminished arterial blood flow.
  - Percuss the patient:

- Percussion does not provide assessment value.
- Auscultate the patient:
  - Use a stethoscope:
    - Diaphragm: Listen for high-pitched sounds.
    - Bell: Listen for low-pitched sounds.
    - Carotid arteries: Listen with the bell of the stethoscope. A buzzing sound (bruit) may indicate formation of arteriosclerotic plaque.
    - Epigastric area: Listen for turbulence over the abdominal aorta, which may indicate an aneurysm.
    - Listen to heart sounds with the patient placed in three positions:
      - Place the patient on his or her back with the head of the bed raised 30 degrees to 45 degrees.
      - Ask the patient to move to a sitting position.
      - Place the patient lying on the left side.
    - Normal heart sounds:
      - S1: Closure of the mitral and tricuspid valves when ventricles contract (systole).
      - S2: Closure of the aortic and pulmonary valves when ventricles relax (diastole).
    - Abnormal heart sounds:
      - S3:
        - Following S2
        - The ventricle requires additional force to accept the volume of blood.
        - Called a ventricular gallop because the rhythm sounds like a galloping horse.
        - Rhythm like "Ken-tuc-ky."
        - Best heard using the bell of the stethoscope at the apex when the patient is lying on the left side (left lateral debcubitus).
        - May indicate:
          - Pulmonary congestion.
          - Heart failure (left or right).
          - Mitral valve insufficiency.
          - Tricuspid valve insufficiency.
          - Myocardial infarction (MI).
          - Intracardiac shunting of blood.
      - S4:
        - Immediately before S1.
        - Called atrial gallop because the rhythm sounds like a galloping horse.
        - Rhythm like "Ten-nes-see."
        - Best heard using the bell of the stethoscope at the apex when the patient is lying in the left lateral position.

- May indicate:
  - Aortic stenosis.
  - Pulmonary hypertension.
  - Acute MI.
  - Angina.
  - Pulmonary embolism.
  - Coronary artery disease (CAD).
  - Hypertension.
  - Increased left ventricular pressure.
  - Fluid volume overload.

- Murmurs:
  - A murmur is a turbulent abnormal sound caused by the flow of blood through the heart during the cardiac cycle.
  - Describe a murmur by:
  - Identify location and when the murmur occurs during the cardiac cycle:
    - Midsystolic:
      - Occurs during the middle of systole; commonly referred to as systolic ejection.
      - Heard over the pulmonary valve (pulmonic stenosis) or over the aortic and suprasternal notch (aortic stenosis).
      - Harsh medium-pitched to high-pitched sound.
    - Holosystolic:
      - Occurs throughout systole; commonly referred to as pansystolic.
      - Heard:
        - Harsh, high-pitched sound over the tricuspid (ventricular septal defect).
        - Blowing high-pitched sound over the tricuspid (tricuspid insufficiency).
        - Blowing high-pitched sound over the mitral (mitral insufficiency).
    - Early diastolic:
      - Occurs at the onset of the diastole.
      - Hard over the midleft sternal edge of the heart (aortic insufficiency) or the pulmonary valve (pulmonic insufficiency).
      - Blowing high-pitched sound.
    - Mid diastolic:
      - Occurs during the middle or toward the end of diastole.
      - Heard over the apex (mitral stensosis) or tricusipid (tricuspid stenosis).
      - Rumbling, low-pitched sound.
    - Pattern
      - Crescendo-decrescendo: The murmur becomes loud then soft.
      - Crescendo: The murmur becomes louder.
      - Decrescendo: The murmur becomes softer.
    - Pitch:
      - High (use diaphragm on stethoscope).
      - Medium (use diaphragm or bell on stethoscope).
      - Low (use bell on stethoscope).

- Intensity grade:
  - Grade I: Faint.
  - Grade II: Soft.
  - Grade III: Loud as normal heart sounds.
  - Grade IV: Louder than a normal heart sound, and a thrill can be palpated at the murmur site.
  - Grade V: Very loud, and a thrill can be palpated at the murmur site.
  - Grade VI: Extremely loud, and a thrill can be palpated at the murmur site. Heard with stethoscope hovering over the site without contact with the chest.
- Quality:
  - Musical.
  - Blowing.
  - Rasping.
  - Rumbling.
  - Machine-like.
  - Harsh.

– Rubs:
  - Scraping, grating sound heard over the lower left sternal border at the third left intercostal space.
  - Occurs throughout the cardiac cycle.
  - May indicate pericarditis or other cardiac infection.

3.3 Critical Care Chest Pain Assessment

- Ask the patient whether he or she is experiencing chest pain.
- Encourage the patient to describe the pain in his or her own words unless the patient is in distress.
- If the patient is in distress, ask the patient to answer yes or no.
- Commonly asked questions:
  - On a scale of 0 to 10, where 0 is no pain and 10 is the worst pain, what number is your pain?
  - Where is the pain?
  - When did the pain begin?
  - What makes the pain worse?
  - What makes the pain better?
  - Is the pain squeezing, burning, or tightening?
  - Does the pain move or remain in one place?
  - Are you nauseous?
  - Do you feel anything unusual with your heart, such as palpitation or your heart skips a beat?
  - Do you feel short of breath?
  - You do have difficulty breathing when you wake up?
  - Do you feel dizzy?

  - Do you faint?
  - Do you get up from sleep to urinate?
- Common cardiac causes of pain:
  - Pulmonary embolus:
    - Sudden stabbing pain over the lung that is worse on inspiration.
    - Administering analgesic improves the pain.
  - Acute MI:
    - Burning, aching pain resulting in pressure or tightness across the chest and radiating to the jaw, arms, back, and neck; worse on exertion.
    - Administer morphine or nitroglycerin to improve the pain.
  - Angina pectoris:
    - Heaviness, burning, squeezing pain over the substernal, radiating to the jaw, arms, back, and neck; may subside within 10 minutes. Pain is worse lying down or with physical activity.
    - Administer nitroglycerin. Rest improves pain in stable angina. Rest does not improve pain in unstable angina.
  - Dissecting aortic aneurysm:
    - Tearing pain in the retrosternal, epigastric, or upper abdominal area, radiating to the shoulders, back, or neck. Blood pressure has different values in left and right arms.
    - Administer analgesic to improve the pain. Surgery may be required to repair the condition.
  - Pericarditis:
    - Sudden onset of sharp and continuous pain over the substernal area, radiating to the left arm, neck, or back; worsens with deep inspiration and lying in the supine position.
    - Administering anti-inflammatory medication and having the patient sit up and forward improve the pain.

3.4 Cardiac Tests

- Cardiac test are used to determine cardiac function and to assess the degree of cardiac malfunction. Some tests, such as an electrocardiogram (ECG) and echocardiography, are not invasive. Other cardiac tests, such as hemodynamic monitoring and cardiac markers, are invasive. Hemodynamic monitoring requires catheterization and cardiac markers require blood samples.

3.4.1 Cardiac markers

- Cardiac markers are enzymes that provide an indication of whether the patient has experienced an acute MI. Cardiac enzymes are contained within cells of cardiac tissues. Cardiac cells rupture as a result of an acute MI, releasing cardiac enzymes into the blood. The amount of cardiac enzymes indicates cardiac damage.
- Cardiac enzymes are:
  - Creatine kinase (CK): Found in muscle tissues.
  - Isoenzyme of creatine kinase with muscle and brain subunits (CK-MB): Found only in cardiac muscle tissues.

- Measurements:
  - CK-MB:
    - CK-MB levels increase 4 hours to 8 hours after an acute MI.
    - Can remain elevated for 72 hours and peak after 20 hours.
  - Troponin:
    - Troponin is used to detect an acute MI that has occurred days before the sample is taken.
    - Troponin elevates 3 hours to 6 hours after an acute MI.
    - Troponin I peaks 14 hours to 20 hours after an acute MI and returns to normal levels in 5 to 7 days.
    - Troponin T peaks 12 hours to 24 hours after an acute MI and returns to normal levels in 10 to 15 days.
  - Ischemia modified albumin (IMA):
    - IMA increases when there is ischemic tissue, which occurs in an acute MI.
    - IMA rises minutes after an acute MI, peaks in 6 hours, and returns to normal levels in 12 hours.
  - Myoglobin:
    - Myoglobin increases between 30 minutes and 4 hours after an acute MI.
    - Myoglobin peaks in 6 hours and returns to normal level 12 hours.
- When working with cardiac markers:
  - Tell the patient that several blood samples will be taken over 24 hours.
  - Do not administer intramuscular (IM) injection or exercise before taking a blood sample. IM injections and exercise can injure muscle tissue, resulting in the release of CK into the blood and leading to invalid results.
  - Do not administer prior to taking a blood sample (notify laboratory if patient was administered these):
    - Lithium (Eskalith).
    - Alcohol.
    - Aminocaproic acid (Amicar).
- Assess the collection of cardiac markers rather than individual test results.

3.4.2 Electrocardiogram

- The ECG shows a graphic representation of the electrical activity of the heart in a three-dimensional perspective. An electrical signal is generated each time the heart contracts. Small pads containing electrodes placed on the surface of the skin detect the electrical signal. Six electrodes are placed on the chest and six electrodes are placed on the arms and legs. Each electrode is connected with wires to an electrocardiograph machine that draws up to 12 different graphical representations of the electrical signal. *Schaum's Outline of ECG Interpretation* provides details on how to administer an ECG and how to interpret the results.
  - P wave: The first deflection is recorded as the P wave and starts when there is electrical activity at the SA node of the heart, indicating atrial contraction (depolarization).
  - PR interval (PRI): The period between the beginning of the P wave and the beginning of the QRS complex is called the PRI. This is the time the electrical impulse takes to travel to the ventricles after atrial relaxation (repolarization).

  - QRS complex: The QRS complex represents ventricle contraction (depolarization).
  - ST segment: The ST segment measures the time from the end of ventricular depolarization to the start of ventricular repolarization.
  - QT interval (QTI): The QTI measures the time from the beginning of ventricular depolarization to the end of ventricular repolarization.

3.4.3 Echocardiogram

- An echocardiogram uses waves to assess the heart. A transducer is placed over an area of the patient's chest that is absent of bone and lung tissue. The transducer generates sounds waves toward the heart and then receives sound waves reflected by the heart. These are converted to an electronic signal that is displayed on a screen or on a strip.
- There are three types of echocardiograms:
  - M-mode: The M-mode generates a thin sound wave to produce a vertical view of cardiac structures.
  - 2-D Mode: The 2-D mode uses a sweeping sound wave to produce a cross-section view of cardiac structures. It is used to record lateral motion of the heart.
  - Transesophageal echocardiograpy (TEE): TEE requires that a small transducer be inserted into the esophagus using a gastroscope, enabling posterior ultrasound images to be taken of the heart.
- During the echocardiogram:
  - Except for TEE, conductive gel is applied to the patient's chest.
  - The patient may experience a little discomfort related to pressure applied to the transducer.
  - The patient must lie still during the test.
  - Excess conductive gel is removed after the test is completed.
- Echocardiogram is used to diagnose:
  - Aortic insufficiency.
  - Mitral stenosis.
  - Pericardial effusion.
  - Endocarditis.
  - Tumors.
  - Intracardiac thrombi.
  - Cardiac abnormalities.

3.4.4 Cardiac catheterization

- Cardiac catheterization is a 1- to 2-hour procedure in which a catheter is passed in an artery or vein in the arm or leg and moved under local anesthetic into the right, left, or both sides of the heart. The procedure may require injection of contrast through the catheter into the heart. The patient is under mild sedation and will be asked to cough and breathe deeply during the procedure. The patient may be administered nitroglycerin during the procedure to dilate coronary arteries.
- Cardiac catheterization is used to:
  - Measure blood flow.
  - Measure blood pressure.
  - Assess ischemia of coronary arteries.
  - Assess blockage of coronary arteries.

- Assess cardiac valves.
- Collect blood samples.
- Perform balloon catheter treatments.
- Assess in calculating cardiac output.

- Preprocedure steps:
  - Assess patient for shellfish and iodine allergies. Contrast material may cause an allergic reaction in these patients.
  - Explain the procedure to the patient.
  - Patient signs consent form.
  - Stop anticoagulant therapy (aspirin, warfarin, Lovenox) prior to the procedure.
  - No food or fluids 6 hours before the test.
  - Open an intravenous (IV) access site.
  - Assess the peripheral pulse.
  - Verify that the patient has normal renal function, which is necessary to excrete the contrast material.
- Postprocedure steps:
  - Monitor for:
    - Chest pain.
    - Bleeding at the insertion site.
    - Shortness of breath.
    - Nausea.
    - Vomiting.
    - Confusion.
    - Sweating.
    - Arrhythmia.
    - Decreased pulse below catheterization puncture site.
    - Cool skin temperature below insertion site.
    - Cyanosis below insertion site.
  - The patient must lie flat with arm or leg used for catheterization extended for:
    - Three hours if the antecubital fossa was used in the arm as the site.
    - Eight hours if the femoral artery is used as the site. Place a sandbag(s) on the catheterization site.
    - Eight hours if catheterization site was not closed using a suture or other device.
    - Two hours if catheterization site was closed using a suture or other device.
  - Monitor vital signs:
    - Every 15 minutes for the first 2 hours.
    - Every 30 minutes for the next 2 hours.
    - Every 4 hours.
    - Every 5 minutes if the patient becomes unstable.
  - Administer IV fluids to flush the contrast material.
  - Complications:
    - Stroke (left side).
    - Arterial embolus (left side).
    - Arrhythmias.

  - Infection.
  - Hematoma.
  - Cardiac tamponade.
  - Pulmonary embolism (right side).
  - Pulmonary edema.
  - MI.
  - Vagal response (right side).
  - Allergic reaction to contract material.
  - Hypovolemia.

3.4.5 Cardiac output monitoring

- Cardiac output is the volume of blood ejected by the heart in 1 minute, which is normally 4 L/min to 8 L/min, and is used to assess cardiac function.
- Several techniques are used for measuring cardiac output. The most commonly used are:
  - Thermodilution:
    - A pulmonary artery (PA) catheter is inserted into the right atrium.
    - A solution is injected into the PA catheter.
    - The solution mixes with the blood and moves through the right ventricle and then into the PA.
    - The catheter's thermistor measures the temperature of blood and calculates the blood flow.
  - Flick method:
    - The Flick method measures oxygen consumption per minute.
    - Oxygen content of blood is measured before (pulmonary/brachial arteries [venous blood]) and after blood passes through the lungs using a spirometer (arterial blood).
    - Cardiac output (L/min) = Oxygen consumption ml/min/ (arterial oxygen content – venous oxygen content ml/min).
  - Dye dilution test:
    - Dye is injected into the blood via IV injection.
    - Blood samples are taken from arteries throughout the body.
    - Cardiac output is calculated based on the rate at which the dye is diluted.
  - Cardiac index:
    - Cardiac index adjusts the value of the cardiac output to the size of the patient, which is measured as body surface area.
    - Cardiac index = cardiac output/body surface area.
    - Cardiac index normal ranges are 2.5 L/min/m^2 to 4.2 L/min/m^2 in adults.
- Sample measurements for cardiac output tests are taken about every 3 hours.
- The patient must remain still during the cardiac output test.
- Chart the patient's position when samples are taken.
- Monitor for signs of decreased perfusion:
  - Decreased level of consciousness.
  - Restlessness.

- Pale skin.
- Fatigue.
- Decreased peripheral pulses.
- Decreased capillary refill.
- Cool skin.

3.4.6 Cardiac function measurements

- Stroke volume:
  - Stroke volume is the volume of blood ejected by contraction of the ventricle.
    - Stroke volume = cardiac output/heart rate.
    - Normal: 60 to 130 ml/heartbeat.
    - Decreased stroke volume caused by:
      - Increased afterload.
      - Hypovolemia.
      - Decreased contractibility.
      - Arrhythmias.
    - Increased stroke volume caused by:
      - Hypervolmeia.
      - Sepsis.
- Stroke volume index:
  - Stroke volume index is the stroke volume adjusted for the patient's body size.
  - Normal: 30 ml/beat/m^2 to 65 ml/beat/m^2.
  - Stroke volume index = stroke volume/body surface area.
  - Changes in stroke volume index values are caused by the same underlying condition as the condition that causes changes in the stroke volume values.
- Systemic vascular resistance:
  - Systemic vascular resistance is measured resistance against the left ventricle.
  - Systemic vascular resistance = mean arterial pressure – central venous pressure/cardiac output × 80
  - Normal: 800 dynes/sec/cm^{-5} to 1400 dynes/sec/cm^{-5}.
  - Decreased systemic vascular resistance caused by:
    - Vasodilation.
    - Shock.
  - Increased systemic vascular resistance caused by:
    - Vasoconstriction.
    - Hyperthermia.
- Pulmonary vascular resistance:
  - Pulmonary vascular resistance is measured resistance against the right ventricle.
  - Normal: 20 dynes/sec/cm^{-5} to 200 dynes/sec/cm^{-5}.
  - Pulmonary vascular resistance = mean pulmonary arterial pressure - pulmonary artery wedge pressure/ cardiac output • 80.

- Decreased pulmonary vascular resistance caused by:
  - Pulmonary vasodilation.
- Increased pulmonary vascular resistance caused by:
  - Pulmonary embolism.
  - Hypoxemia.
  - Hypertension.

3.4.7 Arterial blood pressure monitoring

- Arterial blood pressure monitoring requires the healthcare practitioner to insert a catheter connected to a transducer into the radial or femoral artery. The transducer monitors arterial blood flow, converting the flow into an electronic wave form that is displayed on a screen or recorded on a strip.
- Monitor the insertion site for swelling, bleeding, and redness.

3.4.8 Pulmonary arterial blood pressure monitoring

- Pulmonary arterial blood pressure monitoring measures the amount of pressure required to open the pulmonary valve (systolic pressure) and resistance when the pulmonary valve is closed (diastolic pressure).
- The healthcare practitioner inserts a multilumen catheter into the patient's subclavian vein or internal jugular vein and moves the catheter into the right atrium. The balloon is inflated and floats through the right ventricle into the PA, where the pulmonary artery wedge pressure (PAWP) is measured. The balloon is then deflated and other pressures are measured.
- The catheter contains five lumens:
  - Balloon inflation lumen: Used to inflate a balloon at the tip of the catheter to measure PAWP.
  - Distal lumen: Connects to a transducer to measure PAWP when the balloon is inflated. This lumen is also used to withdraw venous blood samples.
  - Proximal lumen: Used to measure right atrial pressure.
  - Thermistor connector lumen: Contains a temperature-sensitive wire connected to a computer to measure cardiac output.
  - Pacemaker lumen: Used to insert a pacemaker electrode.
- The procedure takes about 30 minutes, and the patient is awake during the procedure.
- Monitor vital signs during the procedure.
- Monitor for swelling, bleeding, and redness.

3.4.9 Central venous blood pressure monitoring

- Central venous blood pressure monitoring requires the healthcare practitioner to insert a catheter connected to a transducer into a vein. The catheter is then moved near the right atrium. The transducer monitors venous blood flow, converting the flow into an electronic wave that is displayed on the screen or recorded on a strip.
- Monitor the insertion site for swelling, bleeding, and redness.

3.5 Cardiac Medication

- Cardiac medication can influence cardiac function, counteracting cardiac malfunction caused by acute or chronic cardiac disorders. Cardiac medications are classified by the medication's effect on the heart. These are:
  - Positive inotropic effect: Medications that increase the force of cardiac contractions.
  - Inotropic agents: Medications that influence the muscular contraction of cardiac muscle.
  - Negative chronotropic effect: Medications that slow the heart rate.
  - Negative dromotropic effect: Medications that decrease the electrical impulse through the AV node.

3.5.1 Cardiac glycosides

- Cardiac glycosides are medications that increase the force of contractions, slow the heart rate, and reduce the electrical impulse through the AV node.
  - Use: Heart failure.
  - Medication:
    - Digoxin (Lanoxin).
  - Considerations:
    - Hold medication if apical pulse is <60 bpm and notify healthcare practitioner.
    - Loading dose is required if immediate effects are required.
    - Measure therapeutic serum level to prevent digoxin toxicity. Therapeutic serum level is 0.5 ng/ml to 2 ng/ml.
- Adverse effects:
  - Digoxin toxicity:
    - Irritability.
    - Abdominal pain.
    - Nausea.
    - Abnormal vision.
  - Anorexia.
  - Arrhythmia.

3.5.2 Phosphodiesterase (PDE) inhibitors

- Phosphodiesterase (PDE) inhibitors are medications that increase contractions by influencing the movement and storage of calcium in cardiac cells.
- Use: Heart failure, vasodilation.
- Medications:
  - Primacor (Milrinone).
  - Inamrinone (Inocor).
- Considerations:
  - Hold medication if serum potassium level is outside normal limits and notify healthcare practitioner.
  - Not used in MI.

- Adverse effects:
  - Chest pain.
  - Headache.
  - Thrombocytopenia.
  - Nausea.
  - Vomiting.
  - Arrhythmia.
  - Fever.
  - Hypokalemia.

3.5.3 Antiarrhythmics medications

- Antiarrhythmic medications are used to correct abnormal cardiac rhythms. There are four major classes of antiarrhythmic medications. Each class is based on the mechanism the medication uses to correct the arrhythmia.
  - Class I: Class I antiarrhythmic medication blocks the sodium channel. Class I is divided into subclasses, reflecting introduction of newer medication.
    - Class IA:
      - Function: Increases conduction rate of the AV node by blocking the parasympathetic nervous system and preventing stimulation of the parasympathetic nervous system, which would decrease the conduction rate of the AV node.
      - Medication:
        - Quinidine sulfate (Quinidex).
        - Procainamide (Procanbid).
        - Quindine gluconate (Quinaglute).
        - Disopyramide (Norpace).
      - Use:
        - Atrial flutter.
        - Ventricular tachycardia.
        - Atrial fibrillation.
      - Considerations:
        - Hold dose if apical pulse rate is very high or very low.
      - Adverse effects:
        - Arrhythmias.
        - Respiratory arrest.
        - Vomiting.
        - Nausea.
        - Diarrhea.
        - Liver toxicity.
    - Class IB:
      - Function: Decreases the refractory period by blocking sodium during cardiac depolarization.

- Medication:
  - Mexiletine (Mexitil).
  - Lidocaine (Xylocaine).
- Use:
  - Ventricular fibrillation.
  - Ventricular tachycardia.
- Considerations:
  - Administer using an IV infusion pump.
  - Can increase the effects of other antiarrhythmic medications.
- Adverse effects:
  - Arrhythmias.
  - Bradycardia.
  - Drowsiness.
  - Hypotension.

- Class IC:
  - Function: Decreases cardiac condition by slowing the action potential of sodium.
  - Medication:
    - Moricizine (Ethmozine).
    - Propafenone (Rythmol).
    - Flecainide (Tambocor).
  - Use:
    - Supraventricular arrhythmias.
    - Ventricular fibrillation.
    - Ventricular tachycardia.
  - Considerations:
    - Monitor ECG before and after administering the dose to detect changes.
    - Hold dose for abnormal electrolyte levels.
  - Adverse effects:
    - Arrhythmias.
    - Heart failure.

- Class II: Class II antiarrhythmic medications block beta-adrenergic receptor sites, decreasing conductivity of the AV node and decreasing cardiac workload. This reduces the oxygen requirement of the heart.
  - Medication:
    - Propranolol (Inderal).
    - Acebutolol (Sectral).
    - Esmolol (Brevibloc).
  - Use:
    - Ventricular arrhythmias.
    - Atrial flutter.
    - Atrial fibrillation.
    - Paroxysmal atrial tachycardia.

- Considerations:
  - Titrate discontinuation of medication. Do not abruptly stop medication.
  - Hold dose for abnormal blood pressure and apical heart rate.
- Adverse effects:
  - Arrhythmias.
  - Heart failure.
  - Bradycardia.
  - Bronchospasm.
  - Hypotension.
  - Nausea.
  - Vomiting.

○ Class III: Class III antiarrhythmic medications' mechanism is not known.

- Medication:
  - Amiodarone (Pacerone).
  - Ibutilide fumurate (Convert).
- Use:
  - Arrhythmias that are life threatening.
- Considerations:
  - Monitor signs of pulmonary toxicity:
    - Pleuritic chest pain.
    - Difficulty breathing (dyspnea).
    - Nonproductive cough.
  - Monitor for changes in cardiac rate and rhythm.
  - Hold dose for abnormal blood pressure and apical heart rate.
  - Risk for digoxin toxicity if patient is also taking digoxin.
- Adverse effects:
  - Arrhythmias.
  - Hypotension.
  - Liver toxicity.

○ Class IV: Class IV antiarrhythmic medications block calcium, slowing cardiac conduction and decreasing the cardiac refractory period.

- Medication:
  - Verapamil (Calan).
  - Diltiazem (Cardizem).
- Use:
  - Supraventricular arrhythmias.
- Considerations:
  - Avoid calcium supplements.
  - Monitor cardiac rhythm and cardiac rate when beginning treatment or increasing the dose.
- Adverse effects:
  - Hypotension.
  - Pulmonary edema.

        - Peripheral edema.
        - Heart failure.
        - Bradycardia.
    - Nonclassified antiarrhythmic: Adenosine (Adenocard) does not fit in classes of antiarrhythmic medications. Adenosine (Adenocard) decreases conductivity of the SA node and AV node.
        - Medication:
            - Adenosine (Adenocard).
        - Use:
            - Paraoxysmal supraventricular tachycardia.
        - Considerations:
            - Administer the medication IV over 2 seconds followed by 20 ml of normal saline (flush).
            - Monitor cardiac rhythm during administration of the medication.
        - Adverse effects:
            - Chest discomfort.
            - Difficulty breathing (dyspnea).

3.5.4 Antiangina medications

- Antiangina medications increase the supply of oxygen to the heart and decrease cardiac oxygen demand for patients who experience chest pain related to angina. During angina, cardiac arteries narrow (ischemia), reducing oxygen to cardiac muscle, resulting in chest pain.
- There are three classes of anti-angina medication:
    - Nitrates cause arteries to dilate, resulting in increased oxygenated blood to cardiac muscles and reducing peripheral vascular resistance (decrease afterload). Nitrates also cause veins to dilate, resulting in less blood return to the heart (preload) and leading to decreased size of workload of the ventricle.
    - Medication:
        - Nitroglycerin (Nitro-Bid).
        - Isosorbide mononitrate (Imdur).
        - Isosorbide dinitrate (Isordil).
    - Use:
        - Prevent angina.
        - Relive chest pains caused by angina.
    - Considerations:
        - Do not administer to patients taking erectile dysfunction medication. Administering both medications can lead to severe hypotension.
        - Administer sublingual or translingual.
        - Monitor blood pressure before administering medication. Administering medication leads to hypotension.
    - Adverse effects:
        - Dizziness.
        - Increased heart rate.

    - Hypotension.
    - Headache.
- Beta-adrenergic blockers decrease cardiac contractions and decrease the heart rate, resulting in decreased cardiac oxygen requirement by blocking beta-adrenergic receptor sites in cardiac muscle.
- Medication:
    - Metoprolol (Lopressor).
    - Propranolol (Inderal).
    - Atenolol (Tenormin).
    - Carvedilol (Coreg).
- Use:
    - Hypertension (first line).
    - Stable heart failure.
    - Prevent angina (long-term).
- Considerations:
    - Monitor blood pressure and heart rate regularly.
    - Can cause hypoglycemic shock in diabetic patients.
- Adverse effects:
    - Hypoglycemia.
    - Fluid retention.
    - Bradycardia.
    - Nausea.
    - Diarrhea.
    - Fainting.
    - Bronchospasm.
    - Heart failure.
- Calcium channel blockers dilate arteries (coronary and peripheral), decreasing the workload of the heart (afterload) by blocking calcium from entering cardiac and smooth muscles.
- Medication:
    - Diltiazem (Cardizem).
    - Amlodipine (Norvasc).
    - Verapamil (Calan).
    - Nifedipine (Adalat).
- Use:
    - Hypertension.
    - Prevent angina (long-term) when other drugs fail to work.
- Considerations:
    - Avoid calcium supplements. Calcium supplements may decrease effect of medication.
    - Monitor vital signs when beginning treatment.
- Adverse effects:
    - Headache.
    - Orthostatic hypotension.

        - Hypotension.
        - Heart failure.
        - Pulmonary edema.
        - Peripheral edema.
        - Arrhythmias.

3.5.5 Antihypertensive medications

- Antihypertensive medications decrease blood pressure using various mechanisms depending on the type of antihypertensive medication prescribed to the patient. Beta adrenergic blockers (see 3.5.4 Anti-angina medications) are the first line of antihypertensive medications, followed by diuretics (See 3.5.6 Diuretic medications). When these medications are ineffective, antihypertensive medications are prescribed.
- There are four categories of antihypertensive medications. These are:
    - Sympoatholytic: Sympatholytic medications cause dilation of peripheral blood vessels by blocking the sympathetic nervous system. This results in decreased cardiac output.
    - Medications:
        - Clonidine (Catapres).
        - Methyldopa (Aldomet).
        - Terazosin (Hytrin).
        - Prazosin (Minipress).
        - Guanabenz (Wytensin).
        - Guanadrel (Hylorel).
    - Use:
        - Hypertension.
    - Considerations:
        - Monitor blood pressure before administering the dose.
    - Adverse effects:
        - Bradycardia.
        - Arrhythmias.
        - Edema.
        - Depression.
        - Hypotension.
        - Liver damage.
    - Vasodilating medication: Vasodilating medications relax smooth muscles of the peripheral vascular system, enabling arteries and veins to dilate, which decreases afterload resistance.
    - Medications:
        - Nitroprusside (Nipride).
        - Diazoxide (Hyperstat).
        - Hydralazine (Apresoline).
    - Use:
        - Hypertensive crisis.
        - Hypertension.

- Considerations:
  - Monitor blood pressure before administering the dose.
- Adverse effects:
  - Angina.
  - Palpitations.
  - Headache.
  - Stevens-Johnson syndrome.
  - Tachycardia.
  - Liver damage.
- Angiotensin-converting enzyme (ACE) inhibitors: ACE inhibitors disrupt the renin-angiotension-aldosterone mechanism, resulting in reduction in aldosterone production. This leads to the excretion of sodium and water, causing blood pressure to decrease.
- Medications:
  - Quinapril (Accupril).
  - Benazepril (Lotensin).
  - Lisinopril (Prinivil).
  - Benazepril (Lotensin).
- Use:
  - Heart failure.
  - Hypertension.
- Considerations:
  - Monitor blood pressure before administering medication.
- Adverse effects:
  - Rash.
  - Cough.
  - Renal insufficiency.
  - Angioedema.
- Angiotensin II receptor blocker (ARB): ARB disrupts the renin-angiotension-aldosterone mechanism, resulting in the same effect as ACE inhibitors.
- Medications:
  - Losartan (Cozaar).
  - Candesartan (Atacand).
  - Valsartan (Diovan).
  - Irbesrtan (Avapro).
- Use:
  - Heart failure.
  - Hypertension.
- Considerations:
  - Monitor blood pressure before administering medication.
- Adverse effects:
  - Rash.
  - Fatigue.

- Hypotension.
- Abdominal pain.

3.5.6 Diuretic medications

- Antihypertensive medications cause water and electrolytes to be excreted by the kidneys, resulting in decreased afterload resistance and decreased blood pressure. There are three categories of diuretics. These are:
  - Loop diuretics: Loop diuretics increase secretion of sodium, chloride, and water, leading to increased concentration of urine in the ascending loop of Henle. This results in a large volume of urine production.
  - Medications:
    - Furosemide (Lasix).
    - Bumetanide (Bumex).
    - Ethacrynic acid (Edecrin).
  - Use:
    - Heart failure.
    - Edema.
    - Hypertension.
  - Considerations:
    - Monitor serum electrolyte levels.
    - Monitor fluid intake and output.
    - Monitor signs of excessive urination.
    - Monitor for signs of hypotension.
  - Adverse effects:
    - Low sodium (hyponatremia).
    - Low potassium (hypokalemia).
    - Dehydration.
    - Rash.
    - Muscle cramps.
    - Hypotension.
    - High uric acid (hyperuricemia).
  - Thiazide diuretics: Thiazide diuretics prevent the absorption of sodium by the kidneys and increase excretion of bicarbonate, potassium, and chloride. This leads to decreased fluid retention and decreased blood pressure.
  - Medications:
    - Methyclothiazide (Enduron).
    - Chlorthalidone (Hygroton).
    - Bendroflumethiazide (Naturetin).
    - Hydroflumethiazide (Saluron).
    - Indapamide (Lozol).

- Use:
  - Edema.
  - Hypertension.
- Considerations:
  - Monitor blood glucose levels.
  - Monitor intake and output.
  - Monitor serum potassium levels.
- Adverse effects:
  - Low sodium (hyponatremia).
  - Low potassium (hypokalemia).
  - Dizziness.
  - Nausea.
  - Hypotension.
- Potassium-sparing diuretics: Potassium-sparing diuretics cause the distal tubule of the kidneys to excrete sodium, water, calcium, and chloride and decreased secretion of potassium and hydrogen. This results in increased urine output and decreased blood pressure.
- Medications:
  - Spironolactone (Aldactone).
  - Triamterene (Dyrenium).
  - Amiloride (Midamor).
- Use:
  - Edema.
  - Hypertension.
  - Cirrhosis.
  - Nephrotic syndrome.
- Considerations:
  - Monitor intake and output.
  - Monitor cardiac rhythm for arrhythmias.
  - Monitor serum potassium levels.
- Adverse effects:
  - Nausea.
  - Rash.
  - Increased serum potassium (hyperkalemia).
  - Headache.

3.5.7 Anticoagulant medications

- Anticoagulant medications decrease blood's ability to clot. There are four classes of anticoagulant medications. These are:
  - Factor Xa Inhibitor: factor Xa inhibitor prevents the formation of thrombin and a blood clot by inhibiting Factor Xa. Factor Xa is the active form of the enzyme that is used in forming block clots.

- Medication:
  - Fondaparinux (Arixtra).
- Use:
  - Acute pulmonary embolism.
  - Deep vein thrombosis (VDT).
- Considerations:
- Monitor anti-Xa levels. Therapeutic level is 0.5 anti-Xa units/ml to 1.0 anti-Xa units/ml.
  - Monitor CBC.
  - Monitor platelet count.
  - Assess for signs of bleeding.
- Adverse effects:
  - Fever.
  - Bleeding.
  - Low platelet count (thrombocytopenia).
- Heparins: Heparins activate antithrombin II, which inhibits the formation of fibrin and thrombin, resulting in the prevention of blood clots' formation. Heparins prevent new blood clots from forming and are used to prevent blood clots in blood from being processed through the cardiopulmonary bypass machine or from blood being filtered during hemodialysis. Heparins do not dissolve existing blood clots.
- Medication:
  - Heparin.
  - Enoxaparin (Lovenox).
  - Dalteparin (Fragmin).
- Use:
  - Disseminated intravascular coagulation (DIC) (heparin).
  - VDT.
  - Prevent embolism.
  - Prevent complications from a MI.
- Considerations:
  - Monitor for signs of bleeding.
  - Use protamine sulfate to reverse the effect of heparin.
  - Monitor partial thromboplastin time (PTT). Therapeutic level is 1.5 to 2.5 normal value.
- Adverse effects:
  - Bleeding.
  - Low platelet count (thrombocytopenia).
- Antiplatelet: Antiplatelet medication interferes with binding of fibrinogen to platelets or blocks the creation of prostaglandin that prevents aggregation of platelets.
- Medication:
  - Aspirin.
  - Ticlopidine (Ticlid).
  - Clopidogrel (Plavix).
  - Dipyridamole (Persantine).

- Use:
  - Lower risk of MI.
  - Lower risk of complications from heart valve replacement.
- Considerations:
  - Dipyridamole (Persantine) is taken an hour before meals with a glass of water.
  - Ticlopidine (Ticlid) and aspirin are taken with food to prevent gastrointestinal upset.
  - Monitor for signs of bleeding.
- Adverse effects:
  - Bleeding.
  - Low platelet count (thrombocytopenia).
  - Gastrointestinal upset.
  - Welts (hives under the skin) (angioedema).
- Oral anticoagulants: Oral anticoagulant medication prevents vitamin K from being synthesized in the liver, which is necessary to create the clotting factor. Oral anticoagulants do not affect the clotting factor already in blood.
- Medication:
  - Warfarin (Coumadin).
- Use:
  - VDT.
  - Atrial arrhythmias.
  - Lower risk of complications from heart valve replacement.
- Considerations:
  - Use vitamin K to reverse the effect .
  - Monitor PTT. Therapeutic level is 1.5 to 2.5 normal values.
  - Monitor international normalization ratio (INR). Therapeutic level is 2 to 3.5 normal values.
- Adverse effects:
  - Diarrhea.
  - Hepatitis.
  - Bleeding.

3.5.8 Thrombolytic medications

- Thrombolytic medications dissolve existing blood clots by converting plasminogen to plasmin, which destroys the blood clot.
- Medications:
  - (Retavase, Reteplasae).
  - Streptokinase (Streptase).
  - Alteplase (Activase).
- Use:
  - Catheter occlusion.
  - Arterial thrombosis.

- Considerations:
  - Monitor for signs of bleeding.
  - Monitor blood pressure manually.
  - Avoid using a tourniquet when getting blood samples.
- Adverse effects:
  - Allergic reaction.
  - Bleeding.

3.5.9 Adrenergic medications

- Adrenergic medications increase cardiac output similar to how the sympathetic nervous system function initiates the fight-or-flight response. There are two classes of adrenergic medications. These are:
  - Catecholamines: Catecholamines combine with alpha receptors, resulting in an excitatory response, and beta receptors, resulting in an inhibitory response.
  - Medications:
    - Dopamine (Intropin).
    - Dobutamine (Dobutrex).
    - Norepinephrine (Levophed).
    - Epinephrine (Adrenalin).
  - Use:
    - Increase cardiac output (norepinephrine [Levophed]).
    - Maintain blood pressure.
    - Hypotension (dopamine [Intropin]).
    - Bronchospasm (epinephrine [Adrenalin]).
    - Anaphylaxis (epinephrine [Adrenalin]).
  - Considerations:
    - Monitor vital signs.
    - Monitor urine output (dopamine [Intropin]).
    - Treat hypovolemia before administering medication.
    - Administer using an infusion pump.
  - Adverse effects:
    - Anxiety.
    - Headache.
    - Increased blood glucose (epinephrine [Adrenalin]).
    - Bronchospasm (dobutamine [Dobutrex]).
    - Arrhythmias.
    - Tissue necrosis if medication leaks onto tissue.
  - Noncatecholamines: Noncatecholamines constrict blood vessels locally or throughout the vascular system to increase blood pressure.
  - Medications:
    - Ephedrine.
    - Phenylephrine (Neo-Synephrine).

- Use:
  - Maintain blood pressure.
  - Hypotension.
- Considerations:
  - Treat hypovolemia before administering medication.
  - Administer using an infusion pump.
  - Monitor vital signs.
- Adverse effects:
  - Anxiety.
  - Headache.
  - Arrhythmias.
  - Dizziness.
  - Tissue necrosis if medication leads onto tissue (phenylephrine Neo-Synephrine]).

3.5.10 Adrenergic blocking medications

- Adrenergic medications decrease cardiac output by blocking the sympathetic nervous system function. There are two classes of adrenergic blocking medications. These are:
  - Alpha-adrenergic blocking: Alpha-adrenergic blocking medications block the alpha-adrenergic receptors, resulting in relaxation of smooth muscles around blood vessels, leading to dilation of blood vessels and decreased blood pressure.
  - Medications:
    - Prazosin (Minipress).
    - Phentolamine (Regitine).
  - Use:
    - Pheochromocytoma.
    - Hypertension.
  - Considerations:
    - Monitor vital signs.
  - Adverse effects:
    - Palpitations.
    - Edema.
    - Orthostatic hypotension.
    - Weakness.
    - Flushing.
  - Beta-adrenergic blocking: Beta-adrenergic blocking medications block the beta-adrenergic receptors, resulting in decreased cardiac consumption of oxygen, slowing impulses between the atria and ventricles and leading to decreased cardiac output. Selective beta-adrenergic blocking medications affect $beta_1$-adrenergic sites. Nonselective beta-adrenergic blocking medications affect all beta-adrenergic sites.
  - Medications:
    - Selective:
      - Metoprolol (Lopressor).

- Acebutolol (Sectral).
- Esmolol (Brevibloc).
- Atenolol (Tenormin).

- Nonselective:
  - Propranolol (Inderal).
  - Carvedilol (Coreg).
  - Sotalol (Betapace).
  - Labetalol (Normodyne).
  - Timolol (Blocadren).

- Use:
  - Angina.
  - Hypertension.
  - Anxiety.
- Considerations:
  - Monitor vital signs.
  - May influence insulin requirements.
- Adverse effects:
  - Hypotension, peripheral vascular insufficiency.
  - Hypoglycemia.
  - Bradycardia.

3.5.11 Antilipemics medications

- Antilipemic medications decrease ipids. Lipids are triglycerides, cholesterol, and phospholipids. There are four classes of antilipemics. These are:
  - Bile-sequestering medication: Bile sequestering medication combines bile acids with low-density lipoproteins (LDLs), which is then excreted in a bowel movement.
  - Medication:
    - Colestipol (Colestid).
    - Cholestyramine (Questran).
    - Colesevelam (Welchol).
  - Use:
    - Decrease serum cholesterol.
  - Considerations:
    - Administer dose before meals.
    - Administer other medication 1 hour before or 6 hours after the dose is administered.
    - Period blood test required.
  - Adverse effects:
    - Headache.
    - Constipation.
    - Joint pain.

  - Bleeding.
  - Nausea.
- Cholesterol absorption inhibitors: Cholesterol absorption inhibitors prevent cholesterol from being absorbed by the intestines.
- Medication:
  - Ezetimide (Zetia).
- Use:
  - Decrease serum LDLs, cholesterol, triglycerides.
- Considerations:
  - Period blood test required.
- Adverse effects:
  - Headache.
  - Cough.
  - Dizziness.
  - Joint pain.
  - Muscle pain.
- Fibric acid derivative medication: Fibric acid derivative medication decreases triglycerides and high-density lipoproteins (HDLs) by decreasing their synthesis.
- Medication:
  - Gemfibrozil (Lopid).
  - Fenofibrate (Tricor).
- Use:
  - High cholesterol.
  - High triglycerides.
- Considerations:
  - Period blood tests.
  - Administer dose with meals.
- Adverse effects:
  - Abdominal pain.
  - Muscle pain.
  - Nausea.
  - Vomiting.
  - Rash.
  - Diarrhea.
  - Impotence.
  - Blurred vision.
- 3-hydroxy-3-methylglutaryl coenzyme A (HMG-CoA) reductase inhibitors: HMG-CoA reductase inhibitors interfere with synthesis of cholesterol, resulting in decreased lipids.
- Medication:
  - Simvastatin (Zocor).
  - Atorvastatin (Lipitor).

    - Rosuvastatin (Crestor).
    - Lovastatin (Mevacor).
    - Fluvastatin (Lescol).
  - Use:
    - High cholesterol.
    - High triglyceride.
    - High LDL levels.
  - Considerations:
    - Periodic blood test.
    - Administer the dose the same time each day.
    - Monitor liver function.
  - Adverse effects:
    - Joint pain.
    - Muscle pain.
    - Headache.
    - Cough.

3.6 Aortic Aneurysm

- Atherosclerosis, degeneration of the middle aortic muscle layer, trauma, infection, or congenital defects can cause weakening of the aortic wall. Pressure from blood flow causes the wall to bulge. Blood becomes turbulent, resulting an increased dilation of the weakened wall. The aneurysm may rupture, causing a drop in circulation, severe hypotension, syncope, and possibly death.

3.6.1 Signs and symptoms

- Asymptomatic.
- Restlessness and anxiety.
- Increased thready pulse and decreased pulse pressure.
- Decreased femoral pulses.
- Abdominal pulsation.
- Back pain radiating to posterior legs.
- Abdominal pain.

3.6.2 Medical tests

- Chest x-ray, abdominal ultrasound, computed tomography (CT) scan, or magnetic resonance imaging (MRI) are used to display the aortic aneurysm
- Accusation of bruit (swishing sound of turbulent blood) over the iliac or femoral arteries or abdominal aorta.

3.6.3 Treatment

- Administer:
  - Morphine sulfate or oxycodone to decrease oxygen demand.
  - Antihypertensives to reduce blood pressure.
  - Analgestics to reduce pain associated with tearing of the aortic wall and pressure the aortic aneurysm is placing on nerves.
- Surgical resection of the aortic aneurysm is commonly performed.

3.6.4 Intervention

- Limit activity and encourage patient to rest in a quiet place to reduce anxiety.
- Listen for abdominal bruits.
- Monitor for:
  - Numbness and tingling.
  - Decrease in temperature of extremities.
  - Increased thready pulse.
  - Change in skin color in extremities.
  - Pale clammy skin, indicating decreased circulation.
  - Restlessness, indicating increased anxiety and decreased oxygenation.
  - Intake and output and urine quality. Low urine output and high specific gravity of urine indicate hypovolemia.
  - Hypovolemic shock:
    - Decreased blood pressure resulting from rupture of the aortic aneurysm.
    - Decreased peripheral pulse resulting from decrease in blood pressure.
    - Increased heart rate as heart tries to meet increased demand for oxygen.
    - Increased respiration resulting from increase demand for oxygen.
  - Decreased pulse pressure resulting from less filling time between cardiac contracts and decreased circulating volume of blood.
  - Severe back pain due to rupture or dissection.

3.7 Angina (Angina Pectoris)

- Arteriosclerosis of the coronary artery narrows blood flow to cardiac muscles. Chest pain, pressure, heaviness, squeezing, or tightness occurs when cardiac muscle demand for oxygen exceeds the supply of oxygen. Three categories of angina are:
  - Stable angina: Chest pain occurs following exercise or stress and is relieved by rest or nitrates.
  - Unstable angina: Chest pain occurs at rest with increasing intensity and duration and not relieved by rest and is slow to respond to nitrates.
  - Prinzmetal's or vasospastic angina: Chest pain occurs at night at rest with minimal exertion.

3.7.1 Signs and symptoms

- Chest pain, pressure, heaviness, squeezing, and tightness for up to 5 minutes radiates to the jaw, back, or arms. Occurs at rest, after exercise, or stress that increases oxygen demand on the heart.
- Shortness of breath (dyspnea) resulting from increased respiration related to increase demand for oxygen.
- Tachycardia resulting from increased need to pump oxygenated blood.
- Increased anxiety resulting from decreased oxygen to cardiac muscles.
- Sweating (diaphoresis) resulting from anxiety and increased cardiac workload.

3.7.2 Medical tests

- ECG during attack:
  - T-wave inverted: First sign of initial ischemia.
  - ST-segment changes: Indicates myocardium injury.
  - Abnormal Q-waves: Indicates myocardium infarction.
- Cardiac panel: troponins, CK-MB, electrolytes.
- Routine blood workup: CBC, blood chemistry, PT/PTT/INR, brain natriuretic peptide (BNP), cholesterol panel.
- Holter monitoring for 24–48 hours provides continuous cardiac monitoring.
- Stress test: Assess cardiac function under pharmacologic or exercise stress.
- Coronary arteriography: Assess arteriosclerosis of the coronary artery.
- Cardiac positron emission tomography (PET): Assess arteriosclerosis of the coronary artery.
- Chest x-ray: Assess for heart failure.
- Echocardiogram or stress echo: Assesses cardiac abnormality caused by ischemia.

3.7.3 Treatment

- Rest: Reduces cardiac demand for oxygen.
- Administer:
  - Two (2) to 4 L of 100% oxygen as necessary using nonrebreather face mask to increase oxygen supply.
  - Analgesic (morphine) to decrease cardiac workload and decrease pain.
  - Nitrates (nitroglycerin) to dilate blood vessels, increasing blood flow to cardiac muscles.
  - Beta-adrenergic blocker to decrease cardiac workload:
    - Inderal (propranolol), Corgard (nadolol), Tenormin (atenolol), Lopressor (metoprolol).
  - Aspirin to reduce formation of platelets.
- Procedures:
  - Percutaneous transluminal coronary angioplasty (percutaneous coronary intervention [PCI]): An inflated balloon within the coronary artery compresses the blockage again the artery wall.
  - Coronary artery stent: a mesh tube is inserted into the coronary artery, reducing the blockage.
  - Coronary artery bypass graft (CABG): A vein from a leg or artery from an arm or chest is graphed to coronary arteries, bypassing the blockage.

- Diet:
  - Low cholesterol.
  - Low sodium.
  - Low fat.

3.7.4 Intervention

- Place patient in a semi-Flowler's position and avoid stress.
- Monitor vital signs:
  - Hold nitrate order if systolic blood pressure <90 mm Hg. Risk of reduced blood to brain.
  - Hold beta-adrenergic blocker if heart rate is less than 60 beats per minute. Risk of low cardiac output.
- Monitor patient with a 12-lead ECG during each attack.
- Monitor intake and output to assess renal function.
- Instruct the patient:
  - Take 1 sublingual dose of nitroglycerin every 5 minutes for maximum of 3 doses at first signs of angina.
  - Rest immediately.
  - Call 911 if signs of angina continue for more than 10 minutes.
  - Avoid stress that brings about angina.
  - Adhere to diet.
  - No smoking.

3.8 Myocardial Infarction (MI)

- Blockage of coronary arteries reduces oxygen supply to cardiac muscle, resulting in necrosis of an area of cardiac muscle known as an infarction. Blockage is caused by atherosclerosis, which results in a buildup of plaque on the wall of the artery.

3.8.1 Signs and symptoms

- Restlessness, feeling of impending doom, anxiety.
- Chest pain radiating to arms, jaw, back and/or neck, which is unrelieved by rest or nitroglycerin, unlike angina.
- Cool, clammy pale skin due to decreased circulation.
- Diaphoresis (sweating) due to anxiety.
- Tachycardia due to pain and low cardiac output.
- Nausea or vomiting possible due to decreased cardiac output.
- Variable blood pressure due to decreased cardiac output.
- Shortness of breath in elderly and women.
- Asymptomatic (silent heart attack) in diabetics.

3.8.2 Medical tests

- Labs
  - Increased white bold cell count (WBC) as the result of inflammatory response to infarction.
  - Elevated CK-MB released by injured tissue. Will follow a predetermined curve, reflecting tissue damage and repair.
  - Elevated troponin I and troponin T-proteins within 1hour of infarction released by injured tissue.
- Urine output: <25 ml/hr due to lack of renal blood flow.
- ECG:
  - T wave: Inversion indicates ischemia.
  - ST segment: Elevated or depressed indicates cardiac tissue injury.
  - Q waves: Significant indicates infarction.
- Decreased pulse pressure due to decreased cardiac output.

3.8.3 Treatment

- Administer:
  - Two (2) to 4 L of 100% oxygen as necessary using a non-rebreather face mask to increase oxygen supply.
  - Aspirin to reduce formation of platelets.
  - Antiarrhythmics to control cardiac arrhythmias:
    - Cordarone (Amiodarone), lidocaine, Pronestyl (procainamide).
  - Antihypertensive to decrease blood pressure:
    - Apresoline (hydralazine).
  - Thrombolytic therapy within 3 hours to 12 hours of an attack to reduce blockage.
    - Activase (alteplase), Streptase (streptokinase), Eminase (anistreplase), Retavase (reteplase).
  - Heparin prevents clots following thrombolytic therapy.
  - Calcium channel blockers for non-Q wave infarction to prevent reinfarction.
    - Isoptin (verapamil), Cardizem (diltiazem).
  - Beta-adrenergic blockers decrease duration of pain.
    - Inderal (propranolol), Corgard (nadolol), Lopressor (metoprolol).
  - Analgesics decrease pain and cardiac workload.
    - Morphine.
  - Nitrates for dilation of blood vessels.
    - Nitroglycerin.
  - Electrical cardioversion in unstable ventricular tachycardia to reestablish sinus rhythm.
  - Percutaneous revascularization to restore cardiac blood flow.

3.8.4 Intervention

- Bed rest without bathroom privileges.
- Place patient in a semi-Flower's position and avoid stress.

- Monitor vital signs.
- Twelve (12)-lead ECG monitoring during an episode.
- Instruct the patient:
  - Eat a low-fat, low-cholesterol, low-sodium diet.
  - Reduce stress, reduce weight, and moderate exercise.
  - Stop smoking.
  - How to identify MI pain and angina pain .
  - When to take nitroglycerine and when to call 911.

3.9 Cardiac Tamponade

- The pericardium fills with fluid, blood, or pus as the result of trauma, postoperative complications, and complications from an MI, cancer, or uremia. Pressure in the pericardium reduces filling of the ventricles, resulting in decreased cardiac output.

3.9.1 Signs and symptoms

- Muffled cardiac sounds due to fluid.
- Sweating (diaphoresis), tachycardia, and difficulty breathing (dyspnea) due to the increased demand for oxygen.
- Restlessness due to decreased oxygen to the brain.
- Pulsus paradoxus (decrease of 15 mmHg or more in systolic blood pressure on inspiration) due to pressure change within the chest on inspiration.
- Fatigue due to increased workload.
- Jugular vein distention due to decreased venous return from the jugular veins.

3.9.2 Medical tests

- Chest x-ray: Assess for enlarged heart.
- Echocardiograph: Ultrasound image of the heart to assess cardiac structure and function.
- ECG: Excludes cardiac disorders.
- Cardiac catheterization.

3.9.3 Treatment

- Pericardiocentesis: Aspirate fluid from the pericardium.
- Administer:
  - Two (2) to 4 L of 100% oxygen as necessary using a nonrebreather face mask to increase oxygen supply.
  - Beta adrenergic blockers decrease duration of pain.
    - Inderal (propranolol), Corgard (nadolol), Lopressor (metroprolol).

3.9.4 Intervention

- Monitor vital signs.

3.10 Cardiogenic Shock

- Cardiac tamponade, myocardial ischemia, myocarditis, or cardiomyopathies result in the heart being unable to pump blood. This results in decreased blood pressure. Blood backs up from the left ventricle into the lungs, causing pulmonary edema. Cardiac rate increases to compensate for the decrease in blood flow. Cardiac muscle oxygenation decreases because the lungs are unable to oxygenate the blood.

3.10.1 Signs and symptoms

- Distended jugular veins caused by fluid overload.
- Hypotension due to decreased blood flow.
- Clammy skin due to tissue deoxygenation.
- Confusion due to poor perfusion of the brain.
- Crackles in lungs, indicating fluid buildup and pulmonary edema.
- Skin pallor (decreased skin temperature) due to decreased circulation.
- Cyanosis due to poor perfusion.
- Arrhythmias due to irritability of cardiac muscle from decreased oxygenation.
- Oliguria (urine output <30 ml/hr) due to decreased kidney perfusion.
- Tachycardia due to increased cardiac demand for blood.

3.10.2 Medical tests

- ECG
  - Q wave: Enlarged due to cardiac failure.
  - ST waves: Elevation due to ischemia.
- Echocardiogram: Ultrasound image of the heart to assess cardiac structure and function.

3.10.3 Treatment

- Swan-Ganz catheterization to measure pressure in the pulmonary artery.
- Labs:
  - Arterial blood gas to assess the acid/base balance of blood.
- Administer:
  - Vasodilator to reduce peripheral arterial resistance and decrease cardiac workload.
    - Nitropress (nitroprusside), nitroglycerin.

- Adrenergic agent to increase blood pressure and cardiac rate.
  - Epinephrine.
- Inotropes to strengthen cardiac contractions.
  - Dopamine, dobutamine, amrinone (inamrinone, inocor), milrinone (Primacor).
- Vasopressor to increase blood flow to the heart and brain and decrease blood flow to other organs.
  - Norepinephrine.

3.10.4 Intervention

- Place patient on bed rest.
- Two (2) to 4 L of oxygen to increase oxygen supply.
- Monitor vital signs. Patient is at risk for respiratory distress.
- Measure fluid intake and output to assess for adequate renal perfusion.
- Daily weights. Notify healthcare provider if weight increases 3 lb. (4.4 kg).
- Instruct the patient:
  - Notify the healthcare provider if the patient is short of breath or shows signs of fluid retention (dependent edema).
  - Eat a low-sodium, low-fat diet.
  - Rest frequently.

3.11 Endocarditis

- An invasive medical procedure or IV drug use can introduce microorganisms into the blood. An infection by a microorganism develops in the inner lining of the heart (endocardium) and heart valves, which results in cardiac inflammation leading to ulceration and necrosis of heart valves. Endocarditis is also secondary to degenerative heart disease and rheumatic heart disease.

3.11.1 Signs and symptoms

- Janeway lesions: On the soles and palms.
- Petechiae: On fingernails and palate.
- Osler nodes: On pads of fingers and feet.
- Fatigue: Related to the infection.
- Murmurs: Due to turbulent blood flow.
- Fever: Related to the infection.

3.11.2 Medical tests

- Echocardiograph: To examine functioning of heart valves.
- TEE: To examine functioning of heart valves.

- Chest x-ray: To examine pulmonary and cardiac abnormalities.
- Blood culture and sensitivity test: three times, 1 hour apart to identify the microorganism and treatment.

3.11.3 Treatment

- Administer antibiotics according to the results of the culture and sensitivity tests.
- Valve replacement when valves are damaged.

3.11.4 Intervention

- Bed rest to reduce cardiac demand.
- Monitor for renal failure:
    - Decreased urine output.
    - Increased blood urea nitrogen (BUN).
    - Increased creatinine clearance.
- Monitor for embolism:
    - Hematuria.
    - *Decrease* mentation.
    - Cough or painful breathing.
- Monitor for heart failure:
    - Weight gain and edema.
    - Distended neck vein.
    - Crackles in lungs.
    - Dyspnea.
    - Tachycardia.
- Instruct the patient:
    - Take all prescribed antibiotics even if the patient is feeling well.
    - Tell a healthcare provider, including a dentist, to administer prophylactic antibiotics before, during, and after an invasive medical procedure.

3.12 Congestive Heart Failure (CHF)

- Ventricles are unable to contract at full capacity, causing decreased circulation and a backup of blood. This is caused by a myocardial infarction, hypertension, valve disorder, or endocarditis. Left-side CHF results in the backup of blood into the lungs. Right-side CHF results in the backup of blood in systemic circulation, causing edema.

3.12.1 Signs and symptoms

- Early signs:
    - Fatigue.
    - S4 heart sound.

  - Nocturia.
  - Dyspnea on exertion.
  - Bilateral rales in lungs.
  - Hepatojugular reflux.
- Advanced signs:
  - Orthopnea.
  - Cardiomegaly.
  - Hepatomegaly.
  - Cough.
  - Anasarca (edema).
  - Cardiac rales.
  - Frothy or pink sputum due to capillary permeability.

3.12.2 Medical tests

- ECG: T-wave sign of ischemia, tachycardia.
- Labs:
  - Increased BNP.
  - Decreased hemoglobin (Hgb).
  - Hematocrit (HCT) less than three times Hgb.
- Increased BUN, increased creatinine clearance, decreased urine output.
- Chest x-ray:
  - Enlarged left ventricle (left-side heart failure).
  - Pulmonary congestion.
  - Pleural effusion (right-side heart failure).
  - Cardiomegaly (right-side heart failure).

3.12.3 Treatment

- Administer:
  - Diuretics: Decrease fluid volume.
    - Lasix (furosemide), Bumex (bumetanide), Zaroxolyn (metolazone) Aldactone (spironolactone) aldosterone antagonist.
  - ACE inhibitors: Decrease pressure in the left ventricle.
    - Prinivil (lisinopril), Capoten (captopril), Vasotec (enalapril)
  - Beta-adrenergic blockers: Decrease cardiac contractions.
    - Inderal (propranolol), Corgard (nadolol), Lopressor (metroprolol).
  - Inotropic agent: Increases cardiac contractions.
    - Dopamine, dobutamine, amrinone (Inamrinone), Primacor (milrinone), digitalis (digoxin).
  - Vasodilator to reduce peripheral arterial resistance and decrease cardiac workload.
    - Nitropress (nitroprusside), nitroglycerin.

- Anticoagulant: Decreases blood coagulation.
  - Heparin, Coumadin (warfarin).

3.12.4 Intervention

- Rest and place in high Fowler's position.
- Administer high-flow oxygen with legs dependent (dangling) and positive end-expiratory pressure (PEEP) by ventilator if necessary.
- Monitor vitals.
- Weigh daily. Notify healthcare provider if weight increases 3 lb. (4.4 kg).
- Measure fluid intake and output.
- Low sodium diet.
- Two (2) to 4 L of oxygen to increase oxygen supply.
- Instruct the patient:
  - Raise legs to reduce dependent edema.
  - Eat foods low in sodium.

3.13 Hypertension and Hypertensive Crisis

- Hypertension occurs when blood vessel pressure increases secondary to an underlying condition or from an unknown cause (idiopathic). Hypertensive crisis occurs when hypertension occurs rapidly, leading to organ damage. Hypertensive crisis is categorized by how significant the end organ damage occurs and the estimation of how quickly the blood pressure must be lowered. Causes can be pheochromocytoma, Cushing's syndrome, abnormal renal function, intracerebral hemorrhage, myocardial ischemia, eclampsia, monamine oxidase inhibitor intraction, and abrupt withdrawal of antihyhpertensive medication.
- Classifications of hypertension:
  - Normal <120 mmHg systolic/ <80 mmHg diastolic.
  - Prehypertension: 120–139 mmHg systolic/80–89 mmHg diastolic.
  - Stage 1 hypertension: 140–159 mmHg systolic/90–99 mmHg diastolic.
  - Stage 2 hypertension: >160 mmHg/systolic >100 mmHg diastolic.
  - Diabetic hypertension: 130 mmHg systolic/80 mmHg diastolic or higher.
- Classification of hypertensive crisis:
  - >120 mmHg diastolic or >180 mmHg systolic.

3.13.1 Signs and symptoms

- Hypertension:
  - Asymptomatic.
  - Dizziness.
  - Headache.

- Hypertensive crisis:
  - Dizziness.
  - Confusion/disorientation.
  - Irritability.
  - Nausea/vomiting.
  - Short of breath on exertion.
  - Blurred vision or double vision.
  - Seizure.
  - Decreased level of consciousness.

3.13.2 Medical tests

- Hypertension: Blood pressure higher than 140/90 mmHg on at least three different occasions lying, sitting, and standing, bilaterally.
- Hypertensive crisis: diastolic pressure >120 mmHg one occasion.

3.13.3 Treatment

- Hypertension:
  - First: Change lifestyle:
    - Decrease caloric intake.
    - Monitor vital signs.
    - Decrease caffeine intake.
    - Decrease alcohol intake.
    - Low-sodium diet.
    - Increase exercise.
    - Stop smoking.
  - Second: Administer medication:
    - Diuretics to decrease circulation:
      - Lasix (furosemide), Bumex (bumetanide), Zaroxolyn (metolazone) Aldactone (spironolactone) (aldosterone antagonist).
      - Beta-adrenergic blocker to decrease cardiac output:
      - Inderal (propranolol), Corgard (nadolol), Lopressor (metoprolol).
    - Calcium channel blockers to increase peripheral vasodilation.
      - Isoptin (verapamil), Cardizem/Dilacor/Tiazac (diltiazem), Cardene (nicardipine).
    - ACE inhibitors to delay renal disease.
      - Prinivil (lisinopril), Capoten (captopril), Vasotec (enalapril).
  - Third: Increase medication dosages.
  - Fourth: Combine medications.
- Hypertensive crisis:
  - Reduce blood pressure slowly over days. Reduce blood pressure no more than 25% of the mean arterial pressure (MAP) within the first 2 hours.

- Administer:
  - Sodium nitroprusside (Nitropress), nitroglycerin (Nitro-Bid), hydralazine (Apresoline) (for preeclampsia).

3.13.4 Intervention

- Hypertension:
  - Measure fluid intake and output.
  - Stress-free environment.
  - Low sodium diet.
  - Instruct the patient:
    - Change lifestyle to avoid being prescribed medication.
    - Decrease weight.
    - On side effects of medications.
- Hypertensive crisis:
  - ECG continuous.
  - Monitor blood pressure every minute while administering medication and then every 15 minutes.
  - Determine MAP.
  - Pulse oximetry.
  - Administer oxygen.
  - Monitor fluid output. Normal is 1 ml/kg per hour. Critical is <0.5 ml/kg per hour.
  - Provide quiet, low-lit environment.
  - Monitor for thiocyanate toxicity if patient is administered Nitropress:
    - Delirium.
    - Blurred vision.
    - Nausea.
    - Fatigue.
    - Tinnitus.

3.14 Hypovolemic Shock

- Decrease in circulation of blood, plasma, or other body fluids, leading to decreased intravascular volume from hemorrhage, dehydration, or flood moving from blood vessels into tissues. This results in inadequate organ perfusion.

3.14.1 Signs and symptoms

- Tachycardia due to cardiac compensation for reduced blood volume.
- Agitation and restlessness due to decreased brain perfusion.
- Hypotension due to decreased blood volume.
- Decreased skin temperature due to decreased circulation, resulting in peripheral vasoconstriction.

- Decreased blood pressure.
- Increased heart rate.
- Urine output less than 25 ml/hr due to decreased kidney perfusion.

3.14.2 Medical tests

- Labs:
  - Decreased Hgb (anemia).
  - Increased BUN.
  - Increased creatinine clearance.
  - Decreased Hct.
  - Arterial blood gas: Decreased pH, increased pCO_2, decreased pO_2.

3.14.3 Treatment

- Administer:
  - Catecholamines to increase blood pressure:
    - Dopamine, epinephrine, and nor epinephrine.
  - Inotropic agent to increase blood pressure.
    - Dobutamine
  - IV use largest catheter (18 G)
  - Crystalloid solutions to expand intravascular and extravascular fluid volume.
    - Use 0.9% normal saline, lactated Ringer's solution (contains electrolytes).
    - Fresh frozen plasma for clotting.
    - Blood replacement (type O negative universal donor).

3.14.4 Intervention

- Monitor vital signs every 15 minutes.
- Administer 2 to 4 L of 100% oxygen as necessary using nonrebreather face mask. Increase oxygen if less than 80 mmHg systolic.
- Measure urine output hourly using indwelling urinary catheter. Increase fluid intake if urine output is less than 30 ml/hr.
- Monitor lungs for crackles and dyspnea due to fluid overflow.
- Instruct the patient:
  - How to avoid hypovolemic shock.

3.15 Myocarditis

- Infection from chronic alcohol abuse, disease, and drug use causes cardiac muscle to become inflamed. Inflammation can degenerate cardiac muscle, leading to CHF.

3.15.1 Signs and symptoms

- Dyspnea related to CHF.
- Chest pain due to infection and inflammation.
- Fever due to infection and inflammation.
- S3 gallop related to CHF.
- Tachycardia due to increased cardiac workload.

3.15.2 Medical tests

- Labs: Increased CK-MB and increased troponins related to cardiac cell injury.
- Chest x-ray shows cardiomegaly.
- Echocardiogram shows cardiomegaly.
- ECG: Abnormal ST segment related to inflammation.
- Endomyocardial biopsy to identify microorganism.

3.15.3 Treatment

- Treat underlying cause.
- Administer:
  - Antiarrhymics to stabilize arrhythmia.
    - Quinidine, Pronestyl (procainamide).

3.15.4 Intervention

- Bed rest.
- No bathroom privileges.
- Monitor vital signs.
- Instruct the patient:
  - Gradually return to normal activities.
  - Avoid competitive activities.

3.16 Pericarditis

- Infection by a microorganism, autoimmune disease, acute MI, or a reaction from medication causes inflammation of the pericardium. Acute pericarditis is typically caused by a viral infection. Chronic pericarditis is typically caused by disease or medication reaction.

3.16.1 Signs and symptoms

- Acute:
  - Anxiety due to pain and respiratory changes.

  - Sharp pain over the percordium, radiating to the neck, shoulders, back, and arm; relieved by leaning forward or sitting up related to common nerve.
  - Pain in the teeth or muscles related to common nerve.
  - Arrhythmias related to irritated heart.
  - Dyspnea related to inflammation.
  - Tachypnea related to increased oxygen demand.
  - Pericardial friction rub due to inflammation.
  - General malaise.
  - Fever and chills.
- Chronic:
  - Hepatomegaly related to decrease in cardiac output and fluid overflow.
  - Ascites related to decrease in cardiac output and liver fluid overflow.
  - Increased fluid retention related to decrease in cardiac output.
  - Pericardial friction rub related to inflammation.

3.16.2 Medical tests

- Chest x-ray shows fluid in pericardium.
- Electrocardiogram shows ST-segment elevation.
- Echocardiograph shows fluid in pericardium.
- Labs:
  - Increased aspartate aminotransferase (AST) and LST due to injury of liver cells.
  - Increased CK due to injury of heart cells.
  - Increased WBC due to inflammation.
  - Increased sedimentation rate due to inflammation.
  - Increased lactic dehydrogenase (LDH) due to tissue damage.

3.16.3 Treatment

- Pericardiocentesis to remove fluid from precordium.
- Pericardial biopsy to identify infecting microorganism.
- Administer:
  - Corticosteroids to decrease inflammation.
    - Medrol (methylprednisolone).
  - Nonsteroidal anti-inflammatory drugs (NSAIDs) to decrease inflammation.
    - Aspirin, indomethacin (indocin).

3.16.4 Intervention

- Rest.
- No bathroom privileges.

- Coughing and deep breathing exercises to decrease discomfort.
- High Fowler's position to ease breathing.
- Instruct the patient:
  - Reduce ongoing fatigue by scheduling rest periods.
  - Slowly resume normal activities.
  - Ease the patient's anxiety by assuring the patient that there will be a recovery.

3.17 Pulmonary Edema

- Decreased pumping action of the left side of the heart causes fluid to build up in the lungs. This is caused by CHF or acute MI.

3.17.1 Signs and symptoms

- Restlessness due to decreased oxygenation of brain.
- Capillary permeability, resulting in frothy/pink sputum.
- Tachypnea due to increased demand for oxygen.
- Cool, clammy skin due to decreased circulation.
- Crackles in lungs due to increased fluid in lungs.
- Distended jugular vein due to fluid overload.
- Cyanosis due to decreased oxygenated blood.
- Dyspnea when sitting upright due to increased fluid in lungs.
- Hypertension.
- Tachycardia.
- Anxiety.

3.17.2 Medical tests

- Chest x-ray shows cardiomegaly.
- Echocardiogram to assess cardiac ejection fraction.
- Oxygen saturation is <90%.

3.17.3 Treatment

- Treat underlying cause.
- Administer:
  - Analgesics to decrease cardiac workload and pain.
    - Morphine.
  - Vasodilator to dilate blood vessels and decrease cardiac workload.
    - Nitropress (nitroprusside), nitroglycerin, Dilatrate (isosorbide dinitrate).

- Inotropes to improve cardiac contractions.
  - Dopamine, dobutamine, (inamrinone), Primacor (milrinone), digitalis (digoxin).
- Bronchodilators to decrease bronchospasms.
  - Albuterol.
- Diuretics to decrease fluid.
  - Lasix (furosemide), Bumex (bumetanide), Zaroxolyn (metolazone), Aldactone (spironolactone).

3.17.4 Intervention

- Monitor vital signs and capillary refill.
- Administer 2 to 4 L of 100% oxygen as necessary using nonrebreather face mask or high-flow oxygen.
- Place patient in full Fowler's position.
- Bed rest.
- Low-sodium diet prevents fluid retention.
- Decrease fluid intake due to existing fluid overload.
- Measure intake and output of fluids to assess renal perfusion.
- Daily weights. Notify healthcare provider if weight increases more than 3 lb. (4.4 kg).
- Instruct the patient:
  - Elevate head when sleeping by placing blocks under the head of the bed frame or use three pillows.
  - Notify the healthcare provider if short of breath and fatigued.

3.18 Thrombophlebitis

- A thrombus (blood clot) in a vein causes inflammation of a vein, usually in the lower extremities. This may be caused by trauma, poor circulation, coagulation disorder, or medication.

3.18.1 Signs and symptoms

- Asymptomatic.
- Cramps caused by decreased blood flow.
- Positive Homans' sign.
- Tenderness and warmth in affected area caused by inflammation.
- Edema due to decrease blood flow.
- Clot moved to lungs:
  - Dyspnea due to clot in lungs.
  - Tachypnea due to clot in lungs.
  - Crackles in lungs due to fluid buildup.

3.18.2 Medical tests

- Photoplethysmography to assess blood flow in affected area.
- Ultrasound to detect blood flow in affected area.

3.18.3 Treatment

- Administer:
  - NSAID to decrease inflammation.
    - Aspirin, Indocin (indomethacin).
  - Anticoagulant to decrease coagulation.
    - Heparin, Coumadin (warfarin), Fragmin (dalteparin), Lovenox (enoxaparin).

3.18.4 Intervention

- Elevate affected area.
- Limit activity: bed rest with bathroom privileges.
- Apply warm, moist compresses on affected area to increase blood flow.
- Monitor therapeutic level of anticoagulant.
- Monitor for tachypnea and dyspnea that may indicate emboli in lungs.
- Instruct the patient:
  - No crossing the legs. It causes decreased circulation.
  - No oral contraceptives due to increase in clotting.
  - Wear support hose.
  - Move frequently once resolved to prevent future clot formation.
  - Contact the healthcare provide if experiencing shortness of breath or signs of bleeding.

3.19 Atrial Fibrillation

- The atria stops beating and quivers, resulting in ineffective contractions. This is caused by abnormal cardiac impulses. It is not life threatening; however, the patient is at risk for strokes and blood clots.

3.19.1 Signs and symptoms

- Asymptomatic.
- Dyspnea due to decreased oxygenation related to decreased circulation.
- Faint feeling and lightheadedness due to decreased circulation.
- Irregular pulse due to arrhythmia.
- Palpitations due to arrhythmia.

3.19.2 Medical tests

- Echocardiogram: Shows structural abnormalities.
- Thyroid function tests to rule out hyperthyroidism.
- ECG:
  - QRS complexes: Irregular.
  - PR interval: Barely visible.
  - P wave: Absent.

3.19.3 Treatment

- Patient unstable: Synchronized cardioversion to reestablish normal sinus rhythm.
- Patient stable:
  - Internal pacemaker.
  - Administer:
    - antiarrhythmics to stabilize arrhythmia.
      - Cordarone (Amiodarone), digitalis (Digoxin), Cardizem Dilacor Tiazac (Diltiazem), Isoptin (Verapamil).
  - After 72 hours administer:
    - Anticoagulant: to decrease coagulation and reduce risk of thromboembolism.
    - Heparin, Coumadin (warfarin), Fragmin (dalteparin), Lovenox (enoxaparin).

3.19.4 Intervention

- Limit activity to decrease cardiac workload.
- Bed rest to decrease cardiac workload.
- Bathroom privileges.
- Monitor for hypoperfusion (cool extremities, increased heart rate, decreased pulse pressure, altered mentation).
- Instruct the patient:
  - Contact the healthcare provider if feeling dizzy.
  - No nicotine, caffeine, or alcohol. These can trigger arrhythmia.

3.20 Asystole

- Cardiac standstill, resulting in no circulation. Asystole can be caused by arrhythmia, cardiac tamponade, pulmonary embolism, sudden cardiac death, acute MI, or hypovolemia.

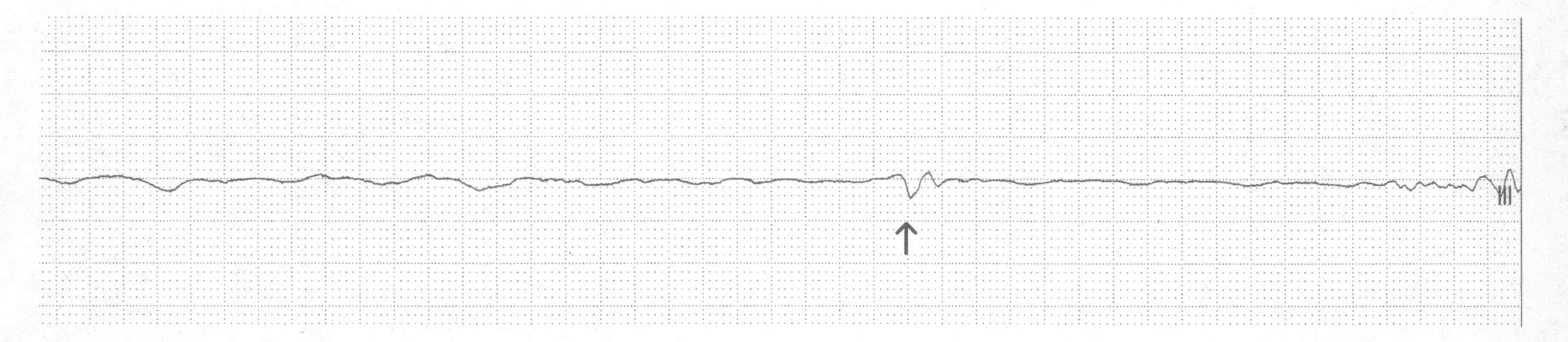

Figure 3.1 Asystole

3.20.1 Signs and symptoms

- No blood pressure.
- No pulse.
- Apnea.
- Cyanosis.

3.20.2 Medical tests

- ECG: No wave.

3.20.3 Treatment

- Cardiopulmonary resuscitation within 2 minutes.
- Advanced cardiac life support within 8 minutes.
- Transcutaneous pacing.
- Endotracheal intubation.
- Administer:
  - Buffering agent to correct acidosis.
    - Sodium bicarbonate.
  - Antiarrhythmics to control arrhythmia.
    - Atropine, epinephrine, vasopressin, and amiodarone.

3.20.4 Intervention

- Cardiopulmonary resuscitation.

3.21 Ventricular Fibrillation

- Erratic impulses cause ventricles to quiver, resulting in disruption of circulation. This is caused by electrolyte disturbances, drug toxicities, ventricular tachycardia, electrical shock, or MI. This rhythm is not compatible with life.

3.21.1 Signs and symptoms

- Apnea.
- No blood pressure.
- No pulse.

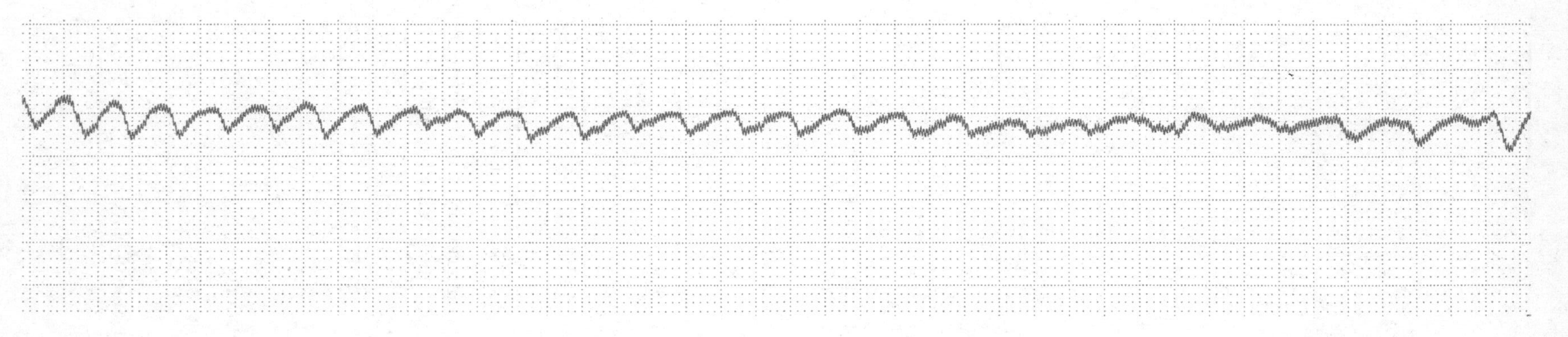

Figure 3.2 Ventricular Fibrillation

3.21.2 Medical tests

- ECG:
    - P wave: Not noticeable.
    - Ventricular rhythm: Chaotic.
    - QRS complex: Irregular and wide.

3.21.3 Treatment

- Cardiopulmonary resuscitation.
- Endotracheal intubation.
- Advanced cardiac life support.
- Defibrillation.
- Administer:
    - Buffering agent to correct acidosis.
        - Sodium bicarbonate.
    - Antiarrhythmics to control arrhythmia.
    - Vasopressin, epinephrine, lidocaine, and amiodarone.

3.21.4 Intervention

- Cardiopulmonary resuscitation.
- Defibrillate.

3.22 Ventricular Tachycardia

- Erratic impulses cause ventricles to contract more than 160 bpm, resulting in inadequate filling of the ventricles and decreased cardiac output. This is caused by mitral valve prolapse, CAD, and acute MI. May suddenly start and stop.

3.22.1 Signs and symptoms

- Hypotension due to decreased circulation.
- Decreased pulse due to insufficient heart rate.
- Decreased breathing.
- Dizziness due to decrease in oxygenation of blood.
- Unconscious.
- Apnea.

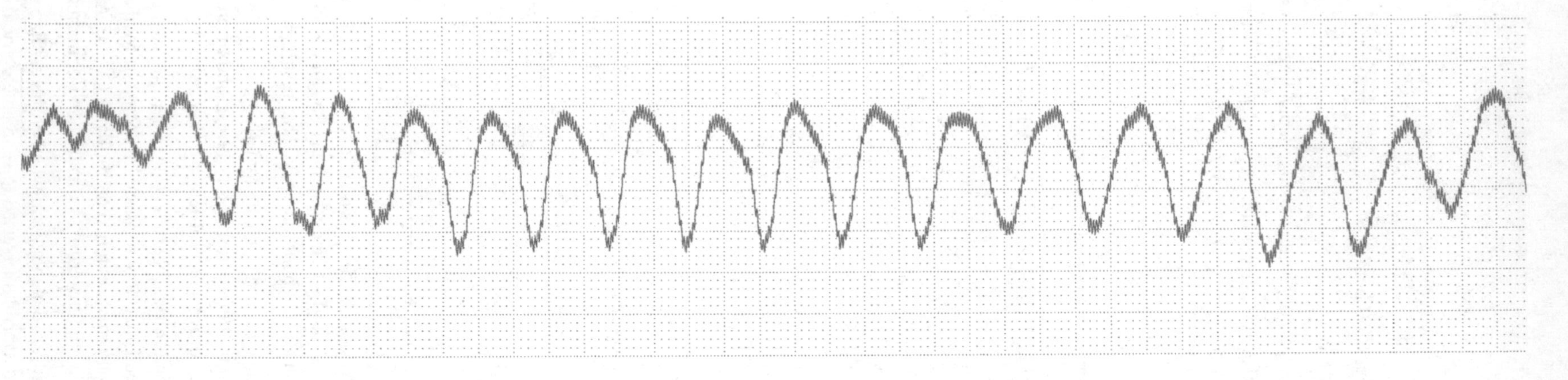

Figure 3.3 Ventricular Tachycardia

3.22.2 Medical tests

- ECG:
  - P wave: Not noticeable.
  - Rhythm: Chaotic, greater than 160 bpm.
  - QRS complex: Abnormal.
  - Ventricular tachycardia may suddenly start and stop, depending on the irritability of the heart.
  - Ventricle contracts greater than 160 per minute.

3.22.3 Treatment

- Treatment consists of establishing a regular rate and rhythm.
- Cardiopulmonary resuscitation.
- Endotracheal intubation.
- Advanced cardiac life support.
- Synchronized cardioversion.
  - Administer:
  - Buffering agent to correct acidosis.
    - Sodium bicarbonate.
  - Antiarrhythmics to control arrhythmia.
    - Vasopressin, epinephrine, lidocaine, procainamide.

3.22.4 Intervention

- Cardiopulmonary resuscitation.
- Synchronized cardioversion.

3.23 Cardiac Arrest

- Cardiac arrest is a condition in which the heart is unable to circulate blood properly as a result of the malfunction of the cardiac muscle. Ineffective circulation of atrial blood leads to a decrease in the oxygenation of tissues and organs throughout the body. This results in necrosis, which is dead tissue.
- Cardiac muscle malfunction can be caused by many underlying conditions, which include myocardial infarction, overdose of medication, trauma, respiratory arrest, and improper impulses leading to ventricular fibrillation (ventricles quiver) or ventricular tachycardia (ventricles beat very fast).
- Treatment for cardiac arrest depends on staff certification. There are two types of certifications. These are Basic Life Support and Advanced Life Support. Basic Life Support focuses on cardiopulmonary resuscitation and the use of the automatic external defibrillator (AED). Advanced Life Support focuses on recognizing ECG patterns and administering medication and/or manually defibrillating the patient.
- The treatment of cardiac arrest differs depending on whether the cardiac rhythm is shockable or not shockable. An AED or manual defibrillator is used to send an electrical impulse through the patient's chest to the heart. The impulse stops the heart suddenly, causing the natural pacemaker cells of the

heart to reestablish a normal rhythm. However, whether the natural pacemaker is not functioning, then the heart is not shocked. The ECG depicts the cardiac wave form that determines whether the natural pacemaker cells are functioning. The AED analyzes the wave to determine whether this is a shockable wave or not. Advanced Cardiac Life Support (ACLS) staff review the ECG to determine whether the wave is shockable (see 3.23.1.2 Advanced Cardiac Life Support).

- As cardiopulmonary resuscitation (CPR) and advanced cardiac life support are performed, look for common causes of cardiac arrest (see Table 3.1). Treating the underlying cause may return the patient to normal cardiac function.

TABLE 3.1 Common Causes of Cardiac Arrest

Acidosis	Hypovolemia	Hypoxia	Hypo/hyperkalemia	Hypoglycemia
Hypothermia	Toxins	Cardiac tamponade	Tension pneumothorax	Thrombosis
Trauma				

3.23.1 Basic life support

- Basic life support requires the following algorithm be performed when presented with a patient who has a sudden loss of consciousness and respirations are absent. This algorithm is provided by the American Heart Association. Consult with the American Heart Association for updates on this algorithm.
- Be sure to push hard and fast, 100 compressions per minute, allowing full chest recoil. One cycle is 30 compressions to two breaths if there is no advanced airway. There should be five cycles every two minutes. Rotate with another person every five cycles.

Step 1

Try arousing the patient by calling the patient by name and rubbing the upper portion of the sternum.

Step 2

Call 911 or send someone to activate the emergency response system.

Step 3

Get an AED or send someone to get an AED.

Step 4

If no response, check for a pulse.

Lightly feeling the carotid artery for a minimum of 5 seconds and maximum of 10 seconds.

Step 5

Bare the patient's chest and position hands for CPR.

Step 6

Deliver first cycle of compression: 100 compressions per minute at depth of at least 2 inches. Allow complete recoil between compressions. Rotate while doing compressions every 2 minutes. Limit interruptions for less than 10 seconds

(Continued)

Step 7

Open the airway.

Tilt the head back if there is no sign of trauma. If there is a sign of trauma, then use a jaw thrust to open the airway.

Step 8

Administer two breaths per 30 compressions.

Make sure the chest rises.

Step 9

Attach AED leads to patient and follow AED's voice instructions.

3.23.2 Advanced cardiac life support

- ACLS is used when the patient experiences cardiac arrest and requires external electric stimulation and/or medication to reestablish cardiac function. ACLS is performed by staff that are ACLS certified and who are permitted to perform ACLS within their scope of practice.
- ACLS requires the following algorithm be performed when presented with a patient who had a sudden loss of consciousness and does not have a pulse. This algorithm is provided by the American Heart Association. Consult with the American Heart Association for updates on this algorithm.

Step 1
- Continue CPR.
- Administer oxygen.
- Attach cardiac monitor.

Step 2
Is there a shockable rhythm?

Step 3
Shockable
- Ventricular fibrillation (fig. 3.2).
- Ventricular tachycardia (fig. 3.2).

Step 4
- Set manual biphasic defibrillator to device-specific setting. If unknown, set to 200 joules.
- Set monophasic defibrillator to 360 joules.
- Call clear.
- Give one shock.
- Give five cycles of CPR.

Step 5
Is there a shockable rhythm?

Step 6
Shockable.
- Call clear.
- Give one shock.
- Give five cycles of CPR over 2 minutes.
- Give during CPR IV/IO epinephrine 1 mg.
- Wait 3 to 5 minutes and give second dose of epinephrine 1 mg.

OR

- Give 1 dose of vasopressin 40 units IV/IO.

Step 7

Is there a shockable rhythm?

Step 8

Shockable.

- Call clear.
- Give one shock.
- Give five cycles of CPR over 2 minutes.
- Give during CPR IV/IO amiodarone 300 mg IV/IO.

IF no conversion:

- Give amiodarone 150 mg IV/IO.

Go to Step 5.

Step 9

Not Shockable

- Asystole/PEA (fig. 3.1).

Step 10

Give five cycles of CPR over 2 minutes.

- Open IV/IO access.
- During CPR:
- Give epinephrine 1 mg IV/VO.
- Wait 3 to 5 minutes.
- Give epinephrine 1 mg IV/VO.
- Wait 3 to 5 minutes.
- Give epinephrine 1 mg IV/VO.

OR

- Give vasopressin 40 units IV/IO. Can replace first or second dose of epinephrine.
- If asystole or slow PEA rate:
- Give atropine 1 mg IV/IO.
- Wait 3 to 5 minutes.
- Give atropine 1 mg IV/IO.
- Wait 3 to 5 minutes.
- Give atropine 1 mg IV/IO.
- Give five cycles of CPR.

Step 11

Is there a shockable rhythm?

Step 12

Not shockable.

- If asystole, go to Step 10.
- If electrical activity, check pulse.

  If no pulse, go to Step 10.

  If pulse, begin postresuscitation treatment.

Step 13

Shockable.

Go to Step 4.

Not Shockable.

Go To Step 12.

3.23.3 Bradycardia treatment

- Bradycardia is a condition in which the heart beats slowly, reducing circulation and resulting in decreased oxygenation of tissues and organs. The American Heart Association recommends the following interventions when treating bradycardia.

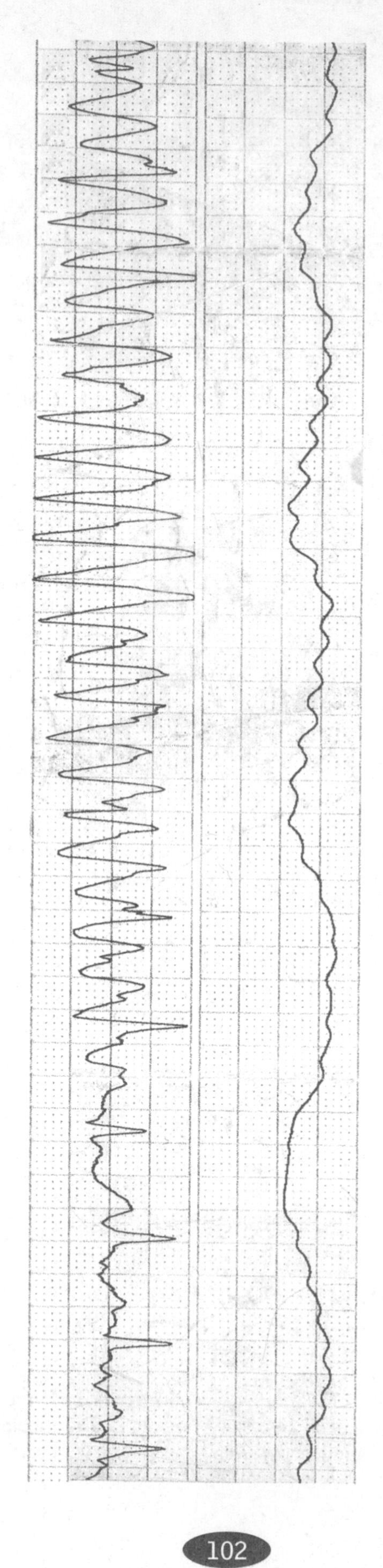

Figure 3.4 Torsades de pointes

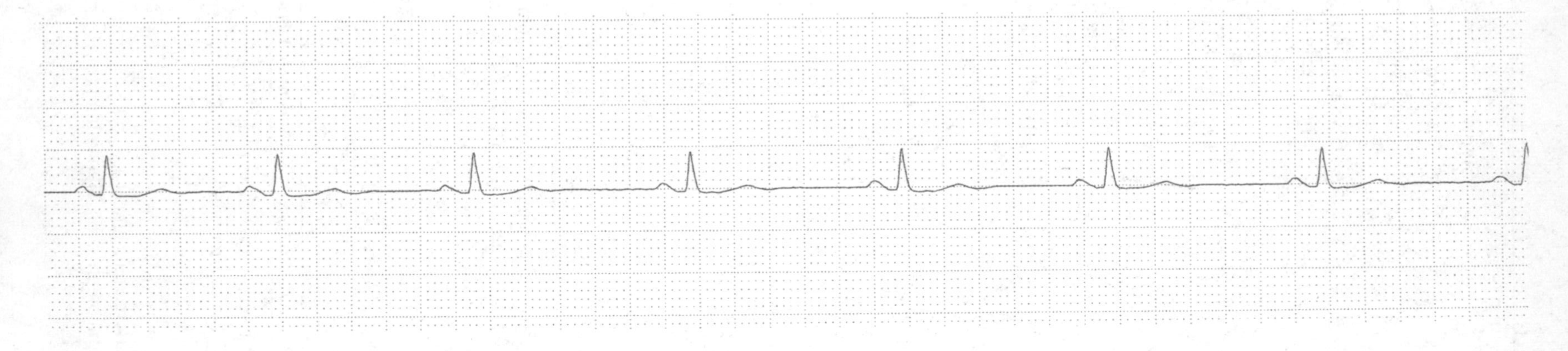

Figure 3.5 Sinus Bradycardia

Step 1

- Maintain a patent airway.
- Assist with breathing.
- Administer oxygen.
- Monitor ECG 12 lead.
- Monitor vital signs.
- Monitor oximetry.
- Establish perfusion.
- Monitor signs of perfusion (shock).
    - Altered mental state.
    - Chest pain.
    - Hypotension.

Step 2

Adequate perfusion.

Step 3

If poor perfusion caused by bradycardia, then go to Step 4.

If poor perfusion not caused by bradycardia, then monitor and observe.

Continue monitoring.

Step 4

- Give Atropine 0.5 mg.
- If ineffective, repeat. No more than 3 mg.
- Give epinephrine 2 μg to 10 μg per min.

OR

- Give dopamine 2 μg per kg to 10 μg per kg per min.

Step 5

- If type II second-degree heart block or third-degree heart block, administer transcutaneous pacing.
- Otherwise, administer transvenous pacing.

Step 6

Treat underlying cause.

Step 7

Treat underlying cause.

3.24 Fibrinolytic Therapy

- Fibrinolytic therapy is used to remove all or a portion of an existing blood clot, resulting in normal blood flow 50% of the time using tissue plasminogen (tPA), reteplase, tenecteplase, or streptokinase. Table 3.2 contains the fibrinolytic checklist used to determine whether the patient is a candidate for fibrinolytic therapy.

TABLE 3.2 Fibrinolytic Check List

Administer Fibrnolytic Therapy	Do Not Administer Fibrnolytic Therapy	
Ischemic chest pain.	Patient presents more than 12 hours after onset of symptoms.	INR > 1.7 PT >15 Platelete count > 100,000 Systolic blood pressure > 185
Persistent ST-segment elevation more than 1 mm in two or more contiguous chest or limb leads.	Arterial puncture at a noncompressible site within past 7 days.	Warfarin in use by patient.

TABLE 3.2 Fibrinolytic Check List (Continued)

Administer Fibrnolytic Therapy	Do Not Administer Fibrnolytic Therapy	
Onset of symptoms within 12 hours of presentation and positive ECG waves.	Active internal bleeding.	Patient received heparin within the past 48 hours.
Onset of symptoms within 12 hours and positive posterior MI (ST-segment depression in early precordial leads).	Witnessed seizure at time of stroke.	Acute trauma.
Age 18 years or older.	Intracranial hemorrhage assessed with noncontrast head CT.	Subarachnoid hemorrhage.
Ischemic stroke with measurable neurologic deficit.	History of intracranial hemorrhage.	AV malformation.
Less than 3 hours since the last time patient seemed normal.		

3.25 Acute Stroke

- A stroke is referred to as a cerebrovascular accident (CVA) that occurs when there is disturbance in blood supply to the brain, resulting in neurologic disturbance. The disturbance can be caused by a blockage that leads to an ischemia, a hemorrhage, or from unknown cause. Decreased blood flow can result in tissue damage in the affected area of the brain. Depending on the area affected, the patient can experience:
  - Weakness in the face, arm, or leg, typically one side of the body.
    - Confusion.
    - Difficulty speaking.
    - Difficulty understanding.
    - Vision problems.
    - Dizziness.
    - Coordination problems.
    - Severe headache from unknown cause.
- A patient can experience a transient ischemic attack (TIA) commonly called a ministroke. A TIA is a brief disturbance of the blood supply. Symptoms resolve once blood supply returns. There is no tissue necrosis (infarction). A patient can also experience a silent stroke where there are no outward symptoms of a stroke. A silence stroke causes lesions on the brain that are identified using an MRI.
- An acute stroke occurs when the patient suddenly shows signs of a stroke. It is critical that the patient receives treatment immediately to minimize the effect of the stroke and reduce tissue necrosis. There are two prehospital stroke assessments. These are the Cincinnati Prehospital Stroke Scale (CPSS) (see table 3.3) and the Los Angeles Prehospital Stroke Scale (LAPSS) (see table 3.4).

TABLE 3.3 Cincinnati Prehospital Stroke Scale

Three Signs Indicate An Acute Stroke		
Sign	**Test**	**Positive Result**
Facial droop	Patient shows teeth.	One side of the patient's face does not move as well as the other side of the face.
Arm drift	Extend both arms palms up for 10 seconds.	One arm moves down.
Abnormal speech	The patient says, "You can't teach an old dog new tricks."	The patient is unable to speak or words are slurred.

TABLE 3.4 Los Angeles Prehospital Stroke Scale

All Signs Present Indicate An Acute Stroke	
Category	**Sign**
Age	>45 years of age.
History	No history of epilepsy or seizures.
Duration	Symptoms started within the past 24 hours.
Ambulatory	Patient is not bedridden or in a wheelchair.
Blood glucose	Between 60 and 400.
Face	Droops.
Grip	Weak or no grip.
Arms	Drift down.

- The following is the algorithm recommended by the American Heart Association to treat an acute stroke.

Start

- Make sure airway, breathing, and circulation are patent.
- Assess vital signs.
- Administer oxygen.
- Open IV access.
- Gather blood samples.
- Assess blood glucose levels.
- Review patient's history.
- Determine when symptoms first presented.
- Administer an ECG.

Perform CT Scan of the Brain

No Hemorrhage

- Assess if patient is a candidate for fibrinolytic therapy (see 3.24 Fibrinolytic Therapy).

Yes

- Administer tPA or appropriate fibrinolytic.
- Do not administer anticoagulants or antiplatelet treatment for 24 hours.

No

- Administer low dose aspirin.
- Transfer to stroke unit for follow-up care.

Hemorrhage

- Consult neurologist/neurosurgeon.

3.26 Acute Coronary Syndrome

- An acute coronary syndrome is reported by the patient as chest discomfort and described as uncomfortable pressure that may extend to the jaw, neck, between the shoulder blades, shoulders, and arms. The patient may experience shortness of breath, nausea, sweating, and lightheadedness that may result in fainting. The acute coronary syndrome may or may not result in chest pain.
- Based on these signs and symptoms, the American Heart Association recommends treatment using the following algorithm.

Start

- Monitor airway, breathing, and circulation.
- Monitor vital signs.
- Administer oxygen 4 L/min to main oxygen saturation level >90%.
- If the patient shows no evidence of recent gastrointestinal (GI) bleed, then
  - If the patient does not have nausea, vomiting, or peptic ulcer, then administer aspirin 160 mg to 325 mg orally and ask the patient to chew the aspirin tablet to increase absorption time.
  - If the patient has nausea, vomiting, or peptic ulcer, then administer aspirin 160 mg to 325 mg rectally.
- If the patient is not hypotensive, bradycardia, or tachycardia and has not taken Viagra or Levitra within 24 hours or Cialis within 48 hours and if the patient is hemodynamically stable, then administer nitroglycerin sublingual, three doses each 3 minutes apart.
- If the patient is unresponsive to nitroglycerin, then administer morphine to reduce the left ventricular preload and cardiac oxygen requirements.
- Administer a 12-lead ECG.
- Open IV access.
- Administer IV fluids if patient is hypotensive.
- Perform fibrinolytic checklist (see 3.24 Fibrinolytic therapy).

(Continued)

- Draw blood sample for cardiac marker levels, electrolyte, and coagulation studies.
- Administer a chest x-ray within 30 minutes of the patient's arrival.

Review ECG
ST Elevation MI (STEMI)
or
Left Bundle Branch Block (LBBB)
Administer

- Beta adrenergic receptor blockers.
- Plavix.
- Heparin.
- If more than 12 hours from onset, then admit patient to the cardiac care unit.
- If 12 hours or less from onset, then
  - Fibrinolytic therapy (within 30 minutes).
  - Percutaneous coronary intervention (PCI) to restore blood to the heart (within 90 minutes).
  - ACE inhibitors angiotension receptor blocker (ARB) (within 24 hours).
  - HMB CoA reductase inhibitor.

Unstable Angina Non-ST Elevation MI (UA/NSTEMI)
Administer

- Nitroglycerin.
- Beta-adrenergic receptor blockers.
- Glycoprotein IIb/IIIa inhibitor.
- Plavix.
- Admit patient to the cardiac care unit.

Normal ST or T Waves

- If troponin positive then administer
  - Nitroglycerin.
  - Beta-adrenergic receptor blockers.
  - Glycoprotein IIb/IIIa inhibitor.
  - Plavix.
- If troponin negative, then
  - If symptoms of ischemia or infarction persist, then
    - Continue monitoring ECG.
    - Admit patient to the cardiac care unit.
- If no symptoms of ischemia or infarction, then discharge patient with appropriate follow-up care.

3.27 Cardiac Contusion

- A cardiac contusion is a blunt trauma injury to the chest that results in bruising of the myocardium, typically the right ventricle.

3.27.1 Signs and symptoms

- Precordial chest pain: Due to bruising.
- Bruising around the sternum: Due to blunt trauma.
- Shortness of breath: Due to cardiac irritability.
- Cardiac arrhythmias: Due to cardiac irritability.
- Bradycardia: Due to cardiac irritability.
- Tachycardia: Due to cardiac irritability.
- Murmurs: Due to cardiac irritability.
- Hemodynamic instability: Due to cardiac irritability.

3.27.2 Medical tests

- Echocardiograph: To assess ejection fraction and ventricular viability.
- Cardiac enzyme level: To assess CK-MB levels and injury to cardiac muscle.
- Cardiac tropoinin I Levels: To assess injury to cardiac muscle.
- ECG: To assess cardiac rhythm.

3.27.3 Treatment

- Administer:
  - IV fluids to provide hemodynamic stability (systolic blood pressure above 90 mm Hg).
  - Digoxin if there are signs of cardiac failure.
  - Lidocaine for ventricular arrhythmias.
  - Inotropic medication to increase cardiac output.
  - Oxygen.

3.27.4 Intervention

- Monitor ECG.
- Assess vital signs each hour until patient is stable, looking for decreased peripheral tissue perfusion.
- Assess respiration, looking for signs of congestion.
- Assess urine output (1 ml/kg/hr).
- Raise head of bed 30 degrees.

3.28 Coronary Artery Bypass Graft (CABG)

- Coronary artery bypass graft involves grafting the saphenous vein from the leg or internal mammary artery to circumvent coronary arteries that are occluded.

- Considerations:
  - Before the CABG:
    - No food or fluids for 8 hours before surgery.
    - Review conditions that the patient will experience following surgery:
      - Indwelling urinary catheterization.
      - Endotracheal tube connected to a ventilator.
      - Epicardial pacing wires.
  - After the CABG:
    - Monitor ECG.
    - Assess for bleeding.
    - Monitor peripherial circulation:
      - Capillary refill.
      - Pedal pulse.
      - Skin temperature.
  - Assess for pulmonary embolism.
  - Monitor:
    - Arterial blood gas every 2 hours and adjust ventilator .
    - Vital signs every 5 minutes.
    - Intake and output.
    - Electrolytes.

3.29 Valve Surgery

- Valve surgery involves repairing or replacing a heart valve to correct stenosis or insufficiency of the valve.
- Considerations:
  - Before surgery:
    - No food or fluids for 8 hours before surgery.
    - Review conditions that the patient will experience following surgery:
      - Indwelling urinary catheterization.
      - Endotracheal tube connected to a ventilator.
      - Epicardial pacing wires.
    - After surgery:
      - Monitor ECG.
      - Assess for bleeding.

- Monitor peripheral circulation:
  - Capillary refill.
  - Pedal pulse.
  - Skin temperature.
- Assess for pulmonary embolism.
- Monitor:
  - Arterial blood gas every 2 hours and adjust ventilator.
  - Vital signs every 5 minutes.
  - Intake and output.
  - Electrolytes.

3.30 Vascular Surgery

- Vascular surgery involves repair of blood vessels (i.e., aortic aneurysm repair), removal of an emboli (i.e., embolectomy), insertion of a filter in the blood vessel (vena cava filter), or circumventing a blocked blood vessel (i.e., bypass graft).
- Considerations:
  - Before surgery:
    - Review conditions that the patient will experience following surgery:
      - Indwelling urinary catheterization.
    - Develop baseline assessment of the patient's vascular system.
    - No food or fluids for 8 hours before surgery.
  - After surgery:
    - Monitor ECG.
    - Assess for bleeding at site.
    - Change dressing.
    - Monitor peripheral circulation:
      - Capillary refill.
      - Pedal pulse.
      - Skin temperature.
    - Assess for pulmonary embolism.
    - Monitor vital signs every 15 minutes.
    - Monitor intake and output.
    - Encourage range-of-motion exercises to prevent formation of thrombus.
    - Encourage ambulation.

3.31 Vascular Assist Device

- A vascular assist device is a device implanted into the patient to increase cardiac output and decrease cardiac workload in patients who experience ventricular failure and are waiting for a heart transplant.
- Considerations:
  - Obtain an informed consent.
  - Monitor cardiac function with ECG.
  - Monitor vital signs every 15 minutes until the patient stabilizes
  - Inspect the incision site for bleeding.
  - Monitor input and output.
  - Monitor for fluid overload.

3.32 Balloon Catheterization

- Balloon catheterization is used to enlarge a narrowing of a blood vessel (percutaneous transluminal coronary angioplasty) or the orifice of a narrowed heart valve (valvuloplasty). Balloon catheterization is also used to increase blood pressure and improve peripheral and coronary perfusion (intra-aortic balloon pump).
- Considerations:
  - Monitor the insertion site for bleeding.
  - Monitor peripheral circulation:
    - Capillary refill.
    - Pedal pulse.
    - Distal pulses.
    - Skin temperature and color.
  - Monitor signs of thrombus:
    - Decreased pedal pulse.
    - Pain.
    - Sensory loss.
    - Sudden weakness.
  - Monitor vital signs.

3.33 Synchronized Cardioversion

- Synchronized cardioversion counter shocks the heart to restore normal cardiac rhythm when a patient is experiencing arrhythmias that do not respond to medication.

- Considerations:
    - Record a baseline ECG before the procedure.
    - No food or fluids for 12 hours before the procedure.
    - Tell the patient that sedation will be administered before the procedure.
    - Tell the patient that there may be soreness in the chest area following the procedure.

3.34 Pacemaker

- A pacemaker is an external or internal device that prevents the heart from beating below a preset cardiac rate. An external pacemaker resides outside the body with electronic leads connecting the external pacemaker to the heart. An internal pacemaker resides inside the body and is permanent. A pacemaker is used for patients who have bradycardia, degenerative heart disease, sick sinus syndrome, or complete heart block.
- Considerations:
    - Record a baseline ECG before the procedure.
    - No food or fluids for 12 hours before the procedure.
    - Monitor the insertion site for bleeding.
    - Monitor vital signs.
    - Monitor ECG after the procedure.
    - Monitor level of consciousness.

Solved Problems

3.1 When is cardiovascular critical care necessary?
Cardiovascular critical care is necessary when cardiovascular reserves are insufficient to sustain circulation, causing the patient to become unstable and requiring mechanical and/or pharmaceutical treatment to supplement cardiovascular reserves.

3.2 What is the goal of cardiovascular critical care?
The goal of cardiovascular critical care is to assist the patient's cardiovascular system to maintain sufficient circulation and blood pressure to perfuse organs.

3.3 What may be indicated by edema in arms or legs?
- Venous insufficiency: Veins are unable to return blood to the heart.
- Left-side heart failure: Insufficient output by the left ventricle.
- Thrombophlebitis: Inflammation of a vein caused by a blood clot.
- Varicosities: Valves in veins deep in the leg malfunction, resulting in pooling of blood that leads to increased venous pressure. This causes surface veins to enlarge.
- Carotid artery: The carotid artery should not be pounding or have a weak pulse and the pulse should remain unchanged when the patient changes position.
- Internal jugular vein: The internal jugular vein pulsating should change when the patient changes position. Jugular vein distention may indicate increased central venous pressure (CVP).

3.4 What may be indicated by no body hair on legs?
This may indicate diminished arterial blood flow.

3.5 What may be indicated by shiny skin?
This may indicate diminished arterial blood flow.

3.6 What is a heart murmur?
A murmur is a turbulent abnormal sound caused by the flow of blood through the heart during the cardiac cycle.

3.7 What is a cardiac rub?
A scraping, grating sound heard over the lower left sternal border at the third left intercostal space that may indicate pericarditis or cardiac infection.

3.8 Why are cardiac markers tested?
Cardiac markers are enzymes that give an indication whether the patient has experienced an acute myocardial infarction. Cardiac enzymes are contained within cells of cardiac tissues. Cardiac cells rupture as a result of an acute myocardial infarction, releasing cardiac enzymes into the blood. The amount of cardiac enzymes indicates cardiac damage.

3.9 What is the value of testing for creatine kinase-MB?
Creatine kinase-MB (CK-MB) is an enzyme found only in cardiac muscle tissues.

3.10 What is an echocardiogram?
An echocardiogram uses sound waves to assess the heart. A transducer is placed over an area of the patient's chest that is absent of bone and lung tissue. The transducer generates sound waves toward the heart and then receives sound waves reflected by the heart that are converted to an electronic signal that is displayed on a screen, on a strip, or recorded.

3.11 What is the purpose of cardiac output monitoring?
Cardiac output is the volume of blood ejected by the heart in 1 minute, which is normally 4 L/min to 8 L/min, and is used to assess cardiac function.

3.12 What is the purpose of monitoring pulmonary arterial blood pressure?
Pulmonary arterial blood pressure measures the amount of pressure required to open the pulmonary valve (systolic pressure) and the resistance when the pulmonary valve is closed (diastolic pressure).

3.13 What is the purpose of administering digoxin?
Digoxin is cardiac glycosides medication that increases the force of contractions, slows the heart rate, and reduces the electrical impulse through the AV node.

3.14 When would you not administer digoxin?
Hold digoxin if apical pulse is < 60 bpm and notify healthcare practitioner.

3.15 What is the purpose of administering propranolol (Inderal)?
Propranolol (Inderal) is a class II antiarrhythmic medication that block beta-adrenergic receptor sites,

decreasing conductivity of the AV node and decreasing cardiac workload. This reduces the oxygen requirement of the heart.

3.16 What is cardiac tamponade?
Cardiac tamponade occurs when the pericardium fills with fluid, blood, or pus as result of trauma, postoperative complications, and complications from an MI, cancer, or uremia. Pressure in the pericardium reduces filling of the ventricles, resulting in decrease cardiac output.

3.17 What is a hypertensive crisis?
Hypertensive crisis is categorized by how significant the end organ damage occurs and the estimation of how quickly the blood pressure must be lowered.

3.18 What is the first treatment for hypertension?

- Change lifestyle:
  - Decrease caloric intake.
  - Monitor vital signs.
  - Decrease caffeine intake.
  - Decrease alcohol intake.
  - Low-sodium diet.
  - Increase exercise.
  - Stop smoking.

3.19 What is hypovolemic shock?
Hypovolemic shock occurs when there is a decrease in the circulation of blood, plasma, or other body fluids, leading to decreased intravascular volume from hemorrhage, dehydration, or flow moving from blood vessels into tissues resulting in inadequate organ perfusion.

3.20 What is pulmonary edema?
Pulmonary edema is decreased pumping action of the left side of the heart, which causes fluid to build up in the lungs. This is caused by congestive heart disease or acute myocardial infarction.

3.21 What is atrial fibrillation?
The atria stops beating and quivers, resulting in ineffective contractions. This is caused by abnormal cardiac impulses. It is not life threatening; however, the patient is at risk for strokes and blood clots.

3.22 What is an acute stroke?
A stroke is referred to as a cerebrovascular accident (CVA) that occurs when there is a disturbance in blood supply to the brain, resulting in neurological disturbance. The disturbance can be caused by a blockage that leads to an ischemia, a hemorrhage, or from unknown cause. Decreased blood flow can result in tissue damage in the effective area of the brain.

3.23 What is acute coronary syndrome?
An acute coronary syndrome is reported by the patient as chest discomfort described as uncomfortable pressure that may extend to the jaw, neck, between the shoulder blades, shoulders, and arms. The patient may experience shortness of breath, nausea, sweating, and lightheadedness that may result in fainting. The acute coronary syndrome may or may not result in chest pain.

3.24 How would you expect the patient to describe angina pectoris?
Heaviness, burning, squeezing pain over the substernal and radiating to the jaw, arms, back, and neck; it may subside within 10 minutes. Pain is worse lying down or with physical activity.

3.25 What would you expect a practitioner to order at the first sign of angina pectoris?
Nitroglycerin sublingual, 1 dose every 5 minutes if symptoms persist.

Respiratory Critical Care

4.1 Definitions

- Respiratory critical care is necessary when respiratory reserves are insufficient to sustain gas exchange. This causes the patient to become unstable, requiring mechanical and/or pharmaceutical treatment to supplement respiratory reserves.
- The respiratory system exchanges carbon dioxide attached to hemoglobin in red blood cells with oxygen in the alveoli.
- Decreased respiratory reserves may result in a cascading failure of systems throughout the body.
- The goal of respiratory critical care is to assist the patient's respiratory system to maintain sufficient gas exchange to oxygenate blood, enabling the cardiovascular system to perfuse organs.
- A patient may be admitted to the critical care unit for a condition other than a respiratory condition. However, a cascading failure of systems other than the respiratory system may result in respiratory instability. Therefore, always carefully monitor the respiratory system for abnormalities.

4.1.1 Respiratory cycle

- Blood flow to and from the heart:
  - Deoxygenated blood returns to the right atrium of the heart from the inferior and superior vena cava.
  - Deoxygenated blood flows from the right atrium to the right ventricle when the right atrium contracts.
  - Deoxygenated blood in the right ventricle flows through the pulmonary arteries into the lungs when the right ventricle contracts.
  - Carbon dioxide, which is attached to the hemoglobin in red blood cells, is replaced by oxygen.
  - Oxygenated blood returns from the lungs to the left atrium through four pulmonary veins.
  - Oxygenated blood flows into the left ventricle when the left atrium contracts.
  - Oxygenated blood flows from the left ventricle through the aorta to the arterial system, providing oxygenated blood to cells throughout the body.

4.1.2 Respiratory assessment

- Assess airway, breathing, and circulation immediately. Begin cardiopulmonary resuscitation (see Chapter 3) if these are not patent.
- Assess for pending respiratory crisis.
  - Is the patient experiencing problems breathing?
  - Is the patient confused or agitated? Decreased oxygenation causes confusion and agitation.
  - Is the patient sweating (diaphoretic)? This is a sign of increased stress.
  - Is the patient cyanotic? This is a sign of decreased circulatory oxygenation.
  - Is the patient pale? This is a sign of decreased circulation.
  - Are the patient's shoulders elevated? This is a sign that the patient is using accessory muscles to supplement the diaphragm to breathe.
- Limit the assessment to identifying the problem area and then direct your assessment to the problem area.
- Stop the assessment if you need to intervene to stabilize the patient.
- Ask the patient to describe the problem.
- Ask questions that help you to quickly identify the problem. Questions should be short and to the point, enabling the patient to answer yes or no. Remember that the patient is typically distressed and is anxious because he or she is experiencing an unusual problem that has not been identified.
  - Are you in pain? Pain might be a sign of pleural inflammation or soreness related to using chest muscles for coughing.
    - Where is the pain?
    - On a scale of 1 to 10, how bad is the pain?
    - Is the pain burning, tight, or squeezing?
    - Does the pain radiate?
    - When did you notice the pain?
    - What were you doing before you noticed the pain?
    - What aggravates the pain?
    - What relieves the pain?
- Do you have a cough? A cough is a reflex action in which short bursts of air are expelled by the lungs to clear the breathing passages.
  - How long have you experienced the cough?
  - Has the cough changed?
  - Is the cough productive?
    - What color is the sputum?
    - Is the sputum liquid or thick?
    - Does the sputum contain blood?
    - How much sputum is produced (e.g., teaspoon)?
  - What time of day do you cough?
  - What aggravates the cough?
  - What relieves the cough?
- Do you have shortness of breath (dyspnea)? This is related to ineffective gas exchange typically associated with an underlying respiratory or cardiac condition and is measured using one of two dyspnea grading scales.

   - On a scale of 1 to 10, where 1 is no shortness of breath and 10 is the worst shortness of breath that you have experienced, how would you rate your current shortness of breath?
   - On a scale of 0 to 4, how would you rate your current shortness of breath?
      - 0 = No shortness of breath.
      - 1 = Shortness of breath when walking up a small hill or walking fast on a level surface.
      - 2 = Shortness of breath causing you to walk slower than others of the same age or you must stop when walking to catch your breath.
      - 3 = Shortness of breath causes you to stop every 100 yards to catch your breath.
      - 4 = Shortness of breath occurs when changing clothes or prevents you from leaving your house.
- Do you have shortness of breath when lying down (orthopnea)?
   - How many pillows do you use when sleeping? Record the answer as two-pillow orthopnea if the patient uses two pillows.
- What aggravates the shortness of breath?
- What relieves the shortness of breath?
- Are you drowsy or irritable during the day? This is a sign of temporary stoppage of breathing during sleep (sleep apnea).
   - Do you sleep throughout the night?
   - Are you told that you snore?
- Do you have allergies?
   - What allergies?
   - Have you recently been exposed to the allergen?
   - How do you react when you are exposed to the allergen?
- Do you smoke?
   - How much do you smoke a day?
   - How long have you smoked?
- Are you exposed to secondary smoke?
   - How long have you been around secondary smoke?
- Do you have any respiratory disease?
- Are you currently or were you previously treated for respiratory disease?
- Were you exposed to environmental conditions that may have caused your current respiratory condition?
- Are you immunocompromised?
- Inspection:
   - Count the respirations. Normal respiration is between 10 and 20 respirations per minute.
   - Look for breathing patterns. A regular breathing pattern is even and unlabored. Signs are normal. Common abnormal breathing patterns are:
      - Biot's respiration: Alternating deep rapid breathing followed by sudden apnea, indicating a problem with the central nervous system.
      - Cheyne-Stokes: A cycle of shallow to deep breathing followed by up to 20 seconds of apnea. This pattern is normal during sleep for some patients. This pattern may indicate kidney or cardiac failure or problems with the central nervous system if the patient is awake.

- Look for signs of cyanosis in extremities, such as nail beds, tip of the nose, and earlobes, which is a sign of deoxygenating of the blood, possibly caused by inadequate gas exchange.
- Look for clubbing of fingers, which is a possible sign of chronic deoxygenating of the blood.
- Look for flaring of the nostrils, which is a sign of respiratory distress.
- Look for pursing of lips, which is a sign that the patient is controlling shortness of breath and improving ventilation because the airway is open longer, decreasing the effort to breathe.
- Look for a symmetrical chest movement on inspiration and expiration. There should be little chest movement. Asymmetrical chest movement may indicate uncoordinated respiration and the use of accessory muscles to breathe.
- Look for a displaced trachea, which may indicate a collapsed lung.
- Look for signs of agitation, which is a sign of decreased oxygenation.
- Look for elevated shoulders, which is a sign that the patient is using accessory muscles to assist in respiration.
- Look for abnormal thoracic cavity, which may inhibit cardiac movement.
- Look at the angle between the ribs and the sternum above the xiphoid process (costal angle). The angle should be less than 90 degrees. An angle 90 degrees or greater may indicate chronic expansion of the lungs related to chronic obstructive pulmonary disease (COPD).

- Palpation:
  - Place the palms of both hands lightly on the patient's bare back in the thoracic region, each hand over the patient's lung.
  - Do not touch the patient with your fingers.
  - Ask the patient to fold his or her arms across chest to reposition scapulae away from the thoracic region.
  - Ask the patient to say 99 several times.
  - You should feel vibrations (tactile fremitus).
    - No or little vibration: A sign of bronchial obstruction or fluid in pleural cavity (pleural effusion).
    - Intense vibration: A sign of tissue consolidation.
    - Less vibration: A sign of pleural effusion, emphysema, or pneumothorax.
  - Repeat the assessment on the front of the patient's chest.
  - Place hands on the front of the patient's chest.
  - Position thumbs in the second intercostal space.
  - Ask the patient to breathe normally.
  - Your thumbs should separate equally and simultaneously.
    - Thumbs separating asymmetrically: Pleural effusion, pneumonia, pneumothorax, or atelectasis.
    - Decreased expansion at the diaphragm: Emphysema, ascites, respiratory depression, paralysis of the diaphragm, obesity, and atelectasis.
  - Repeat the assessment on the patient's back with your thumbs placed at the 10th rib.
- Percussion:
  - Percuss the patient's lung fields by placing one finger on the patient and tapping the finger with a finger from the other hand, causing the patient's lung fields to vibrate.
  - On the front of the chest, begin at the upper right, then move left, down, and to the right. Continue this pattern until the end of the rib cage is reached.
  - On the back, move along the shoulder lines and then move upper right, across to the right, down, and across to the left until the end of the rib cage is reached.

- Hyperresonance: Indicates air in the lungs; common in asthma, emphysema, and pneumothorax.
- Hyporesonance (dull): Indicates decreased air in the lungs; common in atelectasis, pleural effusion, or tumor.

- Auscultation:
  - Listen to air moving through the bronchi with a stethoscope.
  - Over the trachea:
    - Normal: Harsh, discontinuous sounds on inhalation and exhalation.
  - On the front of the chest along the clavicle, begin at the upper right, then move left, down, and to the right. Continue this pattern until the end of the rib cage is reached (see fig. 4.1).
  - On the back, move along the shoulder lines and then move upper right, across to the right, down, and across to the left until the end of the rib cage is reached.

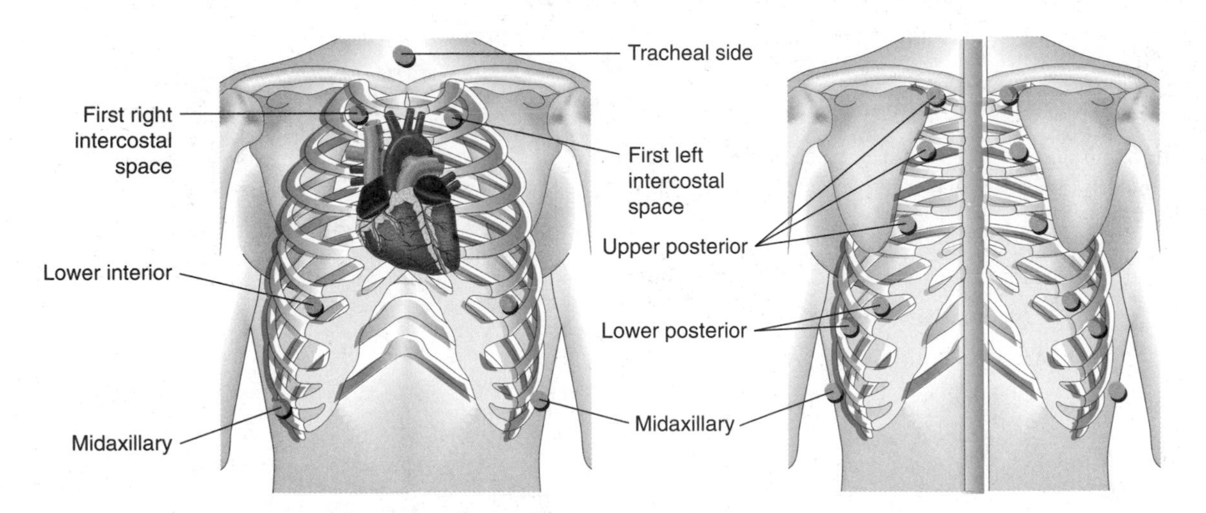

Figure 4.1 Auscultation sites to hear lung sounds.

  - Normal breath sounds:
    - Bronchial (next to the trachea): High-pitched, loud, discontinuous, and loudest on exhalation.
    - Bronchovesicular (between scapulae and upper sternum): Medium-pitched, continuous on inhalation and exhalation.
    - Vesicular (remaining lung area): Low-pitched, soft, prolonged on inhalation, and short on exhalation.
  - Abnormal breath sounds:
    - Crackles: Nonmusical, intermittent sounds on inspiration resembling a crackling sound related to air moving through secretions.
    - Fine crackles: Sound like hair rubbing together.
    - Coarse crackles: Sound like gurgling.
    - Wheezes: High-pitched sound on exhalation or inspiration related to blocked airflow.
    - Rhonchi: Low-pitched sound such as snoring on exhalation that alters when the patient coughs.
    - Stridor: High-pitched, loud sound during inspiration.
    - Pleural friction rub: Painful, low-pitched grating sound on expiration and inspiration.

  - Misplaced breath sounds are normal breath sounds heard in a different area of the lung. For example, normal bronchial sounds in the vesicular area indicate that the vesicular area contains fluid and no air is moving through the vesicular area.
  - Voice sounds are chest vibrations produced when the patient speaks. Listen to voice sounds with a stethoscope. Abnormal voice sounds are:
    - Egophony: Ask the patient to say E.
      - Normal: Muffled.
      - If the lung area is dense (consolidated): Sounds like the patient is saying A.
    - Bronchophony: Ask the patient to say 99.
      - Normal: Muffled.
      - If the lung area is dense: Loud.
    - Whispered pectoriloquy: Ask the patient to whisper 1, 2, 3.
      - Normal: Unable to distinguish the numbers.
      - If the lung area is dense: Numbers are loud and distinct.

4.1.2.1 Signs and symptoms

The respiratory assessment in an emergency situation requires the nurse to recognize common signs and symptoms of underlying causes and then prepare for the anticipated treatment that the practitioner is likely to order.

- Commonly seen signs and symptoms:
  - Stridor (high-pitched wheezing) on inspiration and seesawing or abdominal breathing:
    - Upper airway obstruction.
    - Croup (children).
      - Nebulized epinephrine.
      - Corticosteroids
      - Anaphylaxis.
      - Intramuscular (IM) epinephrine – auto inject.
      - Albuterol.
      - Antihistamine.
      - Corticosteroids.
    - Aspiration of foreign body.
      - Position the patient for comfort.
      - Call the practitioner.
- Stridor (high-pitched wheezing) on expiration:
  - Lower airway obstruction:
    - Asthma (see 4.6 Asthma).
    - Bronchitis (see 4.9 Bronchitis).
- Rapid respiration rate and grunting
  - Lung tissue disease:
    - Pneumonia (see 4.13 Pneumonia).
    - Pulmonary edema (see 4.5 Acute respiratory distress syndrome).
      - Automatic mechanical ventilation.
      - Diuretic medication.
- Disordered control over breathing:
  - Increased intracranial pressure.

  - Medication overdose.
  - Poisoning.
  - Neuromuscular disorder.

4.1.2.2 Pediatric respiratory assessment

At times, infants and children are unable to voice symptoms of respiratory disorders; however, there are signs that indicate a respiratory problem. Here are some common signs of respiratory problems in infants and children.

- Decreased oxygen level:
  - Irritable.
  - Agitated.
  - Decreased response.
  - Listless.
  - Cyanosis.
- Difficulty catching his breath or working to breathe:
  - Nasal flaring indicates respiratory distress.
  - Increased respiration indicates inadequate perfusion.
  - Sepsis shock (wide pulse pressure).
- Respiratory pauses:
  - Disordered control breathing.
- Pale skin indicates:
  - Hypoxemia.
  - Hypercarbia.
  - Increased vascular resistance.
- Change in voice or difficulty breathing on inspiration:
  - Upper airway obstruction.
- Inability to speak more than one word at a time or prolonged forced exhalation:
  - Lower airway obstruction.
- Grunting or breathing oddly:
  - Lung tissue disorder.
  - Respiratory failure.
- Snoring on inspiration:
  - Tongue occlusion.
  - Floppy pharynx.
- Crackles at the base of the lungs:
  - Cardiac shock.

4.2 Respiratory Tests

Respiratory tests are designed to assess the effectiveness of gas exchange and the capability of the respiratory system to function. Some respiratory tests are also used to assess the structural patency of the respiratory system. Emergency department healthcare providers order respiratory tests and results are used to assess the patient and assist the healthcare team to stabilize the patient. Once stabilized, the patient is transferred or referred for follow-up care designed to treat the underlying cause of the current episode, which may require additional respiratory tests. The following respiratory tests are commonly ordered by the emergency department's healthcare providers.

4.2.1 Pulse oximetry

Pulse oximetry estimates the saturation of oxygen in arterial blood by using infrared light passed through a finger, toe, earlobe, or bridge of the nose. A sensor within the pulse oximetry assesses the color absorbed by arterial blood. The test assesses the saturation of oxygen without the need for an arterial blood gas (ABG) test.

- Do not perform the test if the patient is suspected of having carbon monoxide poisoning. Carbon monoxide adheres to hemoglobin and is recorded as oxygen by the pulse oximetry device. In cases of suspected carbon monoxide poisoning, use an ABG test to assess oxygen saturation.
- Administering the test:
  - Assess the patient's pulse prior to administering pulse oximetry.
  - The test can be performed intermittently or continuously.
  - Rotate the pulse oximetry site every 4 hours if used continuously.
  - Some pulse oximetry devices have an audible alarm that sounds when arterial blood saturation levels fall within the abnormal range.
  - Always record whether the patient was on room air or oxygen when the test was performed. If the patient was on oxygen, then note the dose and the delivery method (e.g., nasal cannula).
  - Compare pulse displayed on the device with the pulse that you manually assessed prior to the test. If there is a material difference, then reposition the pulse oximetry and take another reading.
  - Pulse oximetry results are within 2% of saturation results reported from an ABG test.
  - The oxygen saturation level of arterial blood is displayed as a percentage of oxygen to hemoglobin; 100% means that 100% of hemoglobin in the arterial blood contains oxygen.
  - Normal:
    - 95% to 100%.
  - Abnormal:
    - Below 95% may indicate abnormal gas exchange.
    - Patients with COPD or other lung disorders may have consistently abnormal saturation, which is considered normal for the patient. Saturations lower than the patient's abnormal "normal" saturation level may indicate that the lung disorder has worsened.
  - If the oxygen saturation level is abnormal, assess the patient for factors that may interfere with the test:
    - Fingernail polish.
    - Acrylic fingernails.
    - Excessive ambient light.
    - Hypotension.
    - High bilirubin levels in the blood.
    - Patient movement during the test.
    - Administration of vasoconstrictors.

4.2.2 Arterial Blood Gas (ABG)

- The ABG test is a blood test in which an arterial blood sample is taken from the patient and assessed for oxygen (Pao_2), carbon dioxide ($Paco_2$), bicarbonate (HCO_3-), saturation oxygen ($Sao_{2>}$), and pH levels.
  - Normal ranges are:
    - Pao_2: 80 to 100 mmHg.
    - $Paco_2$: 35 to 45 mmHg.
    - HCO_3-: 22 to 26 mEq/L.
    - Sao_2: 95% to 100% of hemoglobin.
    - pH: 7.35 to 7.45.
- The pH value measures the concentration of hydrogen ions in arterial blood.
  - A value greater than 7.45 indicates acidosis, and a value lower than 7.35 indicates alkalosis.
  - The patient's blood must be within normal limits to be considered stabilized.
  - Abnormal values indicate that the patient's body is trying to reestablish the acid-base (alkalosis) balance by having the metabolic system work together with the respiratory system to compensate for the acid-base imbalance.
  - The imbalance could be caused by a problem with the respiratory system. This is referred to as respiratory acidosis or respiratory alkalosis.
  - The imbalance could be caused by a problem with the metabolic system. This is referred to as metabolic acidosis or metabolic alkalosis. The results of the ABG test can help you identify the underlying cause, as shown in table 4.1.

TABLE 4.1 Acid-Base Values

	pH	Pco_2	HCO_{3-}	Signs	Causes
Respiratory acidosis (too much carbon dioxide retained)	<7.35	>45 mmHg	>26 mEq/L (metabolic system compensating)	Flushed face Sweating Restlessness Tachycardia Headache	Hypoventilation Asphyxia Decreased central nervous system function
Respiratory alkalosis (too little carbon dioxide retained)	>7.45	<35 mmHg	< 22 mEq/L	Anxiety Rapid deep breathing Light headedness	Hyperventilation Gram-negative bacteria infection Increased respiratory function related to medication
Metabolic acidosis (too little bicarbonate retained)	<7.35	<35 mmHg (respiratory system compensating)	< 22 mEq/L (metabolic system compensating)	Drowsiness Vomiting Nausea Rapid deep breathing Fruity breath Headache	Diarrhea Renal disease Hepatic disease Medication intoxication Shock Endocrine disorder
Metabolic alkalosis (too much bicarbonate retained)	>7.45	>45 mmHg (respiratory system compensating)	>26 mEq/L	Ringing in the ear Confusion Slow, shallow breathing Irritability	Vomiting Gastric suctioning Steroid administration Diuretic therapy Decreased potassium levels

- It is important that any supplemental oxygen or ventilation assistance that has been administered to the patient shortly before or when the sample is taken is noted on the sample documentation. This enables the lab to adjust the results accordingly.
- Because the sample is taken from an artery, you must apply pressure to the puncture site for 5 minutes and apply a pressure dressing for 30 minutes once the bleeding stops. The site then needs to be monitored regularly to ensure there is no residual bleeding or formation of a hematoma.

4.2.3 End-tidal carbon dioxide monitor

End-tidal carbon dioxide monitoring (see fig. 4.2) uses infrared light to measure carbon dioxide concentration in gas expired from the patient's breath. The end-tidal carbon dioxide monitor is connected to the patient's airway or endotracheal tube. The measurement is typically displayed as a waveform on a monitor, along with other vital signs and can signal the first sign that the patient is having difficulty breathing.

- Normal end-tidal carbon dioxide value is between 35 and 45 mmHg and is usually 2 mmHg to 5 mmHg lower than the corresponding ABG value.
- Greater than10% end-tidal carbon dioxide value: Indicates an increase in carbon dioxide, possibly caused by respiratory depression or partial airway obstruction.
- Less than10% end-tidal carbon dioxide value: Indicates decreased carbon dioxide, possibly caused by a dislodged ventilator or endotracheal tube or complete airway obstruction.

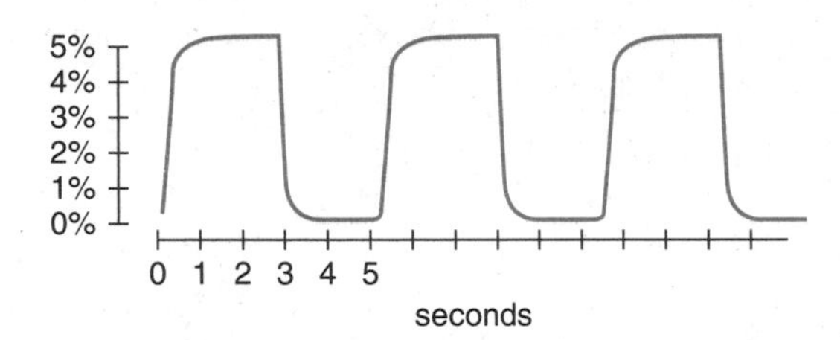

Figure 4.2 Normal waveform from end-tidal carbon dioxide monitoring.

4.2.4 Bronchoscopy

Bronchoscopy is a procedure that enables the healthcare provider to view the patient's larynx, trachea, and bronchi using a bronchoscope. The bronchoscope is a flexible tube that uses fiber optics to display images of the respiratory structure. The healthcare provider uses the bronchoscope to remove airway obstructions including mucus, tumors, and foreign bodies. The bronchoscope is also used to obtain specimens for further testing.

- Bronchoscopy procedure:
  - Administer atropine to decrease secretions.
  - Administer midazolam (Versed) or other sedative and antianxiety medication to help relax the patient.
  - Administer a topical anesthetic to the nasopharynx, vocal cords, and trachea to suppress the gagging reflex.
  - Administer oxygen.
  - Monitor vital signs.
  - Insert the bronchoscope through the mouth or nose.
  - Suction as necessary.

- Remove the obstruction or sample.
- After the bronchoscope is removed, raise the head of the bed 30 degrees or place the patient on his or her side.
- The patient must receive nothing by mouth until the gag response returns.
- Test for the return of the gag response.
- Monitor the patient's vital signs until the gag response returns.

4.2.5 Sputum analysis

Sputum is mucus produced when the patient coughs, and it can contain microorganisms if the patient is experiencing a respiratory infection. Sputum can also contain abnormal lung cells. Sputum analysis is the procedure used to identify cells or microorganisms in the sputum. The color of the sputum may provide a clue as to the underlying infection. Typically sputum colors are:

- Bloody: May indicate tuberculosis.
- Rusty: May indicate pneumonia.
- Yellow-green: May indicate a bacterial infection.
- Frothy pink: May indicate pulmonary edema.
- Foamy white: May indicate edema or a respiratory obstruction.
- White or opaque (milky): May indicate an infection other than bacterial such as a viral infection.
- Sputum collection procedure:
  - The patient takes three deep breaths.
  - Force a deep cough to produce the sputum.
  - Collect sputum in a sterile container. Otherwise, contamination in the container may affect the results of the study.
  - Do not collect saliva: Saliva is bubbly (froth) and has a thinner consistency than sputum.

4.2.6 Chest x-ray

During a chest x-ray the x-ray particles are beamed through the patient's chest onto a photographic film or to a computer. Dense structures such as bone block x-ray particles cause those structures to appear white. Less-dense structures such as fluid, foreign bodies, tumors, and infiltrate block some x-ray particles, causing those structures to appear gray. Lung tissue does not block x-ray particles and appears dark.

- Two common reasons healthcare providers use a chest x-ray to assess the lungs are:
  - To determine whether there are fluid, foreign bodies, tumors, scarring, or infiltrate in the lungs.
  - To compare the current chest x-ray to previous chest x-rays to assess changes that may indicate whether the disorder is getting better or has worsened.
- The chest x-ray procedure:
  - Be sure that the patient is not pregnant.
  - Remove all jewelry in the thoracic area because jewelry may appear on the x-ray image.
  - Assess whether the patient has scars in the thoracic area. If so, note the location of the scar because it may appear on the x-ray image.
  - The patient removes clothes above the waist. Provide the patient with a gown.
  - The patient stands or sits in front of the x-ray machine. An x-ray can also be taken while the patient lies down on the x-ray plate.

- The patient is asked to hold his or her breath while the x-ray is taken.
- Multiple views of the patient's thoracic area may be taken.
- The initial result, called a wet read, provides a relatively superficial assessment of the image. A more thorough reading is taken hours or days later.

4.2.7 Thoracic Computed Tomography (CT) scan

A thoracic CT scan provides a three-dimensional image of the lung using x-rays. It enables the healthcare provider to visualize normal and abnormal structures within the respiratory system. A CT scan can be performed with or without a contrast agent. A contrast agent is iodine based and enhances images of blood vessels and less dense areas of the respiratory system.

- The thoracic CT scan procedure:
  - Assesses whether the patient is allergic to iodine or shellfish if the patient is undergoing a CT scan with contrast. Patients who are allergic to iodine or shellfish have a high likelihood of experiencing an allergic reaction to the contrast agent.
  - Assess whether the patient is claustrophobic. The patient will be placed in an enclosure during the test.
  - Assess whether the patient can remain still for 30 minutes during the CT scan.
  - Administer diphenhydramine (Benadryl) and prednisone (Deltasone) before the CT scan to reduce the risk of an allergic reaction to the contrast agent if the contrast agent is ordered.
  - Administer the contrast agent through an intravenous (IV) tube. The patient may feel flushed and experience a salty or metallic taste in the mouth.
  - The CT scanner encircles the patient for up to 30 minutes.
  - Explain to the patient that the contrast material typically discolors the urine for up to 24 hours after the CT scan. The patient should increase fluid intake after the CT scan to flush the contrast agent from his or her body if the contrast agent is used for the CT scan.

4.2.8 Thoracic Magnetic Resonance Imaging (MRI) Scan

A thoracic MRI provides a three-dimensional view of the respiratory system using radio waves, a strong magnet, and a computer. An MRI is particularly used to assess fluid-filled soft tissue and to identify tumors from other structures within the thoracic area.

- The thoracic MRI procedure:
  - All metal must be removed from the patient.
  - No metal must enter the room containing the MRI scanner. The MRI scanner's magnet is always activated.
  - Assess whether the patient is claustrophobic. If so, then ask the healthcare provider whether an open MRI scanner should be used for the test or whether patient should be sedated before the scan begins.
  - The thoracic MRI scan takes about 30 minutes.
  - The thoracic MRI scan is noninvasive. The patient will not feel any discomfort.

4.2.9 Ventilation perfusion scan

A ventilation perfusion scan assesses the respiratory system's ventilation capacity and perfusion capacity and is used as a less risky alternative to the pulmonary angiograph when evaluating pulmonary function. This test is done to determine whether there is abnormal blood flow or a blood clot in the lungs. However, this test is not performed if the patient is on a mechanical ventilator because it is difficult to perform the ventilation element of the test with a ventilator. The pulmonary angiography is performed in lieu of the ventilation perfusion scan if the patient is on a mechanical ventilator.

- There are two elements of the ventilation perfusion scan:
  - Ventilation: This element determines the ability of air to reach all parts of the lungs.
  - Perfusion: This element determines how well blood circulates within the lungs.
- The ventilation perfusion scan procedure:
  - Assesses whether the patient is allergic to contrast medium (i.e., iodine, shellfish).
  - Keep emergency resuscitation equipment and medication (diphenhydramine [Benadryl] and prednisone [Deltasone]) on hand.
  - Ventilation: A mask is placed over the patient's nose and mouth. The patient breathes gas that contains contrast material and air and the lungs are scanned.
  - Perfusion: The patient lies on a moveable table and contrast material is infused IV while the lungs are scanned.
  - The patient remains on bed rest following the test, during which vital signs are monitored.
  - Signs of an adverse reaction to contrast material are:
    - Tachypnea.
    - Restlessness.
    - Urticaria.
    - Respiratory distress.
    - Nausea and vomiting.
    - Tachycardia.

4.2.10 Pulmonary angiograph

Pulmonary angiograph (pulmonary arteriography) is an x-ray imaging test that uses radioactive contrast dye to assess pulmonary circulation and identify abnormal blood flow in the lungs. A pulmonary angiograph has a higher risk than the ventilation perfusion scan because a catheter is inserted through the heart chambers into the pulmonary artery. This procedure may cause ventricular arrhythmias. However, the pulmonary angiograph produces more reliable results than the ventilation perfusion scan.

- The pulmonary angiograph procedure:
  - Assesses whether the patient is allergic to contrast medium (i.e., iodine, shellfish).
  - Keep emergency resuscitation equipment and medication (diphenhydramine [Benadryl] and prednisone [Deltasone]) on hand.
  - Assesses that renal functions are normal (creatinine and blood urea nitrogen [BUN]).
  - Assesses that bleeding time is normal (prothrombin time [PT], partial thromboplastin time [PTT], international normalized ratio [INR], platelet count).
  - Assesses whether the patient is able to lie still during the test.
  - The patient may feel flushed when the contrast material is infused into him or her.
  - Insert the catheter into the femoral artery.
  - Monitor vital signs during and following the test.
  - Apply a pressure dressing on the insertion site after the test.
  - Compare the insertion site to the opposite leg to assess temperature, sensation, and color. Both legs should have the same assessment. Otherwise, notify the healthcare provider.

- The patient should increase fluid intake either orally or through an IV infusion to flush the contrast material from the body.
- Assess the renal function (creatinine and BUN) after the procedure to ensure that the contrast material has not caused renal malfunction.
- Monitor for signs of an adverse reaction to contrast material:
  - Tachypnea.
  - Restlessness.
  - Urticaria.
  - Respiratory distress.
  - Nausea and vomiting.
  - Tachycardia.

4.3 Respiratory Medication

There are four categories of medication commonly used in respiratory emergencies. These are bronchodilators, anti-inflammatory medication, sedatives, and neuromuscular blocking medications. Bronchodilators relax smooth muscles around the bronchi when the patient experiences bronchospasms. Anti-inflammatory medication is used to reduce the inflammation response around the bronchi. Both of these cause the bronchi to remain open, enabling the flow of air and gas exchange to occur. A sedative is used to reduce anxiety and provide sedation for respiratory medical procedures. A neuromuscular blocking medication is used to inhibit spontaneous breathing when the patient is on a mechanical ventilator.

4.3.1 Bronchodilators

Bronchodilators relax smooth muscles around the bronchi and are used to treat bronchospasms. There are two types of bronchodilators:

- Beta$_2$-adrenergic agonists: Beta$_2$-adrenergic agonists are short-acting medications.
- Use: Acute bronchospasm such as with asthma.
  - Medication:
    - Albuterol (Proventil).
    - Epinephrine (Bronkaid Mist).
    - Pirbuterol (Maxair).
- Considerations:
  - Monitor vital signs.
  - Contraindicated for coronary insufficiency, cerebral arteriosclerosis, and angle-closure glaucoma (epinephrine [Bronkaid Mist]).
  - Risk for paradoxical bronchospasm.
- Adverse effects:
  - Irritability.
  - Palpitations.
  - Tachycardia.
  - Paradoxical bronchospasm.

- Anticholinergic medication: Anticholinergic medications cause bronchodilation by interfering with acetylcholine at the receptor site of smooth muscles.
  - Use: Emphysema and chronic bronchitis.
  - Medication:
  - Ipratropium (Atrovent).
- Considerations:
  - Monitor vital signs.
  - Contraindicated for prostatic hypertropy, angle-closure glaucoma, and bladder neck obstruction.
  - Not for acute respiratory distress.
- Adverse effects:
  - Irritability.
  - Palpitations.
  - Paradoxical bronchospasm.

4.3.2 Anti-inflammatory medication

Anti-inflammatory medication suppresses the immune response to the underlying cause that resulted in the swelling of bronchial tissues. The most commonly used anti-inflammatory medication is corticosteroids. Corticosteroids are categorized by the method that the medication is administered to the patient. These are:

- Inhalation corticosteroids: Inhalation corticosteroids are long acting anti-inflammatory medications used for maintenance treatment of asthma.
- Use: Maintenance treatment for asthma.
- Medication:
  - Fluticasone (Flovent).
  - Salmeterol (Advair).
  - Triamcinolone (Azmacort).
  - Beclomethasone (QVAR).
- Considerations:
  - Rinse mouth after use to prevent oral candidiasis.
  - Not used for acute asthma attack.
  - Monitor vital signs.
  - Use spacer.
- Adverse effects:
  - Oral candidiasis.
  - Dry mouth.
  - Bronchospasm.
  - Hoarseness.
  - Headache.
- Systemic corticosteroids: Systemic corticosteroids are fast-acting anti-inflammatory medications that are initially administered IV and then tapered with oral corticosteroids.

- Use: Acute respiratory distress, COPD, and acute respiratory failure.
- Medication:
  - Methylprednisolone (Solu-Medrol).
  - Prednisone (Deltasone).
  - Dexamethasone (Decadron).
- Considerations:
  - Monitor vital signs.
  - Monitor blood glucose levels.
  - Monitor patients who have renal disease, hypertension, or gastrointestinal ulcers or who have recently experienced myocardial infarction.
- Adverse effects:
  - Edema.
  - Thromboembolism.
  - Circulatory collapse.
  - Arrhythmias.
  - Hyperglycemia.
  - Heart failure.
  - Acute adrenal insufficiency.
  - Hypokalemia.
  - Peptic ulcer.
  - Arrhythmias.
  - Insomnia.

4.3.3 Sedatives

Sedatives (benzodiazepines) are used to reduce anxiety for patients who undergo respiratory tests and for patients who are placed on mechanical ventilators. Patients who are on a mechanical ventilator receive neuromuscular blocking medication that stops spontaneous breathing, enabling the mechanical ventilator to breathe for the patient. However, the patient's level of consciousness remains unchanged. The patient is fully aware that his or her natural breathing is paralyzed, which is distressful. Sedatives are administered to reduce the patient's anxiety.

- Use: Anxiety, mechanical ventilation, conscious sedation, intubation.
- Medications:
  - Lorazepam (Ativan).
  - Propofol (Diprivan).
  - Midazolam (Versed).
- Considerations:
  - Contraindicated for alcohol intoxication, shock, coma, and acute angle-closure glaucoma (lorazepam [Ativan] and midazolam [Versed]).
  - Monitor vital signs.
  - Monitor patients carefully if patient has hyperlipidemia, disabilities, hyperlipoproteinemia, or pancreatitis (propofol [Diprivan]).
  - Do not use with other medications (propofol [Diprivan]).

  - Have resuscitation equipment available.
  - Risk of acute withdrawal syndrome if patient suddenly stops taking medication (lorazepam [Ativan]).
- Adverse effects:
  - Hypotension.
  - Drowsiness.
  - Urine retention (lorazepam [Ativan]).
  - Amnesia (midazolam [Versed]).
  - Bradycardia.
  - Apnea (propofol [Diprivan], midazolam [Versed]).

4.3.4 Neuromuscular blocking medication

Neuromuscular blocking medication is used to prevent a patient from spontaneously breathing in order for a mechanical ventilator to assist the patient to breathe. Although the patient's natural breathing response is blocked, the patient's level of consciousness remains unchanged. The patient is aware that spontaneous breathing is arrested. There are two classifications of neuromuscular blocking medication:

- Depolarizing: Medication causes the plasma membrane of the skeletal muscle fiber to depolarize.
- Use: Endotracheal intubation, mechanical ventilation, skeletal muscle relaxation.
- Medication:
  - Succinylcholine (Anectine).
- Considerations:
  - Contraindicated for penetrating eye injuries, malignant hyperthermia, and acute angle-closure glaucoma.
  - Have resuscitation equipment available.
  - Monitor vital signs.
- Adverse effects:
  - Anaphylaxis.
  - Apnea.
  - Bronchoconstriction.
  - Cardiac arrhythmia.
  - Bradycardia.
- Nondepolarizing: Blocks the acetylcholine receptors, preventing acetylcholine from depolarizing skeletal muscle fiber.
- Use: Endotracheal intubation, mechanical ventilation, and skeletal muscle relaxation.
- Medication:
  - Tubocurarine (curare).
  - Atracurium (Atramed).
  - Pancuronium (Pavulon).
  - Cisatracurium (Nimbex).
  - Vecuronium (Norcuron).

- Considerations:
  - Prolong neuromuscular block in a patient with myasthenic syndrome and myasthenia gravis.
  - Monitor renal function and electrolyte levels to establish a baseline before administering the medication.
  - Monitor for bradycardia.
  - Do not mix with barbiturates using the same syringe.
- Adverse effects:
  - Anaphyalxis.
  - Apnea.
  - Hypotension.
  - Flushing.
  - Arrhythmias.

4.4 Acute Respiratory Distress Syndrome (ARDS)

Acute respiratory distress syndrome is when shock, trauma, or sepsis causes fluid and protein to build up in the alveoli from an inflammatory response. This results in alveolar collapse and impaired gas exchange.

4.4.1 Signs and symptoms

- Dyspnea.
- Pulmonary edema.
- Tachypnea.
- Rales (crackles).
- Hypoxemia.
- Accessory muscle use for respirations.
- Decreased breath sounds.
- Cyanosis.
- Rhonchi.
- Anxiety.
- Tachycardia.
- Restlessness resulting from decreased oxygen levels.

4.4.2 Medical tests

- ABG test shows respiratory acidosis.
- Pulse oximetry shows lowered oxygen levels.
- Chest x-ray shows infiltrates within lung.

4.4.3 Treatment

- Monitor and maintain airway, breathing, and circulatory status.
- Positive end-expiratory pressure mechanical ventilation.
- Continuous positive airway pressure (CPAP) mechanical ventilation.

- Endotracheal intubation.
- Administer:
  - Analgesic to decrease pain.
    - Morphine.
  - Diuretics to decrease fluid.
    - Lasix (furosemide), Edecrin (ethacrynic acid), Bumex (bumetanide).
  - Anesthetic during endotracheal intubation.
    - Diprivan (propofol).
  - Neuromuscular blocking agent during mechanical ventilation.
    - Pavulon (pancuronium), Norcuron (vecuronium).
  - Proton pump inhibitor decreases risk of aspiration and gastric stress ulcer.
    - Zantac (ranitidine), Pepcid (famotidine), Axid (nizatidine), Prilosec (omeprazole).
  - Anticoagulant: decrease coagulation.
    - Heparin, Coumadin (warfarin); Fragmin (dalteparin); Lovenox (enoxaparin).
  - Steroids to decrease inflammation.
    - Hydrocortisone, Medrol (methylprednisolone).
  - Exogenous surfactant.
    - Survanta (beractant).

4.4.4 Intervention

- Bed rest.
- Record intake and output of fluid.
- Monitor for fluid overload.
- Weigh daily.
- No overexertion.
- Instruct the patient:
  - Coughing and deep-breathing exercises.
  - Call healthcare provider at first sign of respiratory distress.

4.5 Asthma

An allergen or nonallergen factor triggers inflammation of the airway and/or bronchospasm, resulting in dyspnea. There are two types of asthma:

- Atopic (extrinsic) asthma caused by allergens.
- Nonatopic (intrinsic) asthma caused by a nonallergy factor such as cold air, humidity, or a respiratory tract infection.

4.5.1 Signs and symptoms

- Asymptomatic between asthma attacks.
- Dyspnea.

- Bronchoconstriction.
- Tachypnea.
- Wheezing on expiration but can also occur on inspiration.
- Cough.
- Use of accessory muscles to breathe.
- Tachycardia.
- Anxiety.
- Sweating (diaphoresis).
- Hyperresonance on percussion related to hyperinflation.

4.5.2 Medical tests

- ABG test show respiratory acidosis.
- Chest x-ray shows hyperinflated lungs.
- Pulse oximetry shows decreased O_2.
- Complete blood cell count shows eosinophils increased.
- Sputum shows positive eosinophils.
- Pulmonary function test shows decreased force on expiration during attack.

4.5.3 Treatment

- Three (3) L of fluid daily to liquefy any secretions.
- Remove allergens and triggers.
- Administer:
    - $Beta_2$-adrenergic bronchodilators.
        - Salmeterol, formoterol, albuterol, pirbuterol, metaproterenol, terbutaline, levalbuterol.
        - Leukotriene modulators anti-inflammatory.
        - Zafirlukast, zileuton, montelukast.
    - Anticholinergic to reduce bronchospasm.
        - Ipratropium inhaler, tiotropium inhaler.
        - Antacid.
        - Aluminum hydroxide/magnesium hydroxide, calcium carbonate.
    - H_2 blockers.
        - Ranitidine, famotidine, nizatidine, cimetidine.
    - Proton pump inhibitor.
        - Omeprazole, lansoprazole, esomeprazole, rabeprazole, pantoprazole.
    - Mast cell stabilizer.
        - Cromolyn, nedocromil.
    - Steroids to decrease inflammation.
        - Hydrocortisone, Medrol (methylprednisolone), prednisolone.
    - Methylxanthines for bronchodilation.
        - Aminophylline, theophylline.

4.5.4 Intervention

- High Fowler's position for comfort.
- Oxygen therapy 1 to 2 L per minute.
- Monitor oxygen saturation.
- Monitor vital signs.
- Instruct the patient:
  - Avoid allergen.
  - Identify signs of asthma attack.
  - How to use inhaler.

4.6 Atelectasis

Atelectasis is a collapsed lung resulting from airway obstruction, pleural space infusion, tumor, anesthesia, immobility, or no deep breathing exercise postoperatively, resulting in decreased gas exchange.

4.6.1 Signs and symptoms

- Decreased breathing.
- Diaphoresis.
- Dyspnea.
- Hypoxemia.
- Tachypnea.
- Tachycardia.
- Cyanosis.
- Anxiety.
- Use of accessory muscle.

4.6.2 Medical tests

- Chest x-ray shows shadows in collapsed area.
- CT scan shows collapsed area.

4.6.3 Treatment

- Administer:
  - $Beta_2$-adrenergic bronchodilators.
    - Salmeterol, formoterol, albuterol, pirbuterol, metaproterenol, terbutaline, levalbuterol.
  - Mucolytics to loosen secretions.
    - Acetylcysteine inhaled, Guaifenesin orally.

4.6.4 Intervention

- Oxygen therapy 1 to 2 L per minute.
- Provide humidified air.
- Monitor breathing.
- Instruct the patient:
    - To use the incentive spirometer.
    - Cough and deep-breathing exercises every 2 hours.

4.7 Bronchiectasis

Bronchiectasis is when the bronchi become obstructed with excessive mucus as a result of abnormal dilation of bronchi and bronchioles related to infection and inflammation. Patient may develop atelectasis and bronchitis.

4.7.1 Signs and symptoms

- Hemoptysis.
- Dyspnea.
- Cyanosis.
- Cough when lying down.
- Foul-smelling cough.
- Crackles on inspiration.
- Rhonchi on inspiration.
- Bronchial infections.
- Weight loss.
- Anemia.

4.7.2 Medical tests

- Pulmonary function test shows decreased vital capacity.
- Chest x-ray shows shadows.
- CT scan shows bronchiectasis.
- Culture and sensitivity of sputum identify microorganism and medication.

4.7.3 Treatment

- Bronchoscopy to remove excessive secretions.
- Postural drainage uses gravity to move mucus from lungs to throat.
- Administer:

  - $Beta_2$-adrenergic bronchodilators.
    - Salmeterol, formoterol, albuterol, pirbuterol, metaproterenol, terbutaline, levalbuterol.
  - Antibiotics to treat infection.

4.7.4 Intervention

- Oxygen therapy 1 to 2 L per minute.
- Chest percussion loosens secretions.
- Monitor vital signs.
- Instruct the patient:
  - Family to perform chest percussion.
  - Family to do postural drainage.

4.8 Bronchitis

In bronchitis, an infection or airborne irritants cause increased mucus production leading to blocked airways and decreased gas exchange.

- Acute bronchitis is reversible within 10 days.
- Chronic bronchitis is not reversible and is classified as COPD.

4.8.1 Signs and symptoms

- Productive cough (acute bronchitis).
- Chronic productive cough for 3 months (chronic bronchitis); annually for at least 2 years.
- Cough due to mucus production and irritation of airways.
- Dyspnea.
- Wheezing.
- Use of accessory muscles to breathe.
- Fever.
- Weight gain due to edema from right-sided heart failure (chronic bronchitis).
- Chest discomfort.
- Fatigue.

4.8.2 Medical tests

- ABG tests show respiratory acidosis.
- Hemoglobin increased.
- Chest x-ray shows infiltrate related to infection.

- Pulmonary function testing shows:
  - Forced vital capacity decreased.
  - Forced expiratory volume in one second (FEV_1) decreased.
  - Residual volume (RV) increased.

4.8.3 Treatment

- Administer:
  - $Beta_2$-adrenergic bronchodilators.
    - Salmeterol, formoterol, albuterol, pirbuterol, metaproterenol, terbutaline, levalbuterol.
  - Steroids to decrease inflammation.
    - Hydrocortisone, Medrol (methylprednisolone), prednisolone.
  - Methylxanthines for bronchodilation.
    - Aminophylline, theophylline.
  - Diuretics to decrease fluid.
    - Lasix (furosemide), Edecrin (ethacrynic acid), Bumex (bumetanide).
  - Proton pump inhibitor decreases risk of aspiration and gastric stress ulcer.
    - Zantac (ranitidine), Pepcid (famotidine), Axid (nizatidine), Prilosec (omeprazole).
  - H_2 blockers.
    - Ranitidine, famotidine, nizatidine, cimetidine.
  - Antacid.
    - Aluminum hydroxide/magnesium hydroxide, calcium carbonate.
  - Expectorant to liquefy secretions.
    - Guaifenesin.
  - Anticholinergic to reduce bronchospasm.
    - Ipratropium inhaler, tiotropium inhaler.

4.8.4 Intervention

- Use incentive spirometer.
- High Fowler's position for comfort.
- Three (3) L of fluid daily to help liquefy secretions.
- Oxygen therapy 1 to 2 L per minute via nasal cannula.
- Monitor vital signs.
- Weigh patient daily. Notify healthcare provider of weight gain of 2 lb in one day.
- Monitor sputum changes.
- Monitor intake and output.
- Increase fluids to keep mucous thinner and easier to expel.
- Instruct the patient:
  - How to administer oxygen.

- Turning, coughing, and deep-breathing exercises.
- Increase calories and protein in diet.
- Increase vitamin C.

4.9 Cor Pulmonale

Cor pulmonale is right-sided heart failure resulting from COPD. It leads to pulmonary hypertension and enlargement of the right ventricle.

4.9.1 Signs and symptoms

- Productive cough.
- Edema.
- Weight gain.
- Orthopnea.
- Dyspnea.
- Tachycardia.
- Cyanosis.
- Fatigue.
- Tachypnea.
- Wheezing.

4.9.2 Medical tests

- Pulse oximetry shows lowered oxygen levels.
- Increased hemoglobin.
- ABGs show respiratory acidosis.
- Chest x-ray shows enlarged right ventricle and enlarged pulmonary arteries.
- Echocardiography shows enlarged right ventricle.
- Pulmonary artery catheterization shows increased pulmonary artery and right ventricular pressure.

4.9.3 Treatment

- Administer:
  - Calcium channel blockers decrease blood pressure and heart rate.
    - Isoptin (verapamil), Cardizem (diltiazem), Tiazac (diltiazem), Procardia (nifedipine), Cardene (nicardipine), Norvasc (amlodipine).
  - Potassium channel activator to dilate pulmonary artery.
    - Diazoxide, hydralazine, nitroprusside.

  - Angiotensin-converting enzyme (ACE) inhibitor.
    - Captopril, enalapril.
    - Diuretics to decrease fluid.
    - Lasix (furosemide), Edecrin (ethacrynic acid), Bumex (bumetanide).
  - Anticoagulant decreases coagulation.
    - Heparin, Coumadin (warfarin), Fragmin (dalteparin), Lovenox (enoxaparin).
  - Cardiac glycoside.
    - Digitalis (digoxin).

4.9.4 Intervention

- Bed rest.
- Monitor vital signs.
- Weigh patient daily. Notify healthcare provider of weight gain of 2 lb in one day.
- No overexertion.
- Oxygen therapy 1 to 2 L per minute via nasal cannula.
- Monitor digoxin level to avoid toxic effect.
- Monitor serum potassium levels if given ACE inhibitors and diuretics.
- Instruct the patient:
  - Low-sodium diet.
  - Limit fluid to 2 L each day.

4.10 Emphysema

Emphysema is chronic inflammation of the lungs that results in decreased flexibility of the alveoli walls and loss of elastic recoil. This leads to overdistention of the alveolar walls and trapped air, causing decreased gas exchange. Linked to smoking. It can be caused by inherited alpha$_1$-antitrypsan deficiency, but this is less frequent.

4.10.1 Signs and symptoms

- Difficulty breathing (dyspnea).
- Use of accessory muscles to breathe.
- Barrel chest.
- Loss of weight.
- Diminished breath sounds.
- Expiratory wheezing.
- Hyperresonance.

4.10.2 Medical tests

- Pulmonary function test shows increased residual volume.
- ABGs show respiratory acidosis.
- Chest x-ray shows flattened diaphragm and overinflated lungs.

4.10.3 Treatment

- Administer:
  - Beta$_2$-adrenergic bronchodilators.
    - Salmeterol, formoterol, albuterol, pirbuterol, metaproterenol, terbutaline, levalbuterol.
  - Anticholinergic to reduce bronchospasm.
    - Ipratropium inhaler, tiotropium inhaler.
  - Methylxanthines for bronchodilation.
    - Aminophylline, theophylline.
  - Steroids to decrease inflammation.
    - Hydrocortisone, Medrol (methylprednisolone), prednisolone.
  - Antacids.
    - Aluminum hydroxide/magnesium hydroxide, calcium carbonate.
  - H_2 blockers.
    - Ranitidine, famotidine, nizatidine, cimetidine.
  - Proton pump inhibitor.
    - Omeprazole, lansoprazole, esomeprazole, rabeprazole, pantoprazole.
  - Expectorant to liquefy secretions.
    - Guaifenesin.
  - Diuretics to decrease fluid.
    - Lasix (furosemide), edecrin (ethacrynic acid), Bumex (bumetanide).
  - Alpha 1 antitrypsin therapy for patients with deficiency.
- Teach patient use of the incentive spirometer to encourage deep breathing and enhance coughing and expelling of mucus.
- Teach patient use of flutter valve to increase the expiration force.
- Nocturnal negative-pressure ventilation for hypercapnic (elevated CO_2 levels) patients.

4.10.4 Intervention

- Oxygen therapy 1 to 2 L per minute via nasal cannula.
- Three (3) L of fluid daily to help liquefy secretions.
- Monitor sputum changes.
- Use incentive spirometer.
- High Fowler's position for comfort.
- Monitor intake and output.
- Monitor vital signs.
- Weigh patient daily. Notify healthcare provider of weight gain of 2 lb in one day.

- Instruct the patient:
  - To administer oxygen.
  - Turning, coughing, and deep-breathing exercises.
  - To avoid infection.
  - To stop smoking.
  - To perform abdominal diaphragmatic breathing exercise with pursed-lip breathing.
  - To avoid pollutants and irritants.

4.11 Pleural Effusion

Pleural effusion is when the pleural sac fills with serous fluid, blood (hemothorax), or pus (empyema) restricting lung expansion, displaying lung tissue, and interfering with gas exchange. Causes include postoperative complication, congestive heart failure, renal failure, pulmonary infarction, embolus, infection, trauma, lupus erythematosis, or cancer.

4.11.1 Signs and symptoms

- Dyspnea.
- Decreased breath sounds.
- Increased respiration.
- Increased pulse.
- Decreased blood pressure (BP) (hemothorax).
- Chest pain if inflamed.
- Fever (empyema).
- Dullness on percussion over the affected area.
- Cough.
- Pleural friction rub.

4.11.2 Medical tests

- Pulse oximeter shows decreased oxygen saturation.
- Chest x-ray shows pleural effusion.
- Chest CT scan shows pleural effusion.
- Chest ultrasound shows pleural effusion.

4.11.3 Treatment

- Thoracentesis to remove fluid.
- Chest tube to drain fluid.
- Administer antibiotics (empyema).

4.11.4 Intervention

- Oxygen therapy 2 to 4 L per minute.
- Monitor chest tube drainage and patency.
- Monitor vital signs.
- Instruct the patient:
  - Turning, coughing, and deep-breathing exercises.

4.12 Pneumonia

Pneumonia is the result of inhalation of bacteria, viruses, parasites, or irritating agents or aspiration of liquids or foods. It leads to infection and inflammation, resulting in increased mucus production, thickening alveolar fluid, and decreased gas exchange.

4.12.1 Signs and symptoms

- Dyspnea.
- Crackles.
- Rhonchi.
- Discolored blood tinged, sputum.
- Cough.
- Fever.
- Chills.
- Pain on respiration.
- Tachypnea.
- Tachycardia.
- Muscle pain (myalgia).
- Hypoxamia.
- Sweating (diaphoresis).
- Wheezing.

4.12.2 Medical tests

- Pulse oximeter shows decreased oxygen saturation.
- Chest x-ray shows infiltration.
- White blood cell count (WBC) elevated.
- ABGs show respiratory acidosis.
- Culture and sensitivity of the sputum.

4.12.3 Treatment

- Chest x-ray.
- Blood culture.
- Sputum culture.
- Administer:
  - Antipyretics when fever >101°F for patient comfort.
    - Tylenol (acetaminophen), Advil, Motrin (ibuprofen).
  - Bronchodilators.
    - Albuterol, metaproterenol, levalbuterol.
  - Antibiotics for bacterial infection.
    - Azithromycin, clarithromycin, levofloxacin, moxifloxacin, amoxicillin/clavulanate, cefotaxime, ceftriaxone, cefuroxime axetil, cefpodoxime, ampicillin/sulbactam, telithromycin.

4.12.4 Intervention

- Oxygen therapy 2 to 4 L per minute.
- Incentive spirometer every 2 hours.
- Monitor intake and output.
- Monitor vital signs.
- Monitor sputum characteristics.
- Place patient in high Fowler's position for comfort.
- Bed rest.
- Increase fluids (hydration) (oral or IV).
- Instruct the patient:
  - Three (3) L of fluid daily to help liquefy secretions.
  - Incentive spirometer every 2 hours.
  - Use nebulizer bronchodilator as needed.

4.13 Pneumothorax

Pneumothorax occurs when air enters the pleural space from an opening in the lung or chest, leading to a partial or complete collapse of the lung. Types of pneumothorax are:

- Open pneumothorax: Penetrating chest wound.
- Closed pneumothorax: Blunt trauma.
- Spontaneous pneumothorax: Caused by underlying disease (e.g., emphysema).
- Tension pneumothorax: Displacement of the mediastinum causes unaffected lung to collapse.

4.13.1 Signs and symptoms

- Sharp chest pain aggravated by coughing.
- Tracheal deviation toward the unaffected side with tension pneumothorax.
- Subcutaneous emphysema.
- Absent breath sounds over the affected area.
- Tachypnea.
- Tachycardia.

4.13.2 Medical tests

- Pulse oximeter shows decreased oxygen saturation.
- Chest x-ray shows infiltration.
- ABGs show respiratory acidosis.

4.13.3 Treatment

- A small-bore chest tube is inserted into the upper chest and connected to a standard water-seal chamber or into a Heimlich valve of a suction device to re-expand the lung.
- Administer analgesic.
  - Morphine.

4.13.4 Intervention

- High Fowler's position.
- Bed rest.
- Oxygen therapy 2 to 4 L per minute.
- Monitor chest tube drainage and patency.
- Monitor vital signs.
- Instruct the patient:
  - Turning, coughing, and deep-breathing exercises.

4.14 Respiratory Acidosis

Respiratory acidosis occurs when blood becomes more acid as a result of acute or chronic respiratory, hypoventilation, asphyxia, or central nervous system disorders. Carbon dioxide (acid) increases, resulting in increased respiration and retention of bicarbonate and sodium and excretion of hydrogen ions by the kidneys to compensate.

4.14.1 Signs and symptoms

- Dyspnea.
- Hypoxemia.
- Headache.
- Irritability.
- Confusion.
- Restlessness.
- Cardiac arrhythmia.

4.14.2 Medical tests

- ABGs:
  - Carbon dioxide (CO_2) >50 mmHg.
  - pH of blood <7.35.

4.14.3 Treatment

- Treat underlying cause.
- Mechanical ventilation.
- Administer:
  - Bronchodilators.
    - Albuterol, metaproterenol, levalbuterol.

4.14.4 Intervention

- Oxygen therapy 2 to 4 L per minute.
- Monitor vitals.
- Monitor blood chemistry.
- Instruct the patient:
  - Turning, coughing, and deep-breathing exercises.

4.15 Tuberculosis

Tuberculosis is a lung infection by the *Mycobacterium tuberculosis* bacteria, transmitted by coughing, sneezing, or talking. It can infect other organs.

- Primary tuberculosis is when the patient is initially infected with the *M. tuberculosis* bacteria.
- Secondary tuberculosis is reactivation of the *M. tuberculosis* bacteria from a previous infection.

- In exposure to *M. tuberculosis* bacteria resulting in negative test results and no symptoms, patients may or may not have tuberculosis.
- Latent tuberculosis results in positive test results and no symptoms.

4.15.1 Signs and symptoms

- Low-grade fever.
- Productive cough persists for 2 weeks.
- Blood-tinged sputum (hemoptysis).
- Fatigue.
- Night sweats.
- Fever.
- Chills.
- Anorexia.
- Weight loss.
- Shortness of breath.

4.15.2 Medical tests

- Positive Mantoux purified protein derivative, or (PPD), skin test.
- Sputum test positive for *M. tuberculosis* bacteria.
- Chest x-ray shows areas of granuloma or cavitation.

4.15.3 Treatment

- Administer:
  - Antitubercular agents.
    - Isoniazid, rifampin, pyrazinamide, ethambutol, streptomycin.

4.15.4 Intervention

- Respiratory isolation.
- Increase carbohydrate, protein, and vitamin C in the diet.
- Monitor vitals.
- Monitor intake and output.
- Instruct the patient:
  - Three (3) L of fluid daily to help liquefy secretions.
  - Schedule rest periods.
  - How to prevent the spread of tuberculosis.

4.16 Acute Respiratory Failure

Acute respiratory failure occurs when there is insufficient ventilation, which reduces adequate gas exchange in the lungs. This results in increased carbon dioxide and decreased oxygen in blood. Acute respiratory failure occurs as a result of depression of the central nervous system resulting from medication or trauma or decompensation of a respiratory illness.

4.16.1 Signs and symptoms

- Dyspnea.
- Orthopnea.
- Tachypnea.
- Coughing.
- Fatigue.
- Diminished breath sounds.
- Hemoptysis.
- Diaphoresis.
- Crackles.
- Rhonchi.
- Cyanosis.

4.16.2 Medical tests

- ABG:
  - Oxygen PaO_2 <60 mmHg
  - Carbon dioxide (CO_2) >50 mmHg.
  - Oxygen saturation (SaO_2) <90%.
  - pH of blood <7.30.
- Pulse oximeter shows decreased oxygen saturation.
- Increased WBC.

4.16.3 Treatment

- Treat underlying cause.
- Mechanical ventilation.
- Administer:
  - Bronchodilators.
    - Albuterol, metaproterenol, levalbuterol.
  - Anticholinergic to reduce bronchospasm.
    - Ipratropium inhaler, tiotropium inhaler.

  - Anesthetic to ease intubation.
    - Propofol.
  - Neuromuscular blocking agent to ease mechanical ventilation ventilator.
    - Pancuronium, vecuronium, atracurium.
  - Steroids to decrease inflammation.
    - Hydrocortisone, methylprednisolone, prednisone.
  - Anticoagulant to decrease coagulation.
    - Heparin, Coumadin (warfarin), Fragmin (dalteparin), Lovenox (enoxaparin).
  - Antacid.
    - Aluminum hydroxide/magnesium hydroxide, calcium carbonate.
  - H2 blockers.
    - Ranitidine, famotidine, nizatidine, cimetidine.
  - Proton pump inhibitor.
    - Omeprazole, lansoprazole, esomeprazole, rabeprazole, pantoprazole.
  - Analgesic for discomfort and decrease myocardial oxygen demand.
    - Morphine.

4.16.4 Intervention

- High Fowler's position.
- Oxygen therapy 2 to 4 L per minute.
- Monitor vitals.
- Change position every 2 hours.
- Monitor intake and output.
- Instruct the patient:
  - Turning, coughing, and deep-breathing exercises.

4.17 Pulmonary Embolism

Gas exchange is impaired because of alveoli collapse from an obstruction of blood flow in the lungs. The obstruction can be caused by thrombus, air emboli, or fat emboli. A small area of atelectasis self-resolves. A large area of atelectasis is fatal. Most common pulmonary embolism results from a thrombus that breaks loose from a deep vein in the legs or pelvis.

4.17.1 Signs and symptoms

- Sudden dyspnea.
- Chest pain.
- Tachypnea.
- Tachycardia.

- Crackles at site of emboli.
- Coughing.
- Hemoptysis.
- Anxiety.
- Leg pain.
- Leg swelling.
- Hypotension
- Decreased level of consciousness.
- Fainting (syncope).

4.17.2 Medical tests

- Lung scan shows ventilation/perfusion mismatch.
- Chest x-ray shows dilated pulmonary artery.
- Pulmonary angiography shows clot.
- Helical CT scan will show clot in pulmonary arteries.
- Arterial blood gases show respiratory acidosis.
- D-dimer will be positive when a thromboembolic event has occurred.
- Pulse oximeter shows decreased oxygen saturation.
- Ultrasound of the lower extremities.

4.17.3 Treatment

- Surgical insertion of a vena cava filter.
- Surgical removal of the emboli.
- Administer:
  - Anticoagulant to decrease coagulation.
    - Heparin, Coumadin (warfarin), Fragmin (dalteparin), Lovenox (enoxaparin).
  - Analgesic for discomfort and to decrease myocardial oxygen demand.
    - Morphine.
  - Thrombolytics to within remove clot within 3 to 12 hours of blockages.
    - Urokinase, alteplase.

4.17.4 Intervention

- Bed rest.
- High Fowler's position.
- Oxygen therapy 2 to 4 L per minute.
- Monitor oxygen saturation levels.

- Monitor vitals.
- Instruct the patient:
    - Turning, coughing, and deep-breathing exercises.
    - No crossing the legs.
    - No sitting and standing for too long.
    - Call healthcare provider at first sign of bleeding.
    - Call healthcare provider at first sign of respiratory increase.

4.18 Respiratory Arrest

Respiratory arrest occurs when gas exchange is ineffective because the patient's respiratory system has failed. The patient has a pulse, indicating the patient's cardiovascular system is functioning, although the patient's heart will stop once the oxygen level decreases and the patient becomes hypoxic.

If you realize the patient is in respiratory arrest, perform the following procedures:

- Try arousing the patient by stimulating the upper sternum with your fingers while calling the patient by his or her first name.
- Call for help and call a code immediately.
- Stay with the patient.
- Open the airway.
- Head tilt-chin lift.
- Jaw lift without head extension if the patient's neck is immobilized.
- Look for the rise and fall of the chest.
- Listen for escaping air during exhalation.
- Feel for the flow of air against your cheek.

If no respirations are felt, then begin rescue breathing:

- Give two breaths, each 1 second long.
- Monitor the carotid pulse for 5 seconds.
- Remember that respiratory arrest quickly becomes cardiac arrest if respirations are not restored.

If the patient has a pulse, then the patient is not in cardiac arrest. Do not begin cardiac compressions. Focus on restoring the patient's respiration.

- Insert an airway or intubate to ensure the airway is patent if the patient is unconscious.
- Use a bag mask to ventilate the patient. Compress the bag once every 5 seconds to provide 10 breaths per minute.
- Monitor end-tidal carbon dioxide (see 4.2.3 End-tidal carbon dioxide monitor) to monitor expired gas in the patient's breath.
- Open IV access.
- Attach electrocardiogram (ECG).
- Monitor pulse oximetry (see 4.2.1 Pulse oximetry). Administer supplementary oxygen if oxygen saturation falls below 90%.
- Identify and treat underlying cause.

4.19 Respiratory Procedures

Several commonly performed respiratory procedures are used in critical care situations to ensure that the patient has an open, unobstructed airway and is adequately exchanging gases so that the patient blood oxygen-carbon dioxide levels are within acceptable range.

4.19.1 Oxygen therapy

Oxygen therapy delivers oxygen to the patient through a nasal cannula, through a mask, or through a mechanical ventilator, to return the patient's blood to an acceptable blood oxygen-carbon dioxide level, thereby reducing the cardiac-respiratory workload related to hypoxemia.

Oxygen is considered a medication and therefore requires a medical order before it can be administered to the patient. Typically in the emergency department, oxygen is ordered with as-needed (PRN) orders or as a standing order. Both types of orders specify the condition under which the order can be carried out and the dose and route to administer to the patient. The nurse assesses the patient and administers oxygen accordingly if the specified patient condition exists.

Types of oxygen therapy systems:

- High-flow system: A high-flow system delivers a precise mixture of oxygen and air through either a Venturi mask or a ventilator.
- Low-flow system: A low-flow system delivers a variable mixture of oxygen and air through a non-Venturi mask or nasal cannula.

Oxygen dose is measured as either liters per minute or a percentage of oxygen concentration delivered to the patient.

- Nasal cannula: 2 to 6 L per minute; 24% to 40% oxygen concentration.
- Simple face mask: 6 to 12 L per minute; 28% to 50% oxygen concentration.
- Venturi mask: 40% oxygen concentration.
- Partial rebreathing mask (has a reservoir bag): 5 to 15 L per minute; 40% to 70% oxygen concentration.
- Nonrebreather mask: 10 L per minute; 60% to 80% oxygen concentration.

When administering oxygen therapy:

- Oxygen therapy can dry mucous membranes. Use an oxygen humidifier if the dose is greater than 3 L per minute except if the Venturi mask is used to deliver the oxygen. The Venturi mask contains valves that might clog if the oxygen is humidified.
- Do not use more than 2 L per minute with patients who are diagnosed with COPD. The level of carbon dioxide in their blood causes the desire to breathe. Decreasing the level of carbon dioxide through oxygen therapy can decrease the respiratory drive in COPD patients. However, a normal amount of oxygen is given if the patient is in respiratory arrest or is intubated because the patient is unable to breathe.
- Monitor the patient's level of consciousness and vital signs. Decreased level of consciousness and increased cardiac and respiratory rates may indicate hypoxemia.

4.19.2 Aerosol therapy

Aerosol therapy is a form of inhalation therapy that delivers liquid medication directly to the patient's are airway, enabling the mucosal member of the respiratory system to absorb the medication. Two devices are used for aerosol therapy. These are metered-dose inhalers and a nebulizer.

Listen to the patient's breath sounds prior to administering the medication and then again after the medication is administered to determine if the medication is effective.

Commonly used medications used for aerosol therapy are:

- Bronchodilators: These relax smooth muscles around the bronchi when the patient experiences bronchospasms.
- Corticosteroids: These decrease inflammation around the bronchi, causing a decrease in swelling, which results in more opened bronchi.
- Mucolytics: These medications make mucus less viscous by dissolving thickened mucous secretions, enabling the patient to easily cough up the mucus.

4.19.3 Continuous positive airway pressure therapy

CPAP is a form of inhalation therapy that mechanically provides positive pressure throughout the respiratory cycle to assist the patient with ventilation. The result of this therapy is increased functional residual capacity and reduced effort to breathe. CPAP therapy is delivered using a mask or nasal mask. CPAP therapy is typically administered by a respiratory therapist.

CPAP therapy can be used instead of:

- Mechanical ventilation.
- Intubation.

CPAP therapy is used for:

- Bronchiolitis.
- Pneumonia.
- Respiratory distress syndrome.
- Atelectasis.
- Pulmonary embolus.
- Pulmonary edema.

During CPAP therapy, monitor the patient for:

- Nausea and vomiting. Patient is at risk for aspiration.
- Swallowing air. The patient might experience gastric distress.
- Decreased cardiac output.

4.19.4 Endotracheal rapid sequence intubation

Endotracheal rapid sequence intubation is an emergency procedure that ensures a patent airway by the insertion of a tube through the mouth between the vocal cords and into the trachea (orotracheal intubation). This prevents aspiration and enables the emergency medical team to suction secretions while providing a stable airway for respiratory resuscitation.

Endotracheal tubes are measured in millimeters; 8 mm is common for men and 7.5 mm for women (see fig. 4.3).

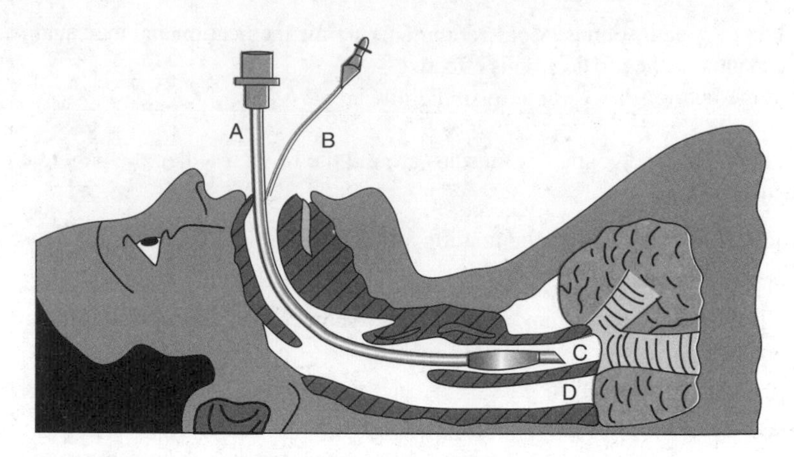

Figure 4.3 The endotracheal tube (A) is inserted into the trachea (C). The tube (B) is inflated to hold the endotracheal tube in position. Be careful not to insert the endotracheal tube into the esophagus (D).

Here are the steps for endotracheal rapid sequence intubation:

- Establish IV access to administer fluids and medication.
- Monitor vital signs continually.
- Administer 100% oxygen using a partial rebreathing face mask for 3 minutes prior to intubation, if time permits.
- Administer a sedative (see 5.4.3 Sedatives), if the patient is conscious.
- Administer:
    - Atropine to maintain cardiac output.
    - Ancetine to reduce the likelihood of facial muscle twitching.
    - Lidocaine to reduce the likelihood of increased intracranial pressure.
    - Administer a neuromuscular blocking medication (see. 4.4.4 Neuromuscular blocking medication), if the patient is conscious.
- Remove dentures, if present.
- Insert the endotracheal tube.
- Inflate the endotracheal tube cuff.
- Verify placement of the endotracheal tube:
    - Observation: The stomach does not inflate. The patient displays normal respirations.
    - Auscultation: Normal respirations are heard over the lung areas. There is absence of sounds in the stomach/abdomen.
    - End-tidal carbon dioxide: Normal end-tidal carbon dioxide values are seen (see 4.2.3 End-tidal carbon dioxide monitor).
    - Chest x-ray: The endotracheal tube is seen in the trachea (see. 4.2.5 Chest x-ray).
- Secure the endotracheal tube with tape.
- Administer mechanical ventilation (see 4.4.5 Mechanical ventilation).
- Continually monitor the patient's vital signs, respiration, and ABGs (see 4.2.2 Arterial blood gas).
- Maintain therapeutic levels of sedation and neuromuscular blocking medication until the endotracheal tube is removed.
- Common complications of endotracheal tube intubation are:

  - Infection: Coughing helps reduce infection. The patient is unable to cough while the endotracheal tube is in place.
  - Spasm: Insertion of the endotracheal tube may stimulate nerves to cause bronchospasm or laryngospasm.
  - Injury: Intubation may damage teeth, vocal cords, mouth, and pharynx.
  - Aspiration: Stomach contents, blood, and other secretions may enter the respiratory system if the endotracheal tube is not in the proper position or if the endotracheal tube becomes dislodged. The patient's normal coughing response is unavailable to expel this content.
  - Cardiac arrhythmias: Insertion of the endotracheal tube may stimulate nerves to cause an abnormal heart beat.
  - Hypoxemia: Decreased oxygenation of the blood can occur if intubation is not performed rapidly. During intubation, respiratory resuscitation stops.
- If there is trauma to the mouth that prevents insertion of the endotracheal tube, then:
  - Insert the endotracheal tube through the nose (nasal intubation). Nasal intubation is also used for elective intubation because this route is more comfortable for the patient, there is less risk of displacement of the endotracheal tube, and there is less risk of tissue damage.

4.19.5 Mechanical ventilation

Mechanical ventilation is a procedure in which a handheld or automated device is used to administer positive or negative pressure to move air into or from the patient's lungs. The mechanical ventilator is connected to the endotracheal tube or tracheostomy tube, depending on which is used with the patient.

- Handheld device: The handheld device is a resuscitation bag that is manually operated by squeezing the bag, forcing air into the patient's lungs. The resuscitation bag can be connected to an oxygen supply (see 4.4.1 Oxygen therapy). The handheld device is used for temporary ventilation during transportation and whenever the automated mechanical ventilator is unavailable. When using a handheld device:
  - Be sure to deliver breaths when the patient inhales and release the bag when the patient exhales.
  - Monitor respirations by observing the rise and fall of the patient's chest, indicating proper ventilation is occurring.
  - Make sure that the handheld device remains properly attached to the tube.
  - Fully squeeze the bag and allow the bag to fully inflate to ensure that the patient is properly ventilated.
  - Document the date and time when the patient was manually ventilated.
- Automated device: An automated device is a mechanical ventilator that uses an electrical pump and other electromechanical components to move air into and from the patient's lungs.
- There are several types of automated ventilators:
  - Volume-cycled ventilator: The volume-cycled ventilator delivers a specific volume of air to the patient, regardless of resistance by the patient's lungs.
  - Time-cycled ventilator: A time-cycled ventilator delivers air for a specified respiratory cycle.
  - Pressure-cycled ventilator: The pressure-cycled ventilator delivers air until a specific pressure is reached. The pressure is resisted by the patient's lungs.
- Automatic mechanical ventilators are typically implemented and maintained by a respiratory therapist. However, the nurse must:
  - Remember that the patient's life depends on the proper functioning of the ventilator.

- Be sure that the ventilator alarms are operational at all times. These alarms signal when there is a problem with the ventilator.
- Make sure that a therapeutic level of sedation and neuromuscular blocking medication is maintained while the patient is on the ventilator.
- Monitor vital signs, including auscultating the respiratory system every 2 hours.
- Be sure that the patient and the patient's family understand that the paralysis is temporary.

4.19.6 Tracheotomy

A tracheotomy is a procedure in which a surgical opening is made into the patient's trachea and an indwelling tube is inserted into the opening to maintain the patient's airway.

In an emergency, the tracheotomy is performed if there is an obstruction in the airway above the trachea, such as with swelling related to an anaphylactic reaction or from a foreign body. In this situation, the tracheotomy tube is open to the environment and the patient is able to breathe normally.

An elective tracheotomy is performed if the patient requires extended use of an automatic mechanical ventilator. If the patient is on an automatic mechanical ventilator (see 4.20.5 Mechanical ventilator), the tracheotomy tube is cuffed to prevent backflow and the automatic mechanical ventilator is connected to the tracheotomy tube.

Make sure that:

- The patient and family members realize that the patient will not be able to speak normally until the tracheotomy tube is removed.
- A respiratory assessment, including ABG test (see 4.2.2 Arterial blood gas) is done before and after the tracheotomy to ensure that the patient's respiration improves because of the procedure.
- Tracheotomy tube assessment and care such as suctioning and cleaning are performed as scheduled.
- The patient is monitored for secretions that must be suctioned.
- The patient is monitored for bleeding around the surgical site.
- Document all secretions suctioned from the patient.

4.19.7 Chest tube

Insertion of a chest tube into the pleural space is an emergency surgical procedure used to drain fluid, blood, or air from the pleural space, restoring negative pressure that enables the lung to reinflate.

The chest tube is typically positioned in the fourth intercostal space.

Chest tubes are used to treat:

- Chylothorax: Lymphatic fluid accumulates in the pleural cavity.
- Empyema: Pus accumulates in the pleural cavity.
- Hemothorax: Blood accumulates in the pleural cavity.
- Pleural effusion: Fluid accumulates in the pleural cavity.
- Pneumothorax: Air accumulates in the pleural cavity.

The chest tube is connected to a water-seal chamber. The water rises on inspiration and decreases on expiration. If the patient is on an automatic ventilator providing positive pressure, then water rises on expiration and decreases on inspiration.

Fluid is collected in a collection chamber. Document the amount of drainage and the type of drainage. Drainage should not exceed 200 ml per hour. If so, then notify the practitioner because the patient might be bleeding. Empty the collection chamber by double-clamping the chest tube close to the insertion site and then remove the collection chamber. Replace the collection chamber and then remove the clamps.

When using a drainage system:

- Make sure the drainage system is below the patient's chest to prevent backflow into the chest tube.
- Do not clamp the chest tube for more than 1 minute, otherwise the patient may experience a tension pneumothorax.
- Monitor the patient's vital signs and respiration for signs of respiratory distress.
- Monitor for chest tube leaks. Bubbles in the water-seal chamber indicate a leak between the patient and the drainage system. Bubbles should stop once the site of the leak is found.
- Tighten and seal loose connections. If the bubbles continue, begin clamping the chest tube.
- Clamp the chest close to the patient. If the bubbles continue, the leak is at the insertion site or inside the patient. Notify the practitioner.
- Clamp the chest farther away from the patient until the bubbles stop. If the bubbles stop, there is a leak in the tube. Notify the practitioner.
- Clamp the chest close to the drainage device. If the bubbles continue, the drainage device needs to be replaced.

4.19.8 Oropharyngeal suctioning

- Administer 100% oxygen before suctioning.
- Measure the catheter before suctioning. The suctioning catheter should be the distance from the patient's tip of the nose to the earlobe.
- Insert the suctioning catheter into the oropharynx beyond the tongue.
- Apply suction by covering the opening in the suctioning catheter.
- Rotate the suctioning catheter.
- Limit suctioning to less than 10 seconds
- Administer 100% oxygen after removing the suctioning catheter.

4.19.9 Endotracheal suctioning

- Use a sterile technique.
- Administer 100% oxygen before suctioning.
- Insert the suctioning catheter into the endotracheal tube:
  - Do not insert the tip of the suctioning catheter beyond the tip of the endotracheal tube.
  - Do not cover the opening in the suctioning catheter when inserting the suctioning catheter into the endotracheal tube.
- Apply suction by covering the opening in the suctioning catheter only when withdrawing the suctioning catheter.
- Rotate the suctioning catheter when suctioning.
- Limit suctioning to less than 10 seconds
- Administer 100% oxygen after removing the suctioning catheter.

Solved Problems

4.1 What may be indicated by a stridor on expiration?

Asthma or bronchitis.

4.2 What may be indicated by rapid respiration and grunting?

Pulmonary edema or pneumonia.

4.3 When may a low oxygen saturation level be considered normal?

Patients with COPD or other lung disorders may have consistently abnormal saturation, which is considered normal for the patient. Saturations lower than the patient's abnormal "normal" saturation level may indicate that the lung disorder has worsened.

4.4 What might be occurring if the patient's blood has an abnormal pH value?

Abnormal values indicate that the patient's body is trying to reestablish the acid-base (alkalosis) balance by having the metabolic system work together with the respiratory system to compensate for the acid-base imbalance.

4.5 What measurement is used to assess the first sign of difficulty breathing?

End-tidal carbon dioxide monitoring.

4.6 What might be indicated if the patient has frothy pink sputum?

May indicate pulmonary edema.

4.7 What might be indicated if the patient has milky sputum?

May indicate a nonbacterial infection.

4.8 What are the two common reasons for a chest x-ray?

- To determine whether fluid, foreign bodies, tumors, scarring, or infiltrate are in the lungs.
- To compare the current chest x-ray to previous chest x-rays to assess changes that may indicate whether the disorder is getting better or has worsened.

4.9 What is the purpose of a ventilation perfusion scan?

A ventilation perfusion scan assesses the respiratory system's ventilation capacity and perfusion capacity and is used as a less risky alternative to the pulmonary angiograph when evaluating pulmonary function. This test is done to determine whether there is abnormal blood flow or a blood clot in the lungs.

4.10 Why is a pulmonary angiograph risky?

A pulmonary angiograph has a higher risk than the ventilation perfusion scan because a catheter is inserted through the heart chambers into the pulmonary artery. This procedure may cause ventricular arrhythmias.

4.11 When might a prescriber order anticholinergic medication?

Emphysema and chronic bronchitis.

4.12 When would a prescriber order benzodiazepines for a respiratory patient?

Sedatives (benzodiazepines) are used to reduce anxiety for patients who undergo respiratory tests and for patients who are placed on mechanical ventilators.

4.13 When would a prescriber order neuromuscular blocking medication for a respiratory patient?

Endotracheal intubation, mechanical ventilation.

4.14 What would you expect the arterial blood gas findings to show in a patient who has acute respiratory distress syndrome ?

Arterial blood gases show respiratory acidosis.

4.15 What causes intrinsic asthma?

Nonatopic (intrinsic) asthma is caused by a nonallergic factor such as cold air, humidity, or a respiratory tract infection.

4.16 Why would a prescriber order 3 L of fluids daily for a patient diagnosed with asthma?

Three liters of fluid daily liquefy any secretions.

4.17 Would you expect to see in a chest x-ray of a patient diagnosed with atelectasis?

The chest x-ray would show shadows in the collapsed area.

4.18 Why would chest percussion be ordered for a patient diagnosed with bronchiectasis?

Chest percussion loosens secretions.

4.19 Why would a patient diagnosed with cor pulmonale need to be weighed daily?

Cor pulmonale is right-sided heart failure resulting from chronic obstructive pulmonary disease (COPD). It leads to pulmonary hypertension and enlargement of the right ventricle. A rapid increase in weight may indicate edema, which is a sign of cor pulmonale.

4.20 What may be the cause of decreased breath sounds, increased respiration, increased pulse and dullness on percussion of the lung area?

Pleural effusion.

4.21 What may be indicated when your patient reports sudden chest pain, difficulty breathing with rapid respiration, and tachycardia?

Pulmonary embolism.

4.22 What is the purpose of continuous positive airway pressure (CPAP) therapy?

CPAP is a form of inhalation therapy that mechanically provides positive pressure throughout the respiratory cycle to assist the patient
with ventilation. The result of this therapy is increased functional residual capacity and reduced effort to breathe.

4.23 What does it mean if bubbles appear in a water-seal chamber of a chest tube drainage system?

There is a leak between the patient and the drainage system.

4.24 What should be done before endotracheal suctioning?

Administer 100% oxygen before suctioning.

4.25 When is an elective tracheotomy performed?

An elective tracheotomy is performed if the patient requires extended use of an automatic mechanical ventilator.

Gastrointestinal Critical Care

5.1 Definitions

- Gastrointestinal critical care is necessary when gastrointestinal reserves are insufficient to sustain ingestion, digestion, and fecal elimination, causing the patient to become unstable and requiring mechanical and/or pharmaceutical treatment to supplement gastrointestinal reserves.
- The respiratory system exchanges carbon dioxide attached to hemoglobin in red blood cells with oxygen in the alveoli.
- Decreased gastrointestinal reserves may result in a cascading failure of systems throughout the body.
- The goal of gastrointestinal critical care is to assist the patient's gastrointestinal system to maintain, ingest, and metabolize nutrients, enabling the gastrointestinal system to supply nutrients to cells throughout the body.
- A patient may be admitted to the critical care unit for a condition other than a gastrointestinal condition. However, a cascading failure of systems other than the gastrointestinal system may result in a gastrointestinal crisis.

5.1.1 Gastrointestinal cycle

- Food is ingested by mouth.
- Chewing breaks down food into small pieces, while saliva moistens the food and breaks down starch. The tongue manipulates food and provides a sense of taste.
- Food moves to the pharynx (throat), where (swallowing) moves food to the esophagus. Muscles in the cricopharyngeal sphincter (opening) relax, allowing food to enter the esophagus.
- The esophagus (tube) connects the pharynx to the stomach. Peristalsis in the esophagus moves food to the stomach.
- The stomach's (collapsible pouch) cardiac sphincter (opening) relaxes to allow food to pass from the esophagus into the stomach. As the stomach increases in size, gastrin is released to stimulate movement of the stomach walls (peristalsis) and to cause the secretion of pepsin (breaks down protein), hydrochloric acid (kills microorganisms in food and provides acid environment for digestive enzymes), proteolytic enzymes (break down protein), and the intrinsic factor (needed to absorb vitamin B12).

- Digested food forms chyme (semifluid). The pyloric sphincter (opening) relaxes to allow chyme to move into the small intestine.
- The small intestine is where most digestion occurs and nutrients are absorbed. There are three segments of the small intestine:
  - Duodenum: Connects to the pyloric sphincter.
  - Jejunum: Shortest segment of the small intestine.
  - Ileum: Connects to the large intestine.
- The small intestine contains:
  - Brunner's glands that secrete mucus to assist movement of chyme.
  - Villi and microvilli, fingerlike projections that assist in moving chyme and absorbing nutrients.
  - Villi are separated by crypts of Lieberkühm glands.
  - Plicae circulares are circular folds in the small intestine.
  - Peyer's patches are lymphatic tissues in the small intestine.
- The large intestine connects to the small intestine at the ileocecal pouch. Chyme in the large intestine consists of undigested food called food bolus. As chyme moves through the large intestine, water and electrolytes are removed, leaving solid-soft food residue called feces, which is then eliminated through the anus.
- There are six segments of the large intestine:
  - Cecum: Receives undigested chyme from the small intestine.
  - Ascending colon: This is the segment of the large intestine located on the right side of the abdomen.
  - Transverse colon: This is the segment of the large intestine located across the top of the abdomen.
  - Descending colon: This is the segment of the large intestine located on the left side of the abdomen.
  - Sigmoid colon: This is the segment of the large intestine that connects the descending colon to the rectum.
  - Rectum: This is the segment of the large intestine that connects to the anus.
- Mucosa throughout the gastrointestinal tract lubricates the intestinal walls and also provides an alkaline protection against bacteria and digestive acids.
- Bacteria in the large intestine:
  - Produce flatus to move stool to the rectum.
  - Synthesize vitamin K.
  - Digest cellulose into carbohydrates.
- The liver assists in metabolizing carbohydrates, proteins, and fat.
- The gallbladder stores bile produced by the liver. Bile is released into the common bile duct, which connects the gallbladder to the duodenum, where bile is used to break down fat and causes the intestine to absorb fatty acids and lipids.
- The pancreas secretes digestive enzymes into the pancreatic duct. The pancreatic duct is connected to the common bile duct, enabling pancreatic digestive enzymes to enter the duodenum.

5.1.2 Gastrointestinal assessment

- Be sure to follow the order of the gastrointestinal assessment:
  - Inspection.
  - Auscultation.

- Percussion.
- Palpation.

- The gastrointestinal assessment interview:
  - Ask open-ended questions:
    - Why did you come to the hospital today?
    - What makes you feel that something is wrong?
  - Look for clues for the underlying cause of the gastrointestinal problem.
    - Do you have allergies?
      - What allergies?
      - What allergic reactions do you experience?
    - Have you taken any medications or herbal supplements recently? Medication can cause gastrointestinal problems such as nausea/vomiting and diarrhea/constipation.
      - What medication or herbal supplement have you taken?
      - When did you take them?
    - Have you recently undergone any medical procedure?
      - What medical procedure?
      - When was the medical procedure performed?
    - What have you eaten recently?
      - What did you eat?
      - When did you eat it?
      - Was there an immediate reaction?
    - What happened prior to you noticing this problem?
    - Do you have irregular bowl movements?
      - Describe the frequency and consistency of your bowl movements.
      - Is there blood in your stool?
        - How much blood?
      - Has the appearance of your stool changed?
        - What changes did you notice?
        - When did you first notice the change?
      - Have you recently traveled out of the country?
        - What country?
        - When did you travel?
        - What did you ingest while you were traveling?
        - Did you notice this problem when you were traveling?
        - Did you receive any vaccinations prior to traveling?
  - Follow-up questions help probe further into the presenting gastrointestinal problem.
    - When did this problem start?
    - How long have you had this problem?
    - Can you describe the problem?
    - How badly does the problem bother you?

        - Where do you feel uncomfortable?
        - Is the problem spreading or remaining in one place?
        - Does anything make the problem worse?
        - Does anything make the problem better?
    - Ask about the patient's lifestyle.
        - Do you drink alcohol?
            - How much alcohol do you drink?
            - When did you start drinking alcohol?
            - Have you ever been treated for alcoholism?
        - Do you use recreational drugs or prescription drugs that are not prescribed to you?
            - What drugs?
            - How much do you use?
            - When did you start using drugs?
            - How you ever been treated for drug abuse?
        - Do you use laxatives?
            - How frequently?
            - Are you able to have a bowl movement without using laxatives?
        - What stressors are in your life?
        - What is your occupation?
        - Do you have any dental problems or problems chewing food?
        - Do you have any dietary restrictions?
        - Do you exercise?
        - Do you use tobacco?
        - Have you been diagnosed with any medical condition?
        - What medical condition?
        - Are you being treated for the medical condition?
            - What is your treatment?
            - Who is treating you?
    - Ask about the patient's family history.
        - Does anyone in your family have or has had colon cancer?
        - Does anyone in your family have or has had Crohn's disease?
        - Does anyone in your family have or has had ulcerative colitis?
- Inspect:
    - Eyes:
        - Abnormal: Yellowing of the sclera.
    - Mouth:
        - Odor:
            - Abnormal: Acetone, unusual odor.
    - Jaw:
        - Abnormal: Asymmetrical, swelling.
    - Bite:
        - Abnormal: Overbite or underbite.

- Teeth:
  - Abnormal: Broken, missing.
- Dentures:
  - Abnormal: Existing, proper fitting.
- Gums:
  - Abnormal: Swelling, bleeding, ulceration, and exudate.
- Lips:
  - Abnormal: Swelling, bleeding, ulceration, and exudate.
- Tongue:
  - Abnormal: Swelling, bleeding, and ulceration.
- Pharynx:
  - Abnormal: Lesions, uvular deviation, plaque, exudate, and abnormal tonsils.
- Abdomen:
- Skin:
  - Abnormal: Striate (pink, blue, silvery white), dilated veins, and scars.
- Surface:
  - Abnormal: Asymmetrical, masses, bulges, peristalsis waves, pulsation

- Auscultation:
  - Abdomen:
    - Turn off suction to abdominal tube or nasogastric tube before auscultating the abdomen.
    - Listen for at least 2 minutes in each quadrant (fig. 5.1).

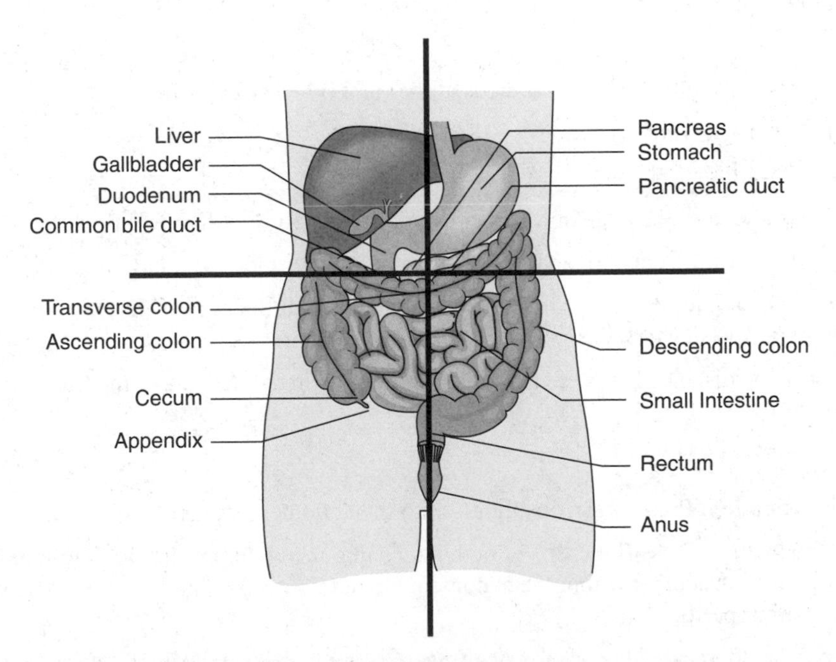

Figure 5.1 The abdomen is divided into four quadrants.

- Use the diaphragm of the stethoscope to listen for bowel sounds.
- Use the bell of the stethoscope to listen for vascular sounds.
- No vascular sounds should be heard in a normal abdomen.

        - Right lower quadrant:
            - Abnormal: Hypoactive bowel sounds, hyperactive bowel sounds.
        - Right upper quadrant:
            - Abnormal: Hypoactive bowel sounds, hyperactive bowel sounds.
        - Left upper quadrant:
            - Abnormal: Hypoactive bowel sounds, hyperactive bowel sounds.
        - Left lower quadrant:
            - Abnormal: Hypoactive bowel sounds, hyperactive bowel sounds.
- Percussion:
    - Abdomen:
        - Do not percuss the abdomen if the patient received a transplanted abdominal organ.
        - Do not percuss the abdomen if you hear a bruit, venous hum, or friction rub over the abdomen.
        - Direct percussion: Strike your finger over the abdomen.
        - Indirect percussion: Rest your finger on the abdomen and strike the finger with the middle finger of your dominant hand.
        - Determine the location and size of abdominal organs.
        - Tympany sound, Clear, hollow sound indicates no organ or hollow organ.
        - Dull sound: Indicates organ or solid mass.
        - Right lower quadrant.
        - Right upper quadrant.
        - Left upper quadrant.
        - Left lower quadrant.
    - Liver:
        - Begin percussing below the umbilicus at the right midclavicular line.
        - Initial sound in tympany.
        - Move upward.
        - Dullness indicates the edge of the liver. Mark this position with a felt-tip pen.
        - Move downward from above the nipple along the right midclavicular line.
        - The sound should be from tympany over the lungs to dullness near the fifth to seventh intercostal space. Mark this position with a felt-tip pen.
        - Measure the distance between these two marks to estimate the size of the liver.
- Palpation:
    - Abdomen:
        - Light palpation: Press fingertips lightly into the abdomen ½ in. to ¾ in.
        - Deep palpation: Press fingertips of both hands into the abdomen 1 ½ in., moving in a circular motion over structures within the abdomen. Do not do deep palpation in patients with suspected aneurysm or perforation.
        - Rebound tenderness: May occur when fingertips are withdrawn from the abdomen.
        - Right lower quadrant.
        - Right upper quadrant.
        - Left upper quadrant.
        - Left lower quadrant.

- Spleen:
    - A normal spleen is not palpable.
    - Ask the patient to stand.
    - Stand on the patient's right side.
    - Place your hand on the back left of the patient's lower rib cage.
    - Ask the patient to take a deep breath.
    - Place your right hand on the patient's abdomen.
    - Press your right hand up to the spleen.
    - Stop palpating if you feel the spleen. Continuing to palpate risks rupturing the spleen.
- Liver:
    - A normal liver is not palpable.
    - Begin at the lower left quadrant.
    - Ask the patient to take and hold a deep breath.
    - Ask the patient to exhale while you move your hands upward to the margin of the liver.

5.1.3 Signs and symptoms

Gastrointestinal assessment in a critical care situation requires the nurse to recognize common signs and symptoms of underlying causes and then prepare for the anticipated treatment that the practitioner is likely to order.

Commonly seen signs and symptoms:

- Rebound tenderness assessment. Rebound tenderness is caused by aggravation of the parietal layer of the peritoneum by stretching or moving.
    - Place patient in the supine position.
    - Flex knees to relax abdominal muscles.
    - Place hand on the right lower quadrant between the umbilicus and the anterior superior iliac spine (McBurney's point).
    - Dip fingers into the abdomen deeply.
    - Release pressure quickly.
    - If pain:
        - Rebound tenderness is present (appendicitis).
        - Do not repeat assessment (risk of rupturing appendix).
- The obturator sign (cope sign) indicates irritation of the obturator internus muscle.
    - Place patient in the supine position.
    - Flex right leg 90 degrees.
    - Hold leg at ankle and above the knee.
    - Rotate leg laterally
    - Rotate leg medially.
    - If pain in hypogastric region:
        - Obturator sign positive (irritation of the obturator muscle).
- The iliopsoas sign (psoas sign) indicates irritation to the iliopsoas group or hip flexors in the abdomen.
    - Place patient in the left side position.

  - Keep legs straight.
  - Exert pressure as the patient raises his or her right leg.
  - Exert pressure as the patient raises his or her left leg.
  - If abdominal pain:
    - Iliopsoas sign positive (irritation of psoas muscle).
- Vomiting.
- Projectile vomiting (hypertrophic pyloric stenosis).
- Diarrhea:
  - If 300 g within 24 hours (virus infection, bacterial infection, or ulcerative colitis).
- Constipation.
- Bleeding:
  - Vomiting red blood (hematemesis) (gums, teeth, esophageal avarices).
  - Vomiting dark blood (coffee ground) (peptic ulcer).
  - Severe retching, coughing blood (Mallory-Weiss syndrome, gastroesophageal laceration syndrome).
  - Low blood pressure.
  - Rapid heart rate.
  - Black tarry stool (melaena) (gastrointestinal bleed).
  - Bloody stool (red) (hemorrhoids).
- Jaundice:
  - Yellowing of sclera (white of the eye).
  - Yellowing of skin.
  - Pale stool.
  - Dark urine.
- Tenderness.
- Abdominal pain:
  - Sudden abdominal pain with rigidity and the pain subsides (perforation).
  - Abdominal rigidity (peritonitis).
  - Acute right upper quadrant pain (acute cholecystitis).
  - Colicky abdominal pain (hernia, adhesion, tumor).
  - Left iliac fossa pain (acute diverticulitis).
  - Right iliac fossa pain (appendicitis).
- Abdominal sounds:
  - Vascular swishing sound (bruits) (arterial obstruction, arterial stenosis).
  - Hypoactive or absent of sound (peritonitis, paralytic ileus).
  - High-pitched rushing with presentment of abdominal cramps (intestinal obstruction).
  - Hyperactive (early intestinal obstruction, hunger, diarrhea).
  - High-pitched tinkling (air or fluid in the intestine).
- Fever.
- Increased white blood cell count (WBC) (leukocytosis) (infection).

5.2 Gastrointestinal Tests

Gastrointestinal tests are designed to assess the effectiveness and the capability of the gastrointestinal system to function. The following are commonly ordered gastrointestinal tests and procedures.

5.2.1 Abdominal x-ray

An abdominal x-ray is commonly called a kidney-ureter-bladder radiography. Besides the kidneys, ureter, and bladder, the x-ray also creates an image of other structures within the abdomen. At least two images are captured: one lying down and the other standing.

- Dense structures, such as bone, block x-ray particles, causing those structures to appear white.
- Less dense structures, such as fat, block some x-ray particles, causing those structures to appear gray. Air does not block x-ray particles; it appears dark. An x-ray image cannot differentiate between fluid and air.
- Common reasons the practitioner orders an abdominal x-ray:
  - Intestinal rupture.
  - Lesions.
  - Tumors.
- The abdominal x-ray procedure:
  - Be sure that the patient's spine is stabilized. Immobilize the spine, if necessary.
  - Be sure that the patient is not pregnant.
  - Remove all jewelry in the area because jewelry may appear on the x-ray image.
  - Assessed whether the patient has scars in the abdominal area. If so, note the location of the scar because it may appear on the x-ray image.
  - The patient removes clothes. Provide the patient with a gown.
  - The patient lies down on the x-ray table, and the x-ray plate is positioned below the table.
  - The patient stands in front of the x-ray table, and the x-ray plate is positioned behind the patient.
  - The initial result, called a wet read, provides a relatively superficial assessment of the image.
  - A more thorough reading is taken hours or days later.

5.2.2 Abdominal computed tomography (CT) scan

An abdominal CT scan provides a three-dimensional image of the abdomen using x-rays. It enables the practitioner to visualize normal and abnormal structures within the abdomen. CT can be performed with or without a contrast agent. A contrast agent is iodine based and enhances images of blood vessels and less dense areas of the brain and spine.

- Common reasons the practitioner orders an abdominal CT scan:
  - Inflammation.
  - Tumor.
  - Occult malignancy.
  - Cysts.
  - Pseudocysts.
  - Blood clots.

  - Abscesses.
  - To differentiate between nonobstructive and obstructive jaundice.
  - Pancreatitis.
- The CT scan procedure:
- Assessed whether the patient is allergic to iodine or shellfish is undergoing a CT scan with contrast. Patients who are allergic to iodine or shellfish have a high likelihood of experiencing an allergic reaction to the contrast agent.
- Assessed whether the patient is claustrophobic. The patient will be placed in an enclosure during the test.
- Assessed whether the patient can remain still for 30 minutes during the CT scan.
- Administer diphenhydramine (Benadryl) and prednisone (Deltasone) before the CT scan to reduce the risk of an allergic reaction to the contrast agent if the contrast agent is ordered.
- Administer the contrast agent through an IV The patient may feel flushed and experience a salty or metallic taste in the mouth.
- The CT scanner encircles the patient for up to 30 minutes.
- Explain to the patient that the contrast material typically discolors the urine for up to 24 hours after the CT scan. The patient should increase fluid intake after the CT scan to flush the contrast agent from the patient's body if the contrast agent is used for the CT scan.

5.2.3 Gastrointestinal magnetic resonance imaging (MRI)

A gastrointestinal system MRI provides a three-dimensional view of the gastrointestinal system using radio waves, a strong magnet, and a computer. An MRI is particularly used to assess fluid-filled soft tissue and to identify tumors from other structures within the gastrointestinal system.

- The gastrointestinal MRI procedure:
  - The patient may need to be NPO (nothing by mouth) for up to 12 hours before the test depending on the site of the MRI.
  - All metal must be removed from the patient.
  - No metal must enter the room containing the MRI scanner. The MRI scanner's magnet is always activated.
  - Assess whether the patient is claustrophobic. If so, ask the healthcare provider whether an open MRI scanner should be used for the test or whether the patient should be sedated before the scan begins.
  - The gastrointestinal MRI scan takes about 30 minutes.
  - The gastrointestinal MRI scan is noninvasive. The patient will not feel any discomfort.

5.2.4 Upper gastrointestinal endoscopy

An upper gastrointestinal endoscopy is also referred to as a gastroscopy and is used to visualize the pharynx, esophagus, lower esophageal sphincter, stomach, pyloric sphincter, and duodenum. An upper gastrointestinal endoscopy is performed to diagnose peptic, gastric, or duodenal ulcers and to obtain biopsies and specimens for *Helicobacter pylori* bacteria.

- The patient will be NPO for up to 12 hours before the procedure.
- The patient will sign an informed consent prior to any anesthesia.
- The patient will receive IV conscious sedation during the procedure. Monitor vital signs to determine whether the patient is tolerating the sedation.
- Assess for loss of teeth.

- Remove dentures.
- The back of the throat is anesthetized, preventing the gag reflex.
- A thin, flexible tube (endoscope) is passed through the pharynx, the stomach, and into the upper part of the small intestine.
- The practitioner will observe, photograph, and obtain biopsies and specimens during the procedure as necessary.
- Monitor vital signs during and after the procedure, including oxygen saturation.
- Place the patient flat on his or her side until the sedation wears off.
- Monitor the patient until the gag reflex returns.
- The patient should be NPO until the gag reflex returns.
- Give the patient ice chips and then sips of water after the gag reflex returns. Gradually increase the patient's intake based on the patient's tolerance.
- Assess for laryngospasm, difficulty swallowing, spitting up blood, black tarry stools, pain, and fever. These can be signs of perforation that occurred during the procedure.

5.2.5 Lower gastrointestinal endoscopy

A lower gastrointestinal endoscopy is also referred to as a colonoscopy, and it is used to assess structures and disorders in the lower gastrointestinal tract. The lower gastrointestinal endoscopy procedure requires the lower bowels to be clean prior to the procedure.

- The lower gastrointestinal endoscopy procedure:
    - The patient must sign an informed consent.
    - The patient should have not eaten or ingested liquids for 6 hours before the procedure, if possible. In emergencies, this may not be possible. However, assess the last time the patient ingested food or liquid.
    - The practitioner may want to perform an electrolyte gastric lavage (see 5.2.6 Gastric lavage) prior to the lower gastrointestinal endoscopy to decrease the risk of aspiration.
    - Clean the bowel with a Fleet enema.
    - Record baseline vital signs.
    - The practitioner may administer conscious sedation prior and during the procedure.
    - Administer oxygen per the practitioner's order.
    - Tell the patient to breathe slowly and deeply as the scope is inserted into the patient.
    - Monitor the patient's vital signs during the procedure.
    - Monitor vital signs every 15 minutes for the first hour.
    - Monitor vital signs every 30 minutes for the next hour.
    - Monitor the patient for rectal bleeding (frank and occult).

5.2.6 Spleen-liver scan

A spleen-liver scan is used to identify abnormalities in the liver and spleen. A radioactive marker is infused intravenously into the patient. A normal liver absorbs most of the marker and the rest is absorbed by the spleen. Lack of absorption indicates an abnormal liver or spleen, which is confirmed by other imaging tests.

- The spleen-liver scan procedure is:
    - Insert an IV line into the patient.

- Instill the radioactive marker.
- Place the patient in the spleen-liver scan.
- Monitor for adverse reactions from the radioactive marker, and report adverse reactions to the practitioner:
  - Difficulty breathing.
  - Fever.
  - Flushed feeling.
  - Light-headedness.

5.2.7 Liver function test

Liver function tests assess hepatic function based on analysis of venous blood obtained through a venipuncture. Normal values for tests are determined by the laboratory that is analyzing the blood sample. Liver function tests include:

- Alanine transaminase (ALT): An enzyme found mainly in liver cells, ALT helps the body metabolize protein. When the liver is damaged, ALT is released in the bloodstream.
- Aspartate transaminase (AST): The enzyme AST plays a role in the metabolism of alanine, an amino acid. An increase in AST levels may indicate liver damage or disease.
- Alkaline phosphatase (ALP): ALP is an enzyme found in high concentrations in the liver and bile ducts, as well as some other tissues. Higher than normal levels of ALP may indicate liver damage or disease.
- Albumin and total protein: Levels of albumin—a protein made by the liver—and total protein show how well the liver is making proteins the body needs to fight infections and to perform other functions. Lower than normal levels may indicate liver damage or disease.
- Bilirubin: Bilirubin is a red-yellow pigment that results from the breakdown of red blood cells. Normally, bilirubin passes through the liver and is excreted in stool. Elevated levels of bilirubin (jaundice) may indicate liver damage or disease.
- Gamma-glutamyl transferase (GGT): This test measures the amount of the enzyme GGT in the blood. Higher than normal levels may indicate liver or bile duct injury.
- Lactate dehydrogenase (LDH): LDH is an enzyme found in many body tissues, including the liver. Elevated levels of LDH may indicate liver damage.
- Prothrombin time (PT): This test measures the clotting time of plasma. Increased PT may indicate liver damage.
- Hepatitis panel: Tests for acute viral hepatitis, including hepatitis B surface antigen (HBsAg), anti-hepatitis A virus (HAV), immunoglobulin M (IgM) anti-hepatitis B core, and anti hepatitis C virus (HCV). Tests for chronic hepatitis include HBsAg and anti-HCV. HAV is confirmed by detecting an IgM antibody to HAV (IgM anti-HAV); hepatitis B virus (HBV) by HBsAg and IgM anti-HBC (when HBeAg is detected, patient is highly infectious); HCV by enzyme-linked immunosorbent assay II (ELISA-II) and recombinant immunoblot assay-2 (RIBA-2); hepatitis delta virus (HDV) by anti-HDV and serologic markers for HBV. For hepatitis E virus (HEV), only research-based tests are available at this time.

5.2.8 Fecal test

A fecal test is used to assess gastrointestinal problems. A fecal sample is taken and sent to the laboratory for analysis. The laboratory results might indicate gastrointestinal abnormalities. Common findings include:

- Hard solid stool: Constipation related to medication or diet.
- Loose stool: Diarrhea related to viral infection or spastic bowel disorder.

- Pasty stool: High fat content related to pancreatic disorder or intestinal malabsorption disorder.
- Greasy stool: High fat content related to pancreatic disorder or intestinal malabsorption disorder.
- Yellow stool: Prolonged diarrhea.
- Green stool: Prolonged diarrhea.
- Black stool: Gastrointestinal bleed, iron supplement ingested.
- Red stool: Rectal bleeding related to hemorrhoids or side effect of drugs or foods.
- White stool: Blockage of hepatic or gallbladder duct or cancer.
- Mucus-containing stool: Bacterial infection.
- Pus-containing stool: Colitis.

5.3 Gastrointestinal Medications

Six categories of medication are commonly used in gastrointestinal critical care. These are antacids, antiemetics, histamine-2 receptor antagonists, proton pump inhibitors, ammonia detoxicants, and antidiuretic hormone. Antacid, histamine-2 receptor antagonists, and proton pump inhibitors reduce acidity in the stomach. Antiemetics prevent nausea. Ammonia detoxicants assist in removing ammonia from blood. Antidiuretic hormone reduces gastrointestinal bleeding.

5.3.1 Antacids

Antacids are medication that increases the pH level in the stomach resulting in decrease stomach acidity.

- Use: Indigestion, heartburn, peptic ulcer disorders.
- Medications:
  - Aluminum hydroxide (Alu-Cap).
  - Aluminum hydroxide and magnesium hydroxide (Maalox).
  - Calcium carbonate (Caltrate).
- Considerations:
  - Wait 2 hours before administering other medications.
  - Not recommended for patients with renal disorders.
- Adverse effects:
  - Nausea/vomiting (calcium carbonate [Caltrate]).
  - Intestinal obstructions (aluminum hydroxide [Alu-Cap]).
  - Constipation (aluminum hydroxide [Alu-Cap]).
  - Diarrhea (aluminum hydroxide and magnesium hydroxide [Maalox]).
  - Hypermagnesemia (aluminum hydroxide and magnesium hydroxide [Maalox]).

5.3.2 Antiemetics

Antiemetics are medications used to treat nausea and vomiting and as adjunct therapy for chemotherapy treatment and post-surgery.

- Use: Prevent nausea/vomiting, increase emptying of the stomach (metoclopramide [Reglan]).
- Medications:
  - Ondansetron (Zofran).

- Dolasetron (Anzemet).
- Metoclopramide (Reglan).

- Considerations:
  - Monitor vital signs.
  - Monitor for extrapyramidal effect (metoclopramide [Reglan]).
  - May cause abnormal liver test results.
- Adverse effects:
  - Arrhythmias.
  - Pruritus.
  - Diarrhea.
  - Seizures (metoclopramide [Reglan]).
  - Restlessness (metoclopramide [Reglan]).
  - Hypertension (metoclopramide [Reglan]).
  - Depression (metoclopramide [Reglan]).

5.3.3 Histamine-2 receptor antagonists

Histamine-2 receptor antagonists are medications that block the action of histamine on the parietal cells in the stomach, reducing the production of acid.

- Use: Treatment of duodenal and gastric ulcers, Zollinger-Ellison syndrome (increased gastrin), gastroesophageal reflux disease (GERD).
- Medications:
  - Famotidine (Pepcid).
  - Ranitidine (Zantac).
- Considerations:
  - Monitor renal function
  - Monitor liver function
  - Give other oral medications 1 hour after administering histamine-2 receptor antagonists.
- Adverse effects:
  - Diarrhea.
  - Constipation.
  - Headache.
  - Palpitations.
  - Blurred vision.
  - Malaise.
  - Leukopenia (decreased WBC).
  - Jaundice.
  - Depression.
  - Confusion.

5.3.4 Proton pump inhibitors

Proton pump inhibitors are medications that block the action of the gastric proton pump of the parietal cells in the stomach, resulting in reduced gastric acid secretion.

- Use: Treatment of duodenal and gastric ulcers, Zollinger-Ellison syndrome (increased gastrin), GERD.
- Medications:
  - Omeprazole (Prilosec).
  - Lansoprazole (Prevacid).
  - Pantoprazole (Protronix).
- Considerations:
  - Monitor liver function.
  - Monitor blood glucose.
- Adverse effects:
  - Hyperglycemia.
  - Constipation.
  - Diarrhea.
  - Dizziness.

5.3.5 Ammonia detoxicant

Ammonia detoxicants are medications used to decrease the ammonia in blood.

- Use: Ammonia detoxification.
- Medication:
  - Lactulose (Chronulac).
- Considerations:
  - Antibiotics may decrease the effectiveness of the medication.
  - Monitor blood ammonia levels.
- Adverse effects:
  - Flatulence.
  - Diarrhea.
  - Abdominal cramps.

5.3.6 Antidiuretic hormone

Antidiuretic hormone is used to decrease bleeding.

- Use: Treating gastrointestinal hemorrhage.
- Medication:
  - Vasopressin (Pitressin).

- Considerations:
  - Monitor intake and output.
  - Monitor cardiac rhythm.
  - Do not use with patients who are diagnosed with chronic nephritis.
  - Monitor water intoxication.
- Adverse effects:
  - Arrhythmias.
  - Bronchospasms.
  - Cardiac arrest.
  - Angina.
  - Small bowel infarction.

5.4 Appendicitis

An obstruction in the vermiform appendix leads to secretion of fluid by the mucosal lining of the appendix, an increase in pressure and decrease in blood flow to the appendix, resulting in gangrene and possibly perforation (rupture) within 36 to 48 hours.

5.4.1 Signs and symptoms

- Guarding of the abdomen.
- Abdominal pain from periumbical to right lower quadrant.
- Abdominal rigidity.
- Rebound pain.
- Right lower quadrant abdominal pain that decreases with right hip flexion indicates perforation.
- Loss of appetite.
- Fever.
- Nausea and vomiting.

5.4.2 Medical tests

- Ultrasound shows enlarged appendix.
- CT scan shows enlarged appendix.
- Blood test:
  - Increased WBC.

5.4.3 Treatment

- Appendectomy.
- Administer:

  - Analgesics for pain.
    - Meperidine.
  - Antibiotics.

5.4.4 Intervention

- NPO.
- Monitor vital signs.
- Monitor intake and output.
- Monitor bowel sounds.
- Assess pain level.
- Instruct the patient:
  - The patient can return to a normal lifestyle following treatment.

5.5 Cholecystitis

Cholecystitis is acute or chronic inflammation of the gallbladder related to cholelithiasis (gallstones). Acute cholecystitis occurs when blood flow to the gallbladder decreases, usually from a blocked cystic duct by a gallstone, leading to difficulty filling and emptying the gallbladder. The gallbladder becomes inflamed, bile is retained, and the gallbladder becomes distended. Chronic cholecystitis occurs when there are recurrent episodes of cholecystitis resulting in chronic inflammation of the gallbladder and leading to obstructive jaundice and an increased risk of gangrene and perforation.

5.5.1 Signs and symptoms

- Pain in the upper right quadrant of the abdomen or epigastric area radiating to the right shoulder.
- Positive Murphy's sign (upper right quadrant abdominal pain increases with palpation on inspiration, resulting in the patient being unable to take a deep breath).
- Increased flatulence.
- Increased eructation (belching).
- Clay-colored stool.
- Foamy, dark urine.
- Nausea and vomiting following ingestion of fatty foods.
- Decreased appetite.
- Fever.
- Icterus.
- Pruritis (itching).
- Jaundice.

5.5.2 Medical tests

- Blood test:
  - Increased bilirubin direct (conjugated).

  - Increased bilirubin indirect (unconjugated).
  - Increased WBC.
  - Increased alkaline phosphatase, AST.
  - Increased lactate dehydrogenase (LDH).
- CT scan shows inflammation of the gallbladder or gallstones.
- Ultrasound of gallbladder shows inflammation of the gallbladder or gallstones.
- HIDA (hepatic iminodiacetic acid) scan shows blocked cystic duct.

5.5.3 Treatment

- Aspirate gallstone.
- Surgical removal of gallbladder.
- Laparoscopic cholecystectomy, open cholecystectomy.
- Insert stent into gallbladder if surgery is not an option

Administer:

  - Antiemetics for nausea and vomiting.
    - Prochlorperazine, trimethobenzamide.
  - Replace fat-soluble vitamins.
    - Vitamins A, D, E, K.
  - Analgesics for pain.
    - Meperidine, no morphine.
  - Antibiotics.

5.5.4 Intervention

- Low-fat diet.
- Monitor vital signs.
- Monitor bowel sounds.
- Assess pain level.
- Instruct the patient:
  - Eat a low-fat diet.

5.6 Cirrhosis of the Liver

Cirrhosis of the liver is chronic inflammation of the liver and necrosis of liver tissue leading to fibrosis and nodule formation. This results in blockage of blood vessels and the bile duct, causing increased portal vein pressure, backup of venous blood to the spleen, enlarged liver, enlarged spleen, and decreased liver function. Common causes are chronic alcohol use, hepatitis, fatty liver (steatohepatitis), metabolic disorders (hemachromatosis), or cystic fibrosis.

5.6.1 Signs and symptoms

- Asymptomatic.
- Fatigue.
- Weight loss.
- Ecchymosis (bruises) related to decreased vitamin K absorption.
- Petechiae.
- Muscle cramps.
- Nausea.
- Pruritus (itching).
- Spider veins.
- Peripheral edema.
- Portal hypertension.
- Jaundice.
- Hepatomegaly (enlarged liver).
- Palmar erythema (red palms).
- Impotence.
- Ascites.
- Dyspnea.
- Glossitis (inflammation of the tongue).
- Encephalopathy (asterixis, tremors, delirium, drowsiness, dysarthria, coma).

5.6.2 Medical tests

- Blood test:
  - Increased:
    - AST.
    - ALT.
    - LDH.
    - Bilirubin direct (conjugated).
    - Indirect (unconjugated).
    - Mean corpuscular volume (MCV).
    - Mean corpuscular hemoglobin (MCH).
    - Ammonia.
    - PT.
  - Decreased:
    - Protein.
    - Albumin.
    - WBC.
    - Platelet count.

- Urine analysis:
  - Increased bilirubin.
- Fecal analysis:
  - Decreased urobilinogen.
- X-ray shows hepatomegaly.
- CT scan shows hepatomegaly and ascites.
- Ultrasound shows hepatomegaly, ascites, and portal vein blood flow.
- Esophagogastroduodenoscopy (EGD) shows esophageal varices.
- Liver biopsy shows fibrosis and regenerative nodules and is the gold standard for the diagnosis.

5.6.3 Treatment

- Paracentesis to remove ascitic fluid.
  - Insert shunt to drain ascitic fluid and divert blood flow.
- Gastric lavage.
- Esophagogastgric balloon tamponade to control esophageal varices bleeding.
- Sclerotherapy to control esophageal variceal bleeding.
- Liver transplant.
- Administer:
  - Vitamins.
    - Folate acid, thiamine, multivitamin.
  - Diuretics to excrete fluids.
    - Furosemide, spironolactone.
  - Lactulose to remove ammonia.
  - Antibiotics to kill flora that produces ammonia.
    - Neomycin sulfate, metronidazole.

5.6.4 Intervention

- Elevate head of bed 30 degrees or greater.
- Elevate feet.
- Monitor for signs of bleeding.
- Monitor for mental status.
- Restrict fluid intake.
- Monitor intake and output.
- Monitor vital signs.
- Check weight daily.
- Measure abdominal girth.
- Monitor electrolytes for imbalance.
- Monitor PT, partial thromboplastin time (PTT), international normalized ratio (INR).
- Monitor for peripheral edema.

- Monitor heart and lung sounds for excess fluid.
- Instruct the patient:
  - Low-sodium diet.
  - No alcohol.

5.7 Crohn's Disease

Crohn's disease is an inflammatory bowel disease that has periods of inflammation of the gastrointestinal GI tract commonly affecting the intestine (terminal ileum and ascending colon) resulting in transmural inflammation (below the superficial mucosal layer), leading to strictures and fistulas.

5.7.1 Signs and symptoms

- Nonbloody diarrhea.
- Fatigue.
- Weight loss.
- Postprandial (bloating after meals).
- Borborygmi (loud, frequent bowel sounds).
- Abdominal cramping.
- Pain in the right lower quadrant of the abdomen.
- Fever.
- Abdominal mass.
- Fistula formation.
- Vomiting.
- Abscesses.

5.7.2 Medical tests

- Blood test:
  - Decreased red blood cells (RBCs).
  - Decreased albumin.
  - Increased erythrocyte sedimentation rate (during exacerbations).
  - Decreased electrolytes.
- CT scan shows thickening of bowel and abscess formation.
- Barium x-ray shows fistula formation, stricture formation.

5.7.3 Treatment

Surgical repair of stricture and fistulas.

- Administer:
  - Vitamins.
    - B12, folic acid.

- Aminosalicylates.
  - Mesalamine, sulfasalazine, olsalazine, balsalazide.
- Glucocorticoids.
  - Hydrocortisone, budesonide.
- Purine.
  - Azathioprine, 6-mercaptopurine.
- Methotrexate.
- Antidiarrheal medications.
  - Diphenoxylate hydrochloride and atropine sulfate.

5.7.4 Intervention

- Dietary restrictions.
- Monitor intake and output.
- Monitor vital signs.
- Instruct the patient:
  - Proper skin care if bowel-skin fistula.
  - Importance of dietary restrictions.
  - Importance of nutritional supplements.

5.8 Diverticulitis

Diverticulitis is a digestive disease particularly found in the large intestine in which undigested food becomes trapped in outpouches (diverticula) along the intestinal track, commonly in the large intestine. This leads to bacterial growth resulting in inflammation of the intestine and risk for bleeding, intestinal perforation, and formation of a fistula within the abdomen.

5.8.1 Signs and symptoms

- Asymptomatic.
- Bloating.
- Rectal bleeding.
- Change in bowel habits.
- Abdominal pain (most common symptom).
- Fever.
- Nausea.
- Vomiting.
- Lower left quadrant pain.
- Fever.

- High WBC (leukocytosis).
- Diarrhea.
- Constipation.

5.8.2 Medical tests

- Blood test:
  - Increased WBC.
- CT scan shows thickening intestinal wall.
- Barium enema shows diverticula (not performed during acute inflammation, when there is a risk of perforation).
- Colonoscopy shows diverticula (not performed during acute inflammation, when there is a risk of perforation).

5.8.3 Treatment

- Surgical repair of intestine.
- Administer:
  - Antibiotics.
    - Ciprofloxacin, metronidazole, trimethoprim-sulfamethoxazole.

5.8.4 Intervention

- NPO to rest bowel.
- Monitor vital signs.
- Monitor intake and output.
- Assess abdomen for bowel sounds and distention.
- Instruct the patient:
  - High-fiber diet when asymptomatic.
  - Low-residue diet during acute during acute inflammation.
  - No lifting during acute inflammation.
  - No laxatives.
  - No enemas.

5.9 Gastroenteritis

Inflammation of the gastric/intestinal mucosa commonly caused by a viral (common), bacterial, parasitic, or protozoal infection or due to an allergic response of toxin exposure.

5.9.1 Signs and symptoms

- Diarrhea.
- Abdominal pain.
- Nausea and vomiting.
- Fever.
- Malaise.
- Headache.
- Dehydration.
- Abdominal distention.

5.9.2 Medical tests

- Blood test:
    - Increased blood urea nitrogen (BUN).
    - Increased creatinine.
    - Electrolyte imbalance.
    - Increased eosinophil count.
    - Increased WBC.
- Stool sample.
- Positive for parasitic infection.

5.9.3 Treatment

- Administer:
    - IV fluids for dehydration.
    - Antiemetic medication.
        - Prochlorperazine, trimethobenzamide.
    - Antidiarrheal medications.
        - Loperamide, diphenoxylate, kaolin-pectin, bismuth subsalicylate.
    - Antimicrobials.
        - Ciprofloxacin, metronidazole.

5.9.4 Intervention

- Monitor vital signs.
- Monitor intake and output.
- Assess for dehydration.
- Replace fluids.
- Instruct the patient:
    - Vomiting and diarrhea are the mechanisms are that the body uses to remove the infecting microorganism.

5.10 Gastroesophageal Reflux Disease (GERD)

GERD occurs when contents (acid) of the stomach enter into the esophagus. This causes pain (heartburn) because the lining of the esophagus is unprotected. It results in damage to the mucosal layer of the esophagus. Pain worsens after eating and when lying down. Scarring may occur, leading to formation of strictures resulting in difficulty swallowing.

Barrett's esophagus: A premalignant esophageal growth resulting from chronic GERD.

5.10.1 Signs and symptoms

- Sour taste.
- Hoarseness.
- Epigastric burning.
- Burping (eructation).
- Cough.
- Nausea.
- Bloating.
- Difficulty swallowing (dysphagia).

5.10.2 Medical tests

- Barium x-ray shows reflux.
- Endoscopy shows irritation.
- Esophageal manometry indicates decreased lower esophageal sphincter tone.

5.10.3 Treatment

- Surgery strengthens lower esophageal sphincter tone.
- Administer:
  - Antacids.
    - Maalox, Mylanta, Tums, Gaviscon.
  - Histamine type 2 blockers.
    - Ranitidine, famotidine, nizatidine, cimetidine.
  - Proton pump inhibitors.
    - Omeprazole, esomeprazole, pantoprazole, rabeprazole, lansoprazole.

5.10.4 Intervention

- Monitor vital signs.
- Elevate head of bed.

- Sleep on left side to reduce nighttime GERD.
- Instruct the patient:
  - Eat six small meals daily.
  - No acidic foods (citrus, vinegar, tomato), peppermint, caffeine, alcohol.
  - Do not lie down after eating.
  - No tight clothing at waist.

5.11 Gastrointestinal Bleeding

Bleeding from the upper or lower gastrointestinal track leads to substantial blood loss. Common causes of upper gastrointestinal bleeding are neoplasms, ulcers, Mallory-Weiss tears related to vomiting, and esophageal varices. Common causes of lower gastrointestinal bleeding are ulcerations, polyps, diverticulitis, fissure formation, colon cancer, and hemorrhoids.

5.11.1 Signs and symptoms

- Pallor.
- Lightheadedness.
- Diaphoresis.
- Orthostatic blood pressure.
- Black, tarry stool (melena).
- Red or maroon rectal bleeding (hematochezia).
- Vomiting maroon, coffee-ground blood (hematemesis).
- Nausea.
- Tachycardia.

5.11.2 Medical tests

- Fecal occult blood test positive.
- Colonoscopy shows site of bleeding.
- Arteriography shows site of bleeding.
- Endoscopy to assess the esophagus.
- Blood test:
  - Decreased hemoglobin.
  - Decreased hematocrit.
  - Decreased RBCs.

5.11.3 Treatment

- Endoscopy to stop bleeding.
- Tamponade with Blakemore-Sengstaken tube for esophageal varices.

- Administer:
  - Isotonic IV fluids.
  - Normal saline.
  - Transfuse packed RBCs.
  - Fresh frozen plasma.
  - Albumin,

5.11.4 Intervention

- Monitor vital signs.
- Monitor intake and output.
- Maintain large-bore IV (16-18 gauge) access.
- Instruct the patient:
  - Treatment will stop the bleeding.

5.12 Gastritis

Gastritis is the inflammation of the stomach lining, leading to malnutrition, gastric cancer, or lymphoma. There are two types of gastritis:

- Erosive gastritis: Caused by stress or medication such as nonsteroidal anti-inflammatory drugs (NSAIDs).
- Atrophic gastritis: Caused by *H. pylori* bacteria, pernicious anemia, and alcohol use.

5.12.1 Signs and symptoms

- Vomiting maroon, coffee-ground blood (hematemesis).
- Nausea.
- Black, tarry stool (melena).
- Epigastric tenderness.
- Anorexia.
- Anemia.
- Abdominal bloating.
- Abdominal pain.

5.12.2 Medical tests

- Endoscopy shows inflammation.
- Gastroscopy.
- Fecal occult blood test positive.

- Blood test:
  - Decreased hemoglobin.
  - Decreased hematocrit.
  - Decreased RBC.
  - *H. pylori* positive.

5.12.3 Treatment

- Administer:
  - Antacids.
    - Maalox, Mylanta, Tums, Gaviscon.
  - Sucralfate.
  - Histamine-2 blockers.
    - Ranitidine, famotidine, nizatidine, cimetidine.
  - Proton pump inhibitors.
    - Omeprazole, esomeprazole, pantoprazole, rabeprazole, lansoprazole.

5.12.4 Intervention

- Monitor stool for occult blood.
- Monitor vital signs.
- Monitor intake and output.
- Instruct the patient:
  - No alcohol, caffeine, or acidic foods.
  - No NSAIDs.
  - No smoking.

5.13 Hepatitis

Hepatitis is inflammation of the liver, commonly caused by a viral infection or exposure to drugs and toxins. Types of hepatitis:

- Hepatitis A: Transmitted orally and related to contaminated water or poor sanitation. Can be prevented by vaccine.
- Hepatitis B: Transmitted percutaneously and related to sexual contact, IV drug use, mother-to-neonate transmission, and transfusion. Can be prevented by vaccine.
- Hepatitis C: Transmitted percutaneously and related to IV drug use and sexual contact (less common). No vaccine available.
- Hepatitis D: Transmitted percutaneously. Needs hepatitis B to spread. No vaccine available.
- Hepatitis E: Transmitted orally and related to water contamination. Acute. No vaccine available.
- Hepatitis G: Transmitted percutaneously. Associated with chronic infection but not liver disease.

5.13.1 Signs and symptoms

- Acute hepatitis:
  - Tenderness in right upper quadrant of abdomen.
  - Jaundice.
  - Dark urine.
  - Hepatomegaly.
  - Diarrhea.
  - Constipation.
  - Malaise.
  - Nausea and vomiting.
  - Low-grade fever.
  - Anorexia.
  - Muscle/joint pain.
- Chronic hepatitis:
  - Asymptomatic.
  - Bleeding.
  - Enlarged spleen.
  - Cirrhosis.
  - Ascites.
  - Esophageal varices.
  - Encephalopathy.
  - Same as acute hepatitis.

5.13.2 Medical tests

- Liver biopsy shows hepatocellular necrosis.
- Urine analysis shows protein and bilirubin.
- Blood test:
  - Increased AST.
  - Increased ALT.
  - WBC count normal to low.
  - IgG anti-HBc shows convalescent or past infection with hepatitis B.
  - IgM anti-HBc shows acute or recent infection with hepatitis B.
  - HBsAg shows current or past infection with hepatitis B.
  - IgM anti-HAV shows acute or early convalescent stage of hepatitis A.
  - IgG anti-HAV shows later convalescent stage of hepatitis A.
  - HBeAg shows current viral replication of hepatitis B and infectivity.
  - HBV DNA shows presence of hepatitis B DNA (most sensitive).
  - Anti-HCV shows hepatitis C infection.

  - HCV RNA shows hepatitis C infection.
  - Anti-HDV shows hepatitis D infection.

5.13.3 Treatment

- Liver transplantation.
- Administer:
  - Interferon or lamivudine (chronic hepatitis B).
  - Interferon and ribavirin (hepatitis C).
  - Prednisone (autoimmune hepatitis).

5.13.4 Intervention

- Remove drug or toxin.
- Activity as tolerated.
- Monitor intake and output.
- Monitor vital signs.
- Schedule rest periods (acute).
- Instruct the patient:
  - No smoking (including secondhand smoke).
  - High-calorie diet.
  - Eat more at breakfast (best tolerated meal).
  - No medications metabolized in the liver (acetaminophen).
  - No alcohol.

5.14 Hiatal Hernia (Diaphragmatic Hernia)

Protrusion of a portion of the stomach through the diaphragm into the chest near the esophagus. There are two types of hiatal hernia:

- Sliding hiatal hernia: The upper portion of the stomach and the lower esophageal sphincter moves throughout the diaphragm. GERD.
- Rolling hiatal hernia: The upper portion of the stomach but not the lower esophageal sphincter moves throughout the diaphragm. No GERD.

5.14.1 Signs and symptoms

- Rolling hernia:
  - Chest pain.
  - Palpitations.

    - Fullness after eating.
    - Difficulty breathing after eating.
- Sliding hernia:
    - Chest pain.
    - Palpitations.
    - Heartburn.
    - Eructation (burping).
    - Dysphagia (difficulty swallowing).

5.14.2 Medical tests

- Barium x-ray shows hiatal hernia.

5.14.3 Treatment

- Surgical repair.
- Administer:
    - Antacids for pain.
        - Maalox, Mylanta, Tums, Gaviscon.
    - Histamine type 2 blockers.
        - Ranitidine, nizatidine, famotidine, cimetidine.
    - Proton pump inhibitors to reduce the production of acid.
        - Omeprazole, esomeprazole, pantoprazole, rabeprazole, lansoprazole.

5.14.4 Intervention

- Elevate head of bed.
- Monitor vital signs.
- Instruct the patient:
    - Eat small, frequent meals.
    - No lying down after eating.
    - No tight clothes at waist.
    - No acidic foods (citrus, vinegar, tomato), peppermint, caffeine, alcohol.
    - No smoking.

5.15 Intestinal Obstruction and Paralytic Ileus

Motility through the intestine is blocked by a mechanical obstruction such as fecal impaction, tumor, or adhesion or caused by a paralytic ileus such as sepsis, diabetic ketoacidosis, or medication.

5.15.1 Signs and symptoms

- Paralytic ileus.
- Diminished or absent bowel sounds.
- Vomiting.
- Constant abdominal pain.
- Abdominal distention.
- Obstruction.
- Vomiting.
- Constipation.
- High-pitched bowel sounds.
- Abdominal tenderness.
- Abdominal cramping.
- Intermittent or constant abdominal pain.
- Abdominal distention.

5.15.2 Medical tests

- Abdominal x-ray shows small bowel dilation.

5.15.3 Treatment

- Administer:
  - Antiemetics after nasogastric (NG) tube insertion.
    - Prochlorperazine, trimethobenzamide.
  - IV fluid replace.
  - Isotonic solution.

5.15.4 Intervention

- NPO.
- NG tube to suction or to remove stomach contents.
- Parenteral nutrition and vitamin supplements.
- Monitor vital signs.
- Monitor intake and output.
- Assess for abdomen tenderness.
- Assess bowel sounds.
- Instruct the patient:
  - That normal lifestyle will return after intestinal motility is restored.

5.16 Pancreatitis

Inflammation of the pancreas as a result of chronic alcohol use, elevated cholesterol, blockage of the pancreatic duct by gallstones, or surgical or abdominal trauma. There are two types of pancreatitis:

- Acute: Autodigestion of the pancreas by pancreatic enzymes and development of fibrosis. Life threatening and a risk of pleural effusion.
- Chronic: Fibrosis resulting in decreased pancreatic function.

5.16.1 Signs and symptoms

- Cullen's sign (bluish gray discoloration of periumbilical area and abdomen).
- Turner's sign (bluish gray discoloration of flank areas).
- Abdominal pain.
- Acute: Radiates to back or left shoulder.
- Chronic: Gnawing continuous pain.
- Epigastric pain.
- Knee-chest position reduces pain.
- Nausea.
- Vomiting.
- Fatigue.
- Hyperglycemia.
- Ascites.
- Weight loss.
- Fever.
- Jaundice.

5.16.2 Medical tests

- CT scan shows inflammation.
- Abdominal ultrasound shows inflammation.
- Blood test:
  - Increased:
    - Amylase.
    - Lipase.
    - WBC.
    - Cholesterol.
    - Glucose.
    - Bilirubin.

5.16.3 Treatment

- Surgical removal of abscess or pseudocyst.
- Administer:
  - No morphine. It causes spasm of the sphincter of Oddi.
  - IV fluids.
  - Total parenteral nutrition.
  - Vitamin supplements.
  - Patient controlled or transdermal analgesia.
  - Insulin (chronic).

5.16.4 Intervention

- NPO (acute).
- NG tube to suction or remove stomach contents if patient is vomiting.
- Monitor intake and output.
- Monitor vital signs.
- Monitor blood glucose.
- Monitor lung sounds for plural effusion.
- Assess abdomen for bowel sounds, tenderness, masses, and ascites.
- Instruct the patient:
  - Schedule rest periods.
  - Take pancreatic enzymes with meals.
  - No alcohol.
  - No caffeine.
  - Bland, low-fat, high-protein, high-calorie diet.
  - Small, frequent meals.
  - Monitor blood glucose.

5.17 Peritonitis

Acute inflammation of the peritoneum (lining of the abdominal cavity), commonly caused by bacterial infection. Life-threatening disease that may lead to septicemia if infection enters the bloodstream.

5.17.1 Signs and symptoms

- Abdominal rebound pain.
- Abdominal distention.
- Rigid abdomen.
- Decreased bowel sounds.

- Fever.
- Tachycardia.
- Nausea.
- Vomiting.
- Decreased urine output.
- Decreased appetite.

5.17.2 Medical tests

- Abdominal x-rays show free air.
- Ultrasound shows underlying cause.
- CT scan shows underlying cause.
- Peritoneal lavage culture and sensitivity to identify microorganism.
- Blood test:
  - Increased WBC.
  - Blood cultures to identify microorganism.

5.17.3 Treatment

- Surgery to correct underlying cause.
- Administer:
  - Broad-spectrum antibiotics.
  - IV fluids.

5.17.4 Intervention

- NPO.
- Elevate head of bed.
- Monitor vital signs.
- Monitor intake and output.
- Get weight daily.
- Instruct the patient:
  - That normal lifestyle will return after inflammation is resolved.

5.18 Peptic Ulcer Disease (PUD)

Erosion of the mucosal layer of the stomach or duodenum, allowing stomach acid to contact epithelial tissues commonly caused by *H. pylori* bacteria or stress. It leads to bleeding, perforation, peritonitis, paralytic ileus, septicemia, shock, ischemia, or ulcerate. There are two types of peptic ulcers:

- Gastric ulcer: Mucosal layer of the stomach is eroded, lessening the curvature of the stomach.
- Duodenal ulcer: Mucosal layer of the duodenal is eroded, resulting in penetration to the muscular layer.

5.18.1 Signs and symptoms

- Bloating.
- Loss of appetite.
- Epigastric pain.
- Worse after eating (gastric ulcer).
- Worse 1 to 3 hours after eating or at night (duodenal ulcer).
- Weight change:
    - Loss (gastric ulcer).
    - Gain (duodenal ulcer).
- Bleeding.
- Vomiting red, maroon bloody (hematemesis) (gastric ulcer).
- Coffee-ground emesis (gastric ulcer).
- Tarry stool (melena) (duodenal ulcer).
- Perforation.
- Sudden, sharp pain relieved with knee-chest position.
- Tender, rigid abdomen.
- Hypovolemic shock.

5.18.2 Medical tests

- Blood test:
    - Decreased RBC.
    - Decreased hemoglobin.
    - Decreased hematocrit.
- Barium x-ray shows ulceration.
- Abdominal x-ray shows free air if perforated.
- Endoscopy shows ulceration.
- Stool occult blood positive.
- *H. pylori* test positive.

5.18.3 Treatment

- Administer :
    - Antacids.
        - Maalox, Mylanta, Amphojel.
    - Histamine-2 blockers.
        - Famotidine, ranitidine, nizatidine.
    - Proton pump inhibitors.
        - Omeprazole, lansoprazole, rabeprazole, esomeprazole, pantoprazole.

- Mucosal barrier fortifiers.
  - Sucralfate.
- Prostaglandin analogue.
  - Misoprostol.
- *H. pylori* medication.
  - Proton pump inhibitor plus clarithromycin plus amoxicillin, proton pump inhibitor plus metronidazole plus clarithromycin, Bismuth subsalicylate plus metronidazole plus tetracycline.

5.18.4 Intervention

- Monitor intake and output.
- Monitor vital signs.
- Monitor bowel sounds.
- Monitor abdomen tenderness, rigidity.
- Instruct the patient:
  - Eat small, frequent meals.
  - No caffeine.
  - No alcohol.
  - No acidic foods.
  - No NSAIDs medication.
  - No smoking.

5.19 Ulcerative Colitis

Inflammation of the mucosal layer of the large intestine, beginning with the colon and rectum and spreading to adjacent tissues. This leads to ulcerations and abscess formation. Periods of exacerbations and remissions. Symptoms increase with each exacerbation. Risk for malabsorption, toxic megacolon, and perforation.

5.19.1 Signs and symptoms

- Chronic bloody diarrhea with pus.
- Tenesmus (spasms of the anal sphincter).
- Weight loss.
- Abdominal pain.

5.19.2 Medical tests

- Double-contrast barium x-ray shows ulceration and inflammation.
- Endoscopy to assess ulceration and inflammation.

- Colonoscopy show ulcerations and bleeding.
- Stool culture.
- Renal function tests.
- Liver function tests.
- Electrolyte test.
- Complete blood test:
  - Decreased RBC.
  - Decreased hemoglobin.
  - Decreased hematocrit.
  - Increased erythrocyte sedimentation rate.

5.19.3 Treatment

- Surgical resection of affected area.
- Administer:
  - Antidiarrheal medications.
    - Loperamide, diphenoxylate hydrochloride and atropine.
  - Salicylate medications.
    - Sulfasalazine, mesalamine, olsalazine, balsalazide.
  - Corticosteroids during exacerbations.
    - Prednisone, hydrocortisone.
  - Anticholinergics.
    - Dicyclomine.

5.19.4 Intervention

- NPO during exacerbations.
- Monitor intake and output.
- Monitor stool output.
- Get weight daily.
- Monitor for signs of toxic megacolon (distended, tender abdomen, fever, distended colon).
- Instruct the patient:
  - Keep stool diary to identify irritating foods.
  - Low-fiber, high-protein, high-calorie diet.
  - Perianal skin care area.
  - Sitz bath.
  - A & D ointment.
  - Apply barrier cream to skin.
  - Witch hazel to soothe sensitive skin.
  - No fragranced products.

5.20 Abdominal Trauma

Abdominal trauma is an injury to the abdominal area, commonly from a motor vehicle accident or a penetrating wound. There are two classifications of abdominal trauma:

- Blunt abdominal trauma: Blunt abdominal trauma is an injury caused by pressure applied to the abdominal area from a motor vehicle accident, fall, or fight with another person or animal. It results in damage to organs within the abdomen (liver, spleen, intestine, pancreas, stomach, or diaphragm) and to the peritoneum.
- Penetrating abdominal trauma: Penetrating abdominal trauma is an injury caused by an object (bullet, knife) puncturing the abdominal area, resulting in lacerations and focused injury to abdominal organs (liver, spleen, intestine, pancreas, stomach, or diaphragm).

5.20.1 Signs and symptoms

- Cullen's signs (discoloration in the umbilicus area).
- Penetrating wound site.
- Abdominal tenderness.
- Abdominal rigidity.
- Abdominal pain.
- Grey-Turner's sign (discoloration along the side).
- Abnormal bowel sounds.
- Pain in right shoulder (referral pain indicating liver injury).
- Kehr's sign (left shoulder pain related to injury to diaphragm).
- The patient guards the abdominal area.

5.20.2 Medical tests

- Abdominal x-rays show injuries.
- Ultrasound show injuries.
- CT scan show injuries
- Blood test:
    - Complete blood count.
    - Blood type and crossmatch.
    - Coagulation test.
    - Electrolyte test.

5.20.3 Treatment

- Stabilize the patient (airway, breathing, circulation).
- Assess for trauma signs.
- Assess for internal bleeding (see 5.11 Gastrointestinal Bleeding).

- Assess neurologic status.
- Monitor vital signs.
- Insert two large-bore IV lines.
- Prepare the patient for surgery, if necessary.
- Oxygen per practitioner's order.
- Administer:
  - Fluids per practitioner's order to maintain hemodynamic status.
  - Normal saline.
  - Lactated Ringer's solution.
  - Pain medication per practitioner's order once a diagnosis is determined.

5.20.4 Intervention

- NPO.
- Monitor intake and output.
- Monitor vital signs continually.
- Instruct the patient:
  - Keep the patient calm by reassuring the patient.
  - Explain each procedure and why the procedure is being performed.

5.21 Gastrointestinal Procedures

Several commonly performed gastrointestinal procedures are used in critical care situations to ensure that the patient's gastrointestinal tract functions properly.

5.21.1 Nasogastric (NG) intubation

An NG tube is inserted into the patient to remove stomach contents either by bulb syringe or suction in cases of intestinal obstruction, bleeding, or other gastrointestinal difficulties where the stomach content places the patient at risk. The nasogastric tube can also be used for feeding.

NG intubation procedure:

- Ask the patient to sit.
- Measure the length of the NG tube:
  - Hold the tip of the tube at tip of the patient's nose.
  - Extend the tube to the patient's earlobe and hold the tube by the patient's earlobe.
  - Extend the tube from the patient's earlobe to the xiphoid process. This is the length of the NG tube.
  - Mark this length on the tube with tape. The tape is the point where you stop inserting the NG tube.
- Assess the patency of each nostril.
- Lubricate the end of the NG tube.

- Ask the patient to place his chin on his or her chest as you insert the NG tube.
- Insert the NG tube into the patient's patent nostril.
- Ask the patient to swallow as the NG tube advances through the pharynx.
- Check placement of the NG tube:
  - Attach a bulb syringe to the NG tube.
  - Aspirate the stomach contents.
  - Place the stomach contents on a pH test strip. The pH test strip should report less than or equal to 5.

5.21.2 Gastric lavage

Gastric lavage is a procedure used to treat gastric hemorrhage and to treat drug overdoses, depending on the nature of the drug. Irrigating fluid is instilled through an NG tube into the upper gastrointestinal system and the gastric content is aspirated through the NG tube.

The gastric lavage procedure:

- Protect the airway from aspiration. Have suction equipment available.
- Monitor vital signs and oxygen saturation every 5 to 10 minutes.
- Insert a large-bore NG tube (see 5.2.5 Nasogastric [NG] intubation).
- Lower the head of the bed 15 degrees.
- Position the patient on his or her left side.
- Fill a syringe with 50 ml of irrigating solution. The practitioner may order a vasoconstrictor added to the irrigating fluid to increase the irrigation performance.
- Instill the contents of the syringe into the NG tube. Continue until 250 ml of irrigating solution is instilled.
- Wait 30 seconds.
- Withdraw the irrigating solution using the syringe or drain the NG tube into an emesis basin.
- Measure the amount of irrigating solution instilled and the volume of fluid withdrawn. If less fluid is withdrawn, then suspect abdominal distention that may result in vomiting.
- Continuously monitor the patient. There is a risk of vomiting, aspiration, bradycardia, electrolyte imbalance, fluid overload, and metabolic acidosis.

5.21.3 Nasogastric decompression

NG decompression is a process used to aspirate intestinal contents and to assist in resolving an intestinal obstruction using an NG decompression tube. NG decompression is also used to prevent nausea and vomiting and reduce the risk of abdominal distention following gastrointestinal surgery. An NG decompression tube contains a balloon filled with water, air, or mercury located at the end of the tube that is inserted into the patient. The NG decompression tube stimulates peristalsis, enabling passage into the intestine.

There are four commonly used NG decompression tubes:

- Cantor tube: Single lumen. Used for aspiration and to reduce bowel obstruction.
- Dennis tube: Three lumen. Used to decompress the intestines for surgery.
- Harris tube: Single lumen. Used to lavage the intestinal tract.

- Miller-Abbott tube: Two lumens. Used for aspiration and to reduce bowel obstruction.
- The NG decompression procedure:
  - Assess the patency of each nostril for septal deviation.
  - Estimate the length of the tube by measuring from the tip of the nose, around the ear, and down just below the costal margin.
  - Position the patient in an upright position with the neck partially flexed.
  - Lubricate the end of the NG tube.
  - Ask the patient to place his chin on his chest as you insert the NG tube.
  - Insert the NG tube into the patient's patent nostril along the floor of the nose.
  - Advance the tube parallel to the nasal floor until the tube reaches the back of the nasopharynx, where resistance will be encountered.
  - Ask the patient to swallow as the NG tube advances through the pharynx until the estimated length is reached.
  - Confirm placement using an x-ray.
  - Connect to suction per practitioner's order.
  - Continuously monitor the patient. There is a risk of vomiting, aspiration, bradycardia, electrolyte imbalance, fluid overload, and metabolic acidosis.
  - Monitor for NG decompression or tube obstruction. If the NG decompression tube is obstructed:
    - Disconnect NG decompression tube from suction.
    - Irrigate the NG decompression tube with normal saline. Drain the normal saline with gravity flow.
    - Carefully pull the NG decompression tube to remove any kinks in the nasogastric decompression tube.
    - Do not pull the NG decompression tube if:
      - The NG decompression tube was difficult to insert.
      - The NG decompression tube was inserted during surgery.

5.21.4 Paracentesis

Paracentesis is a procedure of aspirating fluid from the peritoneal space to decrease intra-abdominal pressure, treat ascites, and to assess for intra-abdominal bleeding. Aspiration is performed by insertion of a needle or cannula through the abdominal wall into the peritoneal space.

The paracentesis procedure:

- The patient must sign an informed consent.
- The patient's bladder must be emptied prior to the procedure, either through urination or insertion of a indwelling urinary catheter.
- Measure the patient's weight and abdominal area.
- The patient is positioned in the supine position in bed.
- A local anesthetic is administered to the insertion site.
- Place the collection container below the level of the patient.
- The needle or cannula is inserted.
- Raise the head of the bed 45 degrees or ask the patient to sit at side of the bed.
- Fluid drains via gravity from the peritoneal space into the collection container.

- No more than 1500 ml should be aspirated during the procedure.
- Monitor the patient every 15 minutes for adverse side effects. If adverse side effects are noticed, then raise the collection container closer to the level of the needle or cannula and report adverse side effects to the practitioner immediately.
    - Hypovolemic shock.
    - Diaphoresis.
    - Tachycardia.
    - Hypotension.
    - Pallor.
    - Dizziness.
- Apply dry sterile pressure dressing to the site once the needle or cannula is removed from the patient.
- Change the dressing every 15 minutes for the first 60 minutes.
- Change the dressing every 30 minutes for the next 2 hours.
- Change the dressing every 4 hours for the next 24 hours.
- Monitor vital signs.
- Monitor signs of shock and hemorrhage.
- Document the patient's weight and abdominal area following the procedure.
- Send the peritoneal fluid to the laboratory for analysis.

Solved Problems

5.1 What might be suspected with abdominal rigidity?

Peritonitis.

5.2 What might be suspected with sudden abdominal pain with rigidity and the pain subsides?

Perforation.

5.3 What might be suspected with red bloody stool?

Hemorrhoids.

5.4 What might be suspected when a patient diagnosed with sclerosis of the liver vomits red blood?

Esophageal varices.

5.5 What would you suspect if a patient vomits dark blood resembling coffee grounds?

Peptic ulcer.

5.6 What might you suspect if the patient has projectile vomiting?

Hypertrophic pyloric stenosis.

5.7 What would you avoid if you discovered rebound tenderness at McBurney's point?

Do not repeat assessment (risk of rupturing appendix).

5.8 What might you suspect if a patient has greasy stools?

High fat content related to pancreatic disorder or intestinal malabsorption disorder.

5.9 What might you suspect if the patient has mucus in the stool?

Bacterial infection.

5.10 What is the function of antacids?

Antacids are medications that increase the pH level in the stomach, resulting in decreased stomach acidity.

5.11 Why would a practitioner prescribe ondansetron before chemotherapy?

To prevent nausea/vomiting.

5.12 What is an adverse effect of aluminum hydroxide?

Intestinal obstructions, constipation.

5.13 What is the function of histamine-2 receptor antagonists?

Histamine-2 receptor antagonists are medications that block the action of histamine on the parietal cells in the stomach, reducing the production of acid.

5.14 Why is lactulose prescribed?

For ammonia detoxification.

5.15 What medication would you expect a prescriber to order for gastrointestinal hemorrhage?

Vasopressin (Pitressin).

5.16 What would you expect would be decreased in a blood test taken from a patient diagnosed with cirrhosis of the liver?

- Protein.
- Albumin.
- WBC.
- Platelet count.

5.17 What causes gastroenteritis?

A viral (common), bacterial, parasitic, or protozoal infection or an allergic response to toxin exposure.

5.18 What are common causes of lower gastrointestinal bleeds?

Common causes of lower gastrointestinal bleeding are ulcerations, polyps, diverticulitis, fissure formation, colon cancer, and hemorrhoids.

5.19 What are common causes of paralytic ileus and intestinal obstruction?

Mechanical obstruction such as fecal impaction, tumor, or adhesion or paralytic ileus such as sepsis, diabetic ketoacidosis, or medication.

5.20 What might be indicated by a positive Cullen's sign and Turner's sign?

Pancreatitis.

5.21 What might you suspect if the patient has chronic bloody diarrhea containing pus?

Ulcerative colitis.

5.22 Why might a practitioner order nasogastric decompression?

Nasogastric decompression is a process used to aspirate intestinal contents and to assist in resolving an intestinal obstruction using a nasogastric decompression tube. Nasogastric decompression is also used to prevent nausea and vomiting and reduce the risk of abdominal distention following gastrointestinal surgery.

5.23 How would you remove the stomach content of the patient?

A nasogastric tube is inserted into the patient to remove stomach contents either by bulb syringe or suction in cases of intestinal obstruction, bleeding, or other gastrointestinal difficulties where the stomach content places the patient at risk.

5.24 What is a common reason for performing paracentesis?

To treat ascites related to liver failure.

5.25 What is the dressing change protocol following removal of the needle or cannula after paracentesis?

Change the dressing every 15 minutes for the first 60 minutes.

Change the dressing every 30 minutes for the next 2 hours.

Change the dressing every 4 hours for the next 24 hours.

Renal Critical Care

6.1 Definitions

- Renal critical care is necessary when urinary system reserves are insufficient to sustain fluid and electrolyte balance, acid-base balance, blood pressure, detoxification of blood and removal of waste, causing the patient to become unstable and requiring mechanical and/or pharmaceutical treatment to supplement urinary system reserves.
- The respiratory system exchanges carbon dioxide attached to hemoglobin in red blood cells with oxygen in the alveoli.
- Decreased urinary system reserves may result in a cascading failure of systems throughout the body.
- The goal of renal critical care is to assist the patient's renal system in filtering blood and creating urine.
- A patient may be admitted to the critical care unit for a condition other than a renal condition. However, a cascading failure of systems other than the renal system may result in a renal system crisis.

6.1.1 The renal cycle

- The kidneys filter 45 gallons of fluids daily, leading to the formation of urine.
- Urine passes from the kidneys through the ureters to the urinary bladder through peristalsis.
- Urine collects in the urinary bladder, which holds between 300 and 500 ml of urine.
- Leading from the urinary bladder is the urethra. At the end of the urethra is a urethral sphincter, consisting of voluntary muscles, that give the person control over urination.
- Detoxification:
  - Blood flows into the glomerulus, where glomerular filtration occurs. Substances such as protein and red blood cells are filtered and reabsorbed. Other substances are not filtered and are excreted in urine.
  - Clearance: Clearance is complete removal of a substance from the blood within a specific time period.
  - Creatinine clearance: Creatinine clearance is a test that determines how well kidneys are working. Creatine is a byproduct of food metabolism. Creatine is broken down into creatinine and excreted by the kidneys in urine. The amount of creatinine remains steady. Creatinine clearance is a measurement of creatinine in urine.

  - Creatinine blood level: Creatinine blood level is the amount of creatinine in blood. A high level indicates that the kidneys may not be functioning properly.
  - Glomerular filtration rate (GFR): The GFR is the rate at which blood is filtered by the kidneys. The normal rate is 120 ml/min. Creatinine clearance is the most accurate measurement of glomerular filtration.
  - If glomerulus function is diminished, then substances normally reabsorbed (i.e., protein, red blood cells, and glucose) are not reabsorbed and are found in urine.
- Fluid and electrolyte balance:
  - Kidneys maintain fluid and electrolyte balance by reabsorbing fluid and specific electrolytes or excreting fluid and specific electrolytes in urine.
  - Antidiuretic hormone (ADH) secreted by the pituitary gland into blood causes the kidneys to reabsorb fluid, leading to decreased urine production. The amount of ADH in the blood correlates to the volume of urine produced by the kidneys.
  - Aldosterone hormone secreted by the adrenal gland into blood causes the kidneys to reabsorb sodium and water, leading to decreased urine production and decreased sodium levels in urine. Aldosterone also controls potassium levels. An increased aldosterone level in blood leads to the excretion of potassium. The amount of aldosterone in the blood correlates to the volume of urine produced by the kidneys and the amount of sodium and potassium reabsorbed and excreted in urine.
- Red blood cells:
  - When oxygen levels decrease in blood, the kidneys secrete erythropoietin hormone and active vitamin D. Erythropoietin causes bone marrow to increase production of red blood cells. Active vitamin D regulates calcium balance, leading to bone metabolism.
- Acid-base balance:
  - The kidneys maintain the acid-base balance of blood by reabsorbing sodium and bicarbonate, secreting hydrogen, producing ammonia, and causing phosphate salts to become acids.
- Blood pressure:
  - Kidneys secrete renin whenever there seems to be a decrease in extracellular fluid.
  - Renin is transformed into angiotensin I, which is converted to angiotensin II. Angiotensin II increases peripheral vasoconstriction and causes the secretion of aldosterone. Increased aldosterone levels in blood lead to increased reabsorption of water and sodium, resulting in increased blood pressure.

6.1.2 Renal assessment

- Be sure to follow the order of the renal system assessment:
  - Inspection.
  - Auscultation.
  - Percussion.
  - Palpation.
- The renal assessment interview:
  - Look for clues for the underlying cause of the renal problem.
    - Do you have allergies?
    - What allergies?
    - What allergic reactions do you experience?

- Have you taken any medications or herbal supplements recently? Medication can cause renal problems.
  - What medication or herbal supplements do you take?
- Have you recently undergone any medical procedure?
  - What medical procedure?
  - When was the medical procedure performed?
- What happened prior to you noticing this problem?
- What color is your urine?
- Does your urine have an odor?
- Do you have urinary hesitation or burning?
  - Describe the frequency and consistency of your urine.
- Is there blood in your urine?
  - How much blood?
- Have there been changes in the appearance of your urine?
  - What changes did you notice?
  - When did you first notice the change?
- Have you recently traveled out of the country?
  - What country?
  - When did you travel?
  - What did you ingest while you were traveling?
  - Did you notice this problem when you were traveling?
  - Did you receive any vaccinations prior to traveling?

- Follow-up questions help probe further into the presenting renal problem.
  - When did this problem start?
  - How long have you had this problem?
  - Can you describe the problem?
  - How badly does the problem bother you?
  - Where do you feel uncomfortable?
  - Is the problem spreading, or does the problem remain in one place?
  - Does anything make the problem worse?
  - Does anything make the problem better?
- Ask about the patient's lifestyle.
  - Do you drink alcohol?
    - How much alcohol do you drink?
    - When did you start drinking alcohol?
    - Have you ever been treated for alcoholism?
  - Do you use recreational drugs or prescription drugs that are not prescribed to you?
    - What drugs?
    - How much do you use?
    - When did you start using drugs?
    - How you ever been treated for drug abuse?

- What stressors are in your life?
- What is your occupation?
- Have you been diagnosed with any medical condition?
- What medical condition?
  - Are you being treated for the medical condition?
    - What is your treatment?
    - Who is treating you?
- Ask about the patient's family history.

- Inspect:
  - Eyes: Abnormal: Periorbital edema.
  - Jugular vein: Abnormal: Distention.
  - Abdomen: Abnormal: Discoloration, enlarged, distention, asymmetric, veins prominent, striae, bruises, scars, lesions.
  - Urethral meatus: Abnormal: Discharge, inflammation, ulceration.
  - Legs: Abnormal: Peripheral edema.
  - Back: Abnormal: Sacral edema.
- Auscultation:
  - Abdomen:
    - Listen in the left and right upper abdominal quadrants.
    - Disconnect suction if patient has nasogastric (NG) tube.
    - Clamp suction tube to abdomen briefly.
    - Use the bell of the stethoscope.
    - Ask patient to exhale deeply.
    - Listen midline to outside.
    - Abnormal: Whooshing sound (systolic bruits) may indicate renal artery stenosis.
- Percussion:
  - Kidneys:
    - Patient should be seated.
    - Place nondominant hand on the patient's back at the 12th rib.
    - Strike hand with your dominant hand.
    - Abnormal: Tenderness, pain.
- Palpation:
  - Bladder:
    - Make sure that the patient has urinated.
    - Ask the patient to lie on his or her back.
    - Press midline 1 to 2 inches above the symphysis pubis.
    - The patient may feel the need to urinate.
    - Abnormal: Tenderness, masses.
  - Kidney:
    - Place left hand under the back between the iliac crest and lower costal margin.
    - Place right hand on the abdomen above the left hand.

- Press right fingertips 1.5 inch above the right iliac crest.
- Press left fingertips upwards.
- Abnormal: Soft, tender, mass, enlarged, unequal bilaterally.

6.1.2.1 Signs and symptoms

Urinary assessment in a critical care situation requires the nurse to recognize common signs and symptoms of underlying causes and then prepare for the treatment that the practitioner is likely to order.

Commonly seen signs and symptoms:

- Not urinating (anuria).
- Excessive urinating (polyuria).
- Producing small amount of urine (oliguria).
- Painful urination (dysuria).
- Hesitancy.
- Involuntary urination (incontinence).
- Getting up from sleep to urinate (nocturia).
- Odor from urine (bacterial infection).
- Cloudy urine (bacterial infection).
- Blood in urine (hematuria).
- Clear urine (overhydrated).
- Dark urine (dehydrated).
- Bladder distended (urine retention).

6.2. Renal Tests

Urinary tests are designed to assess the effectiveness and capability of the urinary system to function. The following are commonly ordered urinary tests.

6.2.1 Urinary computed tomography (CT) scan

A urinary CT scan provides a three-dimensional image of the urinary system using x-rays. It enables the practitioner to visualize normal and abnormal structures. A CT scan can be performed with or without a contrast agent. A contrast agent is iodine based and enhances images of blood vessels and less dense areas.

- Common reasons for the practitioner to order a urinary CT scan are to assess for:
  - Inflammation.
  - Tumor.
  - Cysts.
  - Pseudocysts.
- The CT scan test:
  - Assesses whether the patient is allergic to iodine or shellfish if the patient is undergoing a CT scan with contrast. Patients who are allergic to iodine or shellfish have a high likelihood of experiencing an allergic reaction to the contrast agent.

  - Assesses whether the patient is claustrophobic. The patient will be placed in an enclosure during the test.
  - Assesses whether the patient can remain still for 30 minutes during the CT scan.
  - Administer diphenhydramine (Benadryl) and prednisone (Deltasone) before the CT scan to reduce the risk of an allergic reaction to the contrast agent if the contrast agent is ordered.
  - Administer the contrast agent through an intravenous (IV) tube. The patient may feel flushed and experience a salty or metallic taste in the mouth.
  - The CT scanner encircles the patient for up to 30 minutes.
  - Explain to the patient that the contrast material typically discolors the urine for up to 24 hours after the CT scan. The patient should increase fluid intake after the CT scan to flush the contrast agent from the his or her body, if the contrast agent is used for the CT scan.

6.2.2 Urinary magnetic resonance imaging (MRI)

A urinary MRI provides a three-dimensional view of the urinary systems using radio waves, a strong magnet, and a computer. An MRI is used particularly to assess fluid-filled soft tissue and to identify tumors from other structures within the urinary systems.

- Common reasons for the practitioner to order a urinary MRI are to assess for:
  - Inflammation.
  - Tumor.
  - Cysts.
  - Pseudocysts.
- The urinary MRI test:
  - The patient may need to be NPO (nothing by mouth) for up to 12 hours before the test, depending on the site of the MRI.
  - All metal must be removed from the patient.
  - No metal must enter the room containing the MRI scanner. The MRI scanner's magnet is always activated.
  - Assesses whether the patient is claustrophobic. If so, then ask the healthcare provider if an open MRI scanner could be used for the test or if the patient should be sedated before the scan begins.
  - The musculoskeletal MRI scan takes about 30 minutes.
  - The musculoskeletal MRI scan is noninvasive. The patient will not feel any discomfort.

6.2.3 Kidneys, ureter, and bladder (KUB) radiography

KUB radiography provides an x-ray view of the kidneys, ureter, and bladder without using contrast. No special preparation is necessary. This test is typically performed at bedside using a portable x-ray machine.

- Common reasons for the practitioner to order a KUB radiography are to assess for:
  - Lesions.
  - Calculi.
  - The position of the kidneys.
- The KUB radiography test:
  - The patient lies on his or her back.
  - The x-ray machine is positioned.
  - Images are recorded.

6.2.4 Urinary ultrasound

A urinary ultrasound provides a view of the kidneys, ureter, and bladder using high-frequency sound waves. No special preparation is necessary. This test is can be performed at bedside or in an imaging room.

- A common reason for the practitioner to order a urinary ultrasound is to:
  - View underlying structures.
- The urinary ultrasound test:
  - If the bladder is being examined, then the patient's bladder must be full during the test.
  - The patient lies on his or her back or stomach, depending on which structure is being examined.
  - A conductive gel is placed on the site and on the ultrasound transducer.
  - The ultrasound transducer is moved over the site.

6.2.5 Renal scan

A renal scan provides a functional view of the kidneys. A radioactive tracer is injected into the patient's vein and is traced as the tracer flows through the kidney. The renal scan is an alternative to the intravenous pyelogram (IVP).

- Common reasons for the practitioner to order a renal scan are to assess for:
  - Kidney function.
  - Blood flow through the kidneys.
- The renal scan test:
  - The patient drinks three glasses of water before the test.
  - The patient lies on his back.
  - A radioactive tracer is injected into the patient's vein.
  - The renal scan camera is positioned.
- Function study:
  - An image is taken every 3 minutes for 30 minutes.
  - The patient may be administered a diuretic to increase kidney function during the test.
- Perfusion study:
  - A renogram is created, showing movement of the tracer throughout the kidneys.
  - Following the test, the patient drinks a lot of water to flush the tracer from his body.
  - For 2 days following the renal scan, the patient must flush the toilet quickly after urinating and defecating. The radioactive tracer remains in urine and feces for 2 days.

6.2.6 Intravenous pyelogram (IVP)

An IVP provides an x-ray view of the kidneys, ureters, and bladder. A contrast material is injected into the patient's vein. Images are taken periodically for up to 5 minutes as the contrast material flows through the urinary system.

- Common reasons for the practitioner to order an IVP are to assess for:
  - Obstructions.
  - Tumors.
  - Cysts.

- The IVP test:
  - The patient drinks at least three glasses of water before the test.
  - The patient lies on his back.
  - Contrast material is injected into the patient's vein.
  - The x-ray machine is positioned.
  - Several images are taken over a 5-minute period.

6.2.7 Renal angiograph

A renal angiograph provides a fluoroscopy view using x-rays of the arterial and venial blood flow in the kidneys. A contrast material is injected into the patient's vein. Images are taken continually as the contrast material flows through the kidneys.

- Common reasons for the practitioner to order a renal angiograph are to assess for:
  - Blood clots.
  - Narrowing of blood vessels in the kidneys (renal stenosis).
  - Aneurysm.
  - Pyelonephritis.
  - Kidney disorders.
- The renal angiograph procedure:
  - The patient lies on his back.
  - The injection site near the groin is cleaned.
  - Contrast material is injected into the patient's artery through a catheter.
  - Fluoroscopy images are taken.
  - Pressure is applied to the site for 15 minutes after the catheter is removed.
  - The patient must keep the leg used for the test straight for 6 hours following the test.
  - Monitor the patient's serum creatinine and BUN levels (see 6.2.8 Renal blood tests) following the test for signs of renal failure related to the contrast material.

6.2.8 Renal blood tests

Practitioners use blood studies to assist in diagnosing urinary disorders. A practitioner may order one or multiple of the following blood studies.

- Blood urea nitrogen (BUN): BUN levels are compared with serum creatinine levels to assess whether an increase in the BUN level is caused by a renal disorder. Renal disorder is suspected if both BUN and serum creatinine levels are increased.
  - Increased levels may indicate:
    - Glomerulonephritis.
    - Obstruction.
    - Oliguria.

- Serum creatinine: Positively correlates with GFR.
  - Increased levels may indicate:
    - Renal disorder.
- Serum osmolality:
  - Increased levels may indicate renal disorder if urine osmolality decreases.
  - Decreased distal tube reaction to ADH may indicate decrease ability to concentrate urine.
- Serum proteins:
  - Decreased levels may indicate:
    - Nephrosis.
    - Nephritis.
- Creatinine clearance: Positively correlates with GFR.
  - Decreased levels may indicate:
    - Pyelonephritis.
    - Glomerulonephritis.
    - Tubular necrosis.
    - Nephrosclerosis.
    - Decreased renal blood flow.
    - Renal lesion.
    - Decreased renal blood flow.
- Uric acid:
  - Increased levels may indicate:
    - Decreased renal function.
  - Decreased levels may indicate:
    - Tubular absorption disorder.
- Urea clearance:
  - Decreased levels may indicate:
    - Glomerulonephritis.
    - Nephrosclerosis.
    - Pyelonephritis.
    - Renal blood flow disorder.
    - Tubular necrosis.
    - Dehydration.
    - Renal lesion.
    - Ureteral obstruction.
- Complete blood count (CBC):
  - White blood cell count (WBC):
    - Increases may indicate:
      - Infection.

- Red blood cell count (RBC):
  - Decreases may indicate:
    - Chronic renal insufficiency.
- Hemoglobin (Hgb):
  - Decreases may indicate:
    - Chronic renal insufficiency.
- Hematocrit (Hct):
  - Decreases may indicate:
    - Chronic renal insufficiency.

- Electrolytes:
  - Calcium:
    - Decreased levels may indicate:
      - Renal failure.
  - Phosphorus:
    - Increased levels may indicate:
      - Renal failure.
  - Chloride:
    - Increased levels may indicate:
      - Renal failure.
      - Tubular necrosis.
      - Dehydration.
    - Decreased levels may indicate:
      - Pyelonephritis.
  - Potassium:
    - Increased levels may indicate:
      - Acidosis.
      - Renal insufficiency.
      - Renal failure.
    - Decreased levels may indicate:
      - Tubular disorder.
  - Sodium:
    - Decreased levels may indicate:
      - Renal failure.

6.2.9 Urine analysis

Practitioners use urine analysis to assist in diagnosing genitourinary disorders. A practitioner may order one or more of the following urine studies. Table 6.1 contains information about common urine studies.

TABLE 6.1 Common Urine Studies

Study	Abnormal Results	May Indicate
pH	Alkaline (>8.0)	Urinary tract infection
		Chronic renal disease
		Respiratory alkalosis
		Metabolic alkalosis
	Acidic (<4.5)	Acidosis
		Tuberculosis
		Phenylketonuria
Specific gravity	Decrease	Renal failure
		Glomerulonephritis
		Diabetes insipidus
		Alkalosis
		Pyelonephritis
	Increase	Nephrosis
		Dehydration
Ketones	Found	Starvation
		Diabetes mellitus
		Vomiting
		Diarrhea
Protein	Found	Renal disease
Odor/color	Fruity odor	Starvation
		Dehydration
		Diabetes mellitus
	Turbid	Renal infection
	Cloudy	Infection
	Dark	Dehydration
Epithelial cells	Many found	Tubular degeneration
Red blood cells	Many found	Urinary tract infection
		Trauma
		Renal hypertension
		Inflammation
		Obstruction
		Hydronephrosis
		Tuberculosis
		Glomerulonephritis
		Pyelonephritis
		Bladder infection
Glucose	Found	Diabetes mellitus

TABLE 6.1 Common Urine Studies

Study	Abnormal Results	May Indicate
Crystals	Calcium oxalate	Hypercalcemia
	Cystine crystals	Metabolic disorder
White blood cells	Many found	Urinary tract infection
		Pyelonephritis
		Cystitis
Creatinine clearance	Decrease	Renal artery obstruction
		Glomerulonephritis
		Renal lesion
		Dehydration
		Nephrosclerosis
		Heart failure
		Tubular necrosis
Yeast cells	Found	Vaginitis
		Prostatovesiculitis
		Urethritis
		Contaminated sample
Casts	Red blood cell casts	Renal infarction
		Bacterial endocarditis
		Malignant hypertension
		Sickle cell anemia
		Collagen disorder
		Glomerulonephritis
	White blood cell casts	Renal infection
	Many hyaline casts	Inflammation
		Trauma
		Renal parenchymal disorder
	Waxy casts	Chronic renal disease
		Diabetes mellitus
		Nephrotic syndrome
	Epithelial casts	Nephrosis
		Chronic lead intoxication
		Tubular disorder
		Eclampsia
	Many casts	Renal disease
Parasites	Found	Contaminated sample
Nitrites	Found	Urinary tract infection

6.3. Urinary Medication

There are four categories of medication commonly used in urinary critical care. These are adrenergics, loop diuretics, a sulfonate cation-exchange resin, and an alkalinizing agent.

Adrenergic medication is used to profuse the kidneys. Loop diuretics increase urine production. A sulfonate cation-exchange resin lowers potassium levels in blood related to renal failure. An alkalinizing agent is used to treat metabolic acidosis.

6.3.1 Adrenergic medication

Adrenergic medication is used to increase blood flow to the kidneys, enabling sufficient perfusion to create urine. This results in sufficient excretion of waste. The most commonly prescribed adrenergic medication is:

- Dopamine
- Use: Renal failure.
- Considerations:
  - Administer as IV using large vein and IV pump after fluid volume is restored.
  - Monitor vital signs.
- Adverse effects:
  - Extravasation may occur, resulting in dopamine entering the extravasation space.
    - Stop infusion.
    - Administer phentolamine (Regitine) to the extravasation site.
  - Palpitations.
  - Hypotension.
  - Hypertension.
  - Nausea/vomiting.
  - Arrhythmias.

6.3.2 Diuretics

Diuretic medications cause water and electrolytes to be excreted by the kidneys, resulting in decreased afterload resistance and decreased blood pressure. There are three categories of diuretics. These are:

- Loop diuretics: Loop diuretics increase secretion of sodium, chloride, and water, leading to increased concentration of urine in the ascending loop of Henle. This results in a large volume of urine production.
- Medications:
  - Furosemide (Lasix).
  - Bumetanide (Bumex).
  - Ethacrynic acid (Edecrin).
- Use:
  - Heart failure.
  - Edema.
  - Hypertension.

- Considerations:
  - Monitor serum electrolyte levels.
  - Monitor fluid intake and output.
  - Monitor signs of excessive urination.
  - Monitor for signs of hypotension.
- Adverse effects:
  - Low sodium (hyponatremia).
  - Low potassium (hypokalemia).
  - Dehydration.
  - Rash.
  - Muscle cramps.
  - Hypotension.
  - High uric acid (hyperuricemia).
- Thiazide diuretics: Thiazide diuretics prevent the absorption of sodium by the kidneys and increases excretion of bicarbonate, potassium, and chloride. This leads to decreased fluid retention and decreased blood pressure.
- Medications:
  - Methyclothiazide (Enduron).
  - Chlorothalidone (Hygroton).
  - Bendroflumethiazide (Naturetin).
  - Hydroflumethiazide (Saluron).
  - Indapamide (Lozol).
- Use:
  - Edema.
  - Hypertension.
- Considerations:
  - Monitor blood glucose levels.
  - Monitor intake and output.
  - Monitor serum potassium levels.
- Adverse effects:
  - Low sodium (hyponatremia).
  - Low potassium (hypokalemia).
  - Dizziness.
  - Nausea.
  - Hypotension.
- Potassium-sparing diuretics: Potassium-sparing diuretics cause the distal tubule of the kidneys to excrete sodium, water, calcium, and chloride and decrease secretion of potassium and hydrogen. This results in increased urine output and decreased blood pressure.
- Medications:
  - Spironolactone (Aldactone).
  - Triamterene (Dyrenium).
  - Amiloride (Midamor).

- Use:
  - Edema.
  - Hypertension.
  - Cirrhosis.
  - Nephrotic syndrome.
- Considerations:
  - Monitor intake and output.
  - Monitor cardiac rhythm for arrhythmias.
  - Monitor serum potassium levels.
- Adverse effects:
  - Nausea.
  - Rash.
  - Increased serum potassium (hyperkalemia).
  - Headache.

6.3.3 Sulfonate cation-exchange resin

Sulfonate cation-exchange resin is used to treat increased levels of potassium (hyperkalemia).

- Medications:
  - Sodium polystyrene sulfonate (Kayexalate).
- Use: Lower potassium levels in blood related to renal failure.
- Considerations:
  - Monitor vital signs.
  - Risk of sodium overload.
  - Do not mix medication with orange juice (high potassium level).
  - Monitor for electrolyte imbalance.
- Adverse effects:
  - Risk of constipation (elderly).
  - Hypocalcemia.
  - Nausea/vomiting.
  - Diarrhea.
  - Anorexia.

6.3.4 Alkalinizing agent

An alkalinizing agent is used to treat metabolic acidosis.

- Medications:
  - Sodium bicarbonate.
- Use: Decrease acid (metabolic acidosis) related to renal failure.
- Considerations:
  - Monitor vital signs.
  - Monitor for electrolyte imbalance.

- Adverse effects:
  - Extravasation may occur, resulting in sodium bicarbonate entering the extravasation space. This results in local irritation.
  - Hypernatremia.
  - Hypokalemia.
  - Metabolic alkalosis.

6.4 Acute Glomerulonephritis

This kidney infection, also known as acute nephritic syndrome, results from an ascending urinary infection or infection from elsewhere in the body.

6.4.1 Signs and symptoms

- Oliguria.
- Hematuria.
- Peripheral edema.
- Blood pressure: Elevated.

6.4.2 Medical tests

- BUN: Elevated.
- Albumin: Decreased.
- GFR: Decreased.
- 24-hour urine: Elevated protein.
- Urinalysis: Shows RBC casts.
- Renal biopsy: Identifies cause of infection.

6.4.3 Treatment

- Administer:
  - Diuretic.
  - Plasmapheresis, if cause is an autoimmune disorder.

6.4.4 Intervention

- Monitor vital signs.
- Monitor intake and output.
- Weigh daily.
- Monitor extremities for edema.
- Instruct the patient:
  - Decrease fluid intake.

6.5 Kidney Trauma

Kidney trauma is damage to the kidney caused by either a blunt or penetrating injury. A blunt injury is commonly caused by a motor vehicle accident, assault, fall, or sports injury. A penetrating injury is commonly caused by a blast, knife, or gunshot. Kidney trauma is classified by a five-grade scale as illustrated in table 6.2.

TABLE 6.2 Classification of Kidney Trauma

Grade	Description
1	Superficial laceration of the renal cortex.
	Bruising (contusion) of the parenchyma.
2	Hematoma of the kidney that does not expand.
	Laceration less than 1 cm of the parenchyma.
3	Laceration 1 cm or more of the parenchyma. Collecting system intact.
4	Thrombosis in a portion of the renal artery.
	Bleeding of the renal artery and veins that is controllable.
	Laceration 1 cm or more of the collecting system.
	Leaking of fluid (extravasation) around and within the kidney.
5	Fractured kidney.
	Tearing of the renal artery or vein.
	Thrombosis of the renal artery.

6.5.1 Signs and symptoms

- Sign of wound.
- Flank bruising or hematoma.
- Blue-red-purple or green-brown flank discoloration (Turner's sign).
- Flank tenderness or pain.
- Blood in the urine (hematuria).
- Blood clots in urine.
- Hypotension related to bleeding (grades 3, 4, or 5).
- Hypovolemic shock (grade 5).

6.5.2 Medical tests

- KUB: Shows wound and kidney damage.
- IVP: Used to stage the trauma.
- Renal angiograph: Shows arterial damage.
- Blood test:
  - CBC: Shows blood loss and clotting ability.

- Urinalysis: Shows presence of RBCs.
- Ultrasound: Shows renal damage.
- CT scan with contrast: Shows renal damage.
- MRI: Shows renal damage.

6.5.3 Treatment

- Stabilize airway, breathing, cardiovascular, hemodynamics.
- Administer:
  - Oxygen.
  - Lactated Ringer's solution or normal saline.
  - Antibiotic.
  - Analgesic for symptom relief.
- Surgical repair of kidney.

6.5.4 Intervention

- Apply direct pressure on wound to control bleeding.
- Cover the wound.
- Insert two large-bore saline/heparin locks.
- Monitor vital signs every 15 minutes.
- Monitor for abdominal distention.
- Instruct the patient:
  - On the need to rest.

6.6 Kidney Stones (Renal Calculi)

Kidney stones are also known as renal calculi and nephrolithiasis. Slow urine flow enables crystals to form from calcium, uric acid, cysteine, or struvite in the kidneys or in the urinary tract. The crystal may block the ureter, causing hydronephrosis and swelling. There is a genetic predisposition to kidney stones.

6.6.1 Signs and symptoms

- Unilateral extreme flank pain (renal colic) may radiate to lower abdomen, groin, scrotum, or labia.
- Hematuria.
- Blood pressure elevated with pain.
- Nausea.
- Vomiting.

6.6.2 Medical tests

- Urinalysis: Shows leukocytosis.
- Ultrasound: Shows stones.
- X-ray of KUB: Shows stones.
- CT scan: Shows stones.
- MRI: Shows stones.

6.6.3 Treatment

- Lithotripsy: Shock waves break the stone into pieces so the stone can pass.
- Surgical removal of the stone.
- Surgical insertion of stent.
- Administer:
    - Narcotics.
    - Morphine.
    - Nonsteroidal anti-inflammatory drugs (NSAIDs).
    - Ketorolac.

6.6.4 Intervention

- Monitor intake and output.
- Strain urine.
- Instruct the patient:
    - Increase fluid intake.
    - Dietary modification based on makeup of stone.

6.7 Pyelonephritis

Infection of the kidneys commonly from *Escherichia coli, Klebsiella, Enterobacter, Proteus, Pseudomonas*, and *Staphylococcus saprophyticus* related to ascending urinary tract infection.

6.7.1 Signs and symptoms

- Flank pain.
- Fever.
- Chills.

- Urinary frequency.
- Urinary urgency.
- Costovertebral angle (CVA) tenderness.
- Nausea.
- Vomiting.
- Diarrhea.

6.7.2 Medical Tests

- Urinalysis: Shows RBCs.
- Urine culture and sensitivity: Identify organism and medication to treat the illness.
- CBC: Shows leukocytosis.

6.7.3 Treatment

- Administer:
  - Antibiotics:
    - Nitrofurantoin, ciprofloxacin, levofloxacin, ofloxacin, trimethoprim-sulfamethoxazole, Ampicillin, Amoxicillin.
  - Antipyretics:
    - Phenazopyridine.

6.7.4 Intervention

- Monitor vital signs.
- Monitor intake and output.
- Increase fluid intake.
- Instruct the patient:
  - Phenazopyridine will cause orange-colored urine.

6.8 Renal Failure

Renal failure is decreased renal function. There are five types of renal failure. These are:

- Acute: Sudden decrease in renal function.
- Prerenal: Caused by diminished renal perfusion.
- Hypovolemia: Caused by blood or fluid loss.
- Postrenal: Caused by urinary tract obstruction.
- Chronic: Progressive decrease in renal function due to irreversible renal disease.

6.8.1 Signs and symptoms

- Decreased urinary output.
- Peripheral edema.
- Abdominal bruit.
- Weight loss.
- Uremic pruritis.

6.8.2 Medical tests

- Renal ultrasound: Shows decrease in renal size.
- Blood test:
  - BUN: Elevated.
  - Creatinine: Elevated.
  - Creatinine clearance: Decreased.
  - RBCs: Decreased.
  - Hgb: Decreased.
  - Urinalysis: Shows proteinuria.
  - GER: Decreased.

6.8.3 Treatment

- Dialysis.
- Stent placement or catheter to allow for drainage of urine.
- Administer:
  - Phosphate binders to reduce phosphate levels.
  - Sodium polystyrene sulfonate to reduce potassium levels.
  - Erythropoetin to treat anemia.
  - Antibiotics for pyelonephritis.

6.8.4 Intervention

- Monitor vital signs.
- Monitor intake and output.
- Monitor electrolyte levels.
- Monitor blood glucose levels.
- No contrast dye tests.
- No nephrotoxic medication.
- Instruct the patient:
  - Restrict potassium, phosphate, sodium, and protein in the diet.

6.9 Urinary Tract Infection

An infection of the urinary tract, typically due to a gram-negative bacteria such as *E. Coli* found on the skin of the genital area or introduced by an invasive procedure.

6.9.1 Signs and symptoms

- Dysuria.
- Low back pain.
- Feeling of fullness in suprapubic area.
- Urinary frequency.
- Urinary urgency.

6.9.2 Medical tests

- Urinalysis: Shows leukocytes, nitrites, and RBCs.
- Urine culture and sensitivity: Identifies microorganism and medication to treat microorganism.

6.9.3 Treatment

- Administer:
  - Antibiotics:
    - Nitrofurantoin, ciprofloxacin, levofloxacin, ofloxacin, trimethoprim-sulfamethoxazole, ampicillin, amoxicillin.
  - Phenazopyridine.

6.9.4 Intervention

- Increase fluid intake.
- Monitor intake and output.
- Monitor vital signs.
- Instruct the patient:
  - Phenazopyridine will cause orange-colored urine.
  - Drink cranberry juice to acidify urine.

6.10 Bladder Cancer

Bladder cancer is typically a nonaggressive cancer that occurs in the transitional cell layer of the bladder. It is recurrent in nature. Less frequently, bladder cancer is found invading deeper layers of the bladder tissue. In these cases, the cancer tends to be more aggressive. Exposure to industrial chemicals (paints, textiles), history of cyclophosphamide use or smoking increases the risk of bladder cancer. The more aggressive the cancer cell type, the greater the risk of metastasis of the disease. Patients may have advanced disease at the time of diagnosis. The more advanced the disease at the time of diagnosis and the more aggressive the tumor, the greater the risk of death for the patient.

6.10.1 Signs and symptoms

- Fatigue, due to increased cell growth.
- Hematuria: Blood in urine, may be microscopic.
- Change in urinary pattern.

6.10.2 Medical tests

- Urinalysis: Shows RBCs in urine.
- Cystoscopy: Used to identify tumor site and obtain biopsy.
- Bladder biopsy: Shows cancer cell type.
- CT scan: Shows metastasis or invasion of tumor.

6.10.3 Treatment

- Surgical removal of tumor:
    - May be removal of superficial tumor from bladder wall with transurethral approach or removal of part or all of the bladder.
    - If all of the bladder is removed, a stoma is created on the surface of the abdomen or an ileal reservoir is created internally to collect the urine.
- Instillation of bCG (bacilli Calmette-Guérin) into bladder to decrease chance of recurrence.
- Radiation therapy.
- Chemotherapy.

6.10.4 Intervention

- Monitor vital signs.
- Monitor intake and output.
    - Document amount and color of drainage from all drains.
- Monitor color of urine.
- Monitor stoma for color, checking adequate blood flow to tissue.
- Monitor abdomen for bowel sounds, pain, and distention.
- Monitor skin for signs of breakdown, redness.
- Monitor for side effects of medications.
- Instruct the patient:
    - Proper skin care postoperatively.
    - Catheterization of ileal reservoir, if needed.

6.11 Kidney Cancer

Kidney cancer occurs when cancer cells create a tumor within the kidney. Exposure to chemicals, lead, and smoking all increase the risk of developing kidney cancer. Identification of a renal cancer is integral to a favorable outcome. Patients often have vague symptoms and may not seek health care until later in the disease, when the cancer is well developed. Metastatic disease has the worst prognosis.

6.11.1 Signs and symptoms

- Weight loss.
- Anemia due to altered erythropoietin production.
- Hematuria.
- Elevated blood pressure due to increase in renin production.
- Flank pain, dull or aching, occurs in a small number of patients.

6.11.2 Medical tests

- CBC: May show either anemia or erythrocytosis.
- Urinalysis: Shows RBCs.
- Erythrocyte sedimentation rate: Elevated.
- Ultrasound: Shows renal mass.
- CT scan with contrast: Shows renal mass.
- MRI: Shows renal mass.

6.11.3 Treatment

- Surgical removal by nephrectomy.
- Tumor destruction by radiofrequency ablation.
- Chemotherapy.
- Hourly urine output monitoring for first 24 to 48 hours postoperatively.
- Monitor Hgb and Hct as scheduled.
- Monitor for signs of infection postoperatively.

6.11.4 Intervention

- Monitor vital signs for changes.
- Monitor intake and output.
- Monitor operative site for redness, swelling, and bleeding.
- Monitor pain level postoperatively.

6.12 Acute Tubular Necrosis

Acute tubular necrosis occurs when the tubular segment of the nephron is inoperable. This is caused by interruption of blood flow to the kidneys (ischemic injury) or nephrotoxicity and leads to uremia and renal failure. Acute tubular necrosis can result in infection (septicemia), gastrointestinal hemorrhage, and hypercalcemia.

6.12.1 Signs and symptoms

- Asymptomatic (early stage).
- Decreased urine output.
- Agitation.
- Edema.
- Confusion.
- Bleeding.
- Arrhythmias.
- Muscle weakness.
- Vomiting blood.

6.12.2 Medical tests

- Blood tests show:
    - Increased BUN.
    - Increased creatinine.
    - Increased potassium.
    - Decreased RBCs.
    - Decreased Hgb.
    - Decreased serum protein.
- Urinalysis shows:
    - Low osmolality.
    - High sodium level.
    - Diluted urine.
    - Casts.
    - RBCs.
- Electrocardiography (ECG): Shows arrhythmia.

6.12.3 Treatment

- Administer:
    - Diuretics to remove casts.
    - Dopamine to increase renal flow.

- ○ Calcium channel blockers to treat nephrotoxicity.
- ○ Prostaglandins to treat nephrotoxic.
- ○ Antibiotics to treat infection.
- ○ Pack RBC transfusion for anemia.
- ○ Dialysis to treat uremia and electrolyte imbalance.

6.12.4 Intervention

- Monitor vital signs for changes.
- Monitor intake and output.
- Restrict protein intake.
- Ensure the patient is well hydrated.

6.13 Renal Procedures

Several commonly performed renal procedures are used in critical care situations to ensure that the patient's urinary tract functions properly.

6.13.1 Calculi basketing

Calculi basketing is a procedure in which a basketing device is inserted into the ureter using an ureteroscope or cystoscope to remove a ureteral calculus.

- A common reason for the practitioner to order a calculi basketing is to assess for:
  - ○ Removing a stone (calculi) that is too large to pass through the ureter.
- The calculi basketing procedure:
  - ○ The patient lies on his or her back.
  - ○ Ureterscope or cystocope is inserted into the ureter.
  - ○ The basketing device is inserted into the ureterscope or cystocope.
  - ○ The calculi is removed, as are the basketing device and ureteroscope or cystocope.
  - ○ An indwelling urinary catheter is inserted into the ureter.
  - ○ The patient is administered IV fluids for up to 48 hours.
  - ○ Fluid intake and output are measured.
  - ○ The indwelling urinary catheter is removed within 48 hours.

6.13.2 Extracorporeal shock wave lithotripsy (ESWL)

ESWL is a procedure in which a high-energy shock wave is administered to the patient to break up calculi. The calculi then pass naturally through the ureter.

- A common reason for the practitioner to order a calculi basketing is to assess for:
  - ○ Breakup of a stone (calculi) that is too large to pass through the ureter.

- The ESWL procedure:
  - The patient receives an anesthetic.
  - The patient lies on his or her back.
  - Shock waves are applied.
  - An indwelling urinary catheter is inserted into the ureter.
  - The patient is told to increase fluid intake to increase urine output.
  - The patient is told to ambulate.
  - The patient is told to urinate in a container. Urine is then strained for calculi.
  - The patient is told that there might be a small amount of blood in the urine for several days following the procedure.
  - The patient should contact the practitioner immediately if there is persistent bleeding, persistent pain, fever, chills, nausea, vomiting, or an inability to urinate.

6.13.3 Hemodialysis

Hemodialysis uses a mechanical/chemical process that replaces the kidney function. It removes urea, uric acid, creatinine, and excess water from the patient's blood.

- Common reasons for the practitioner to order hemodialysis:
  - Renal failure.
  - Restore electrolyte balance.
  - Restore acid-base balance.
- Hemodialysis procedure:
  - The patient is weighed.
  - Vital signs are taken. Do not use arm that contains the site for blood pressure or venipuncture.
  - The patient lies on his or her back.
  - The vascular site is assessed for bruit or thrill.
  - A vascular access site is open:
    - Atrioventricular (AV) fistula: An artery and vein in the wrist or lower forearm are sutured together, forming a common opening.
    - AV graft: A synthetic or natural graft connects an artery and vein in the wrist or lower forearm.
    - Subclavian vein catheterization: A catheter is inserted into the subclavian vein.
    - Femoral vein catheterization: A catheter is inserted into the femoral vein.
  - The hemodialysis equipment is connected to the vascular site according to the manufacturer's protocol.
  - Blood circulates from the patient into the hemodialysis equipment, where waste and excess water are removed before the blood returns to the patient.
  - During hemodialysis:
    - Assess for disequilibrium syndrome (rapid fluid removal):
      - Arrhythmias.
      - Muscle twitching.
      - Nausea.
      - Vomiting.
      - Headache.

        - Assess for internal bleeding:
            - Paleness.
            - Clammy skin.
            - Restlessness.
            - Thready pulse.
            - Increased respiration.
        - Monitor dialyzer lines for blood clots.
    - After hemodialysis:
        - Monitor site for bleeding.
        - Assess site for circulation.

6.13.4 Peritoneal dialysis

Peritoneal dialysis uses a chemical process that replaces the kidney function and removes urea, uric acid, creatinine, and excess water from the patient's blood. No dialysis machine is used. The patient's peritoneal membrane is used as the dialyzing membrane.

- Common reasons the practitioner orders peritoneal dialysis:
    - Renal failure.
    - When hemodialysis is ineffective.
    - The patient may choose peritoneal dialysis over hemodialysis.
- The peritoneal dialysis procedure:
    - The patient is asked to urinate to empty the bladder.
    - The patient is weighed.
    - Vital signs are taken.
    - The patient lies on his or her back.
    - The dialysate is instilled into the peritoneum through a catheter, causing excess fluid, electrolytes, and waste to exit the semipermeable peritoneal membrane into the peritoneum.
    - The dialysate is drained.
    - The process is repeated several times until all the excess fluid, electrolytes, and waste are removed.
    - During peritoneal dialysis, assess:
        - Vital signs every 10 minutes until stabilized, then every 2 hours.
        - Catheter obstruction.
        - Hypotension.
        - Hypovolemia.
        - Measure the drained solution. Always use gloves and protective eyewear.
        - Monitor tubing for obstruction.
        - Encourage the patient to:
            - Change position.
            - Breathe deeply and cough.
            - Perform passive range-of-motion exercise.

- After peritoneal dialysis:
  - Monitor site for bleeding and leakage.
  - Monitor for infection.
  - Calculate the patient's fluid balance.

Solved Problems

6.1 What should the patient do before you examine his or her bladder?

Urinate.

6.2 What might be suspected if you hear a whooshing sound when auscultating the abdomen?

Renal artery stenosis.

6.3 How do the kidneys maintain acid-base balance?

The kidneys maintain the acid-base balance of blood by reabsorbing sodium and bicarbonate, secreting hydrogen, producing ammonia, and causing phosphate salts to become acids.

6.4 How do the kidneys increase the production of red blood cells?

When oxygen levels decrease in blood, the kidneys secrete erythropoietin hormone and active vitamin D. Erythropoietin causes bone marrow to increase production of red blood cells. Active vitamin D regulates calcium balance, leading to bone metabolism.

6.5 What might a high level of creatinine in blood indicate?

Creatinine blood level is the amount of creatinine in blood. A high level indicates that kidneys may not be functioning properly because kidneys excrete creatinine.

6.6 Why might you suspect kidney problems if red blood cells and protein appear in a urine sample?

The kidneys filter and reabsorb red blood cells and protein.

6.7 What should you do before auscultating the abdomen of a patient who has an NG tube to suction?

Disconnect the suction.

6.8 What are abnormal findings when palpating the kidney?

Soft, tender, mass, kidney enlarged, unequal bilaterally.

6.9 What are common reasons for ordering a CT scan of the urinary tract?

To assess for:

- Inflammation.
- Tumor.
- Cysts.
- Pseudocysts.

6.10 What is KUB radiography?

KUB radiography provides an x-ray view of the kidneys, ureter, and bladder without using contrast. No special preparation is necessary. This test is typically performed at bedside using a portable x-ray machine.

6.11 Why is a KUB radiograph ordered?

To assess for:

- Lesions.
- Calculi.
- Position of kidneys.

6.12 What is a renal scan?

A renal scan provides a functional view of the kidneys. A radioactive tracer is injected into the patient's vein and is traced as the tracer flows through the kidney.

6.13 What are the reasons for ordering an intravenous pyelogram (IVP)?

To assess for:

- Obstructions.
- Tumors.
- Cysts.

6.14 Why might a renal angiograph be ordered?

To assess for:

- Blood clots.
- Narrowing of blood vessels in the kidneys (renal stenosis).
- Aneurysm.
- Pyelonephritis.
- Kidney disorders.

6.15 What might a decrease in creatinine clearance indicate?

A decrease may indicate:

- Pyelonephritis.
- Glomerulonephritis.
- Tubular necrosis.
- Nephrosclerosis.
- Decreased renal blood flow.
- Renal lesion.

6.16 What is the importance of the creatinine clearance test?

The results of the creatinine clearance test positively correlates with the glomerular filtration rate (GFR).

6.17 What is a common reason for an increase in urine specific gravity?

Dehydration.

6.18 What might be indicated by cloudy urine?

Infection.

6.19 Why would sodium polystyrene sulfonate (Kayexalate) be prescribed to a patient with renal disorder?

The kidneys maintain the electrolyte balance. A patient with a kidney disorder may have high levels of potassium (hyperkalemia). Sodium polystyrene sulfonate (Kayexalate) lowers potassium levels.

6.20 What are renal calculi?

Slow urine flow enables crystals to form from calcium, uric acid, cysteine, or struvite in the kidneys or in the urinary tract. The crystal may block the ureter, causing hydronephrosis and swelling. There is a genetic predisposition to kidney stones.

6.21 What is pyelonephritis?

Infection of the kidneys commonly from *E. coli*, *Klebsiella*, *Enterobacter*, *Proteus*, *Pseudomonas*, and *Staphylococcus saprophyticus* related to an ascending urinary tract infection.

6.22 What are common ways for a patient to contract a UTI?

An infection of the urinary tract typically is caused by a gram-negative bacteria such as *E. coli* found on the skin of the genital area or introduced by an invasive procedure.

6.23 How would you remove the stomach contents of the patient?

A nasogastric (NG) tube is inserted into the patient to remove stomach contents either by bulb syringe or suction in cases of intestinal obstruction, bleeding, or other gastrointestinal difficulties in which the stomach content places the patient at risk.

6.24 What is calculi basketing?

Calculi basketing is a procedure in which a basketing device is inserted into the ureter using an ureteroscope or cystoscope to remove a ureteral calculus.

6.25 What is the purpose of the ESWL procedure?

Extracorporeal shock wave lithotripsy (ESWL) is a procedure in which a high-energy shock wave is administered to the patient to break up calculi. The calculi then pass naturally through the ureter.

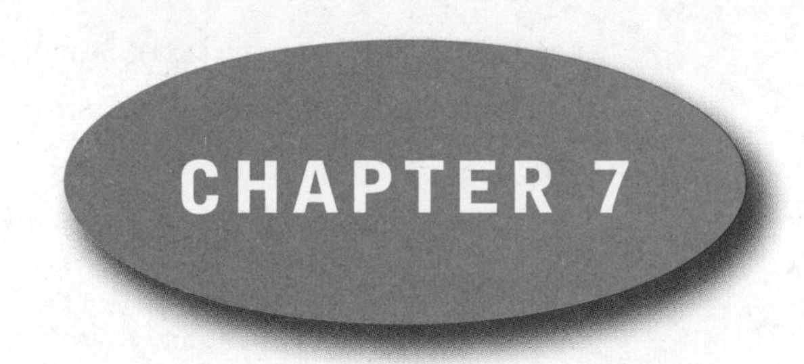

Endocrine Critical Care

7.1 Definitions

- Endocrine critical care focuses on conditions that alter glands, hormones, and hormone receptors. These conditions result in the patient becoming unstable.
- Endocrine physiology can be disrupted by an inflammation, infection, or trauma, leading to life-threatening conditions that compromise other systems.
- Endocrine critical care requires immediate, quick assessment and intervention.

7.1.1 Endocrine cycle

- Glands secrete hormones into the bloodstream.
- Hormones are chemical transmitters that stimulate organs to perform a specific physiological action.
- Receptors are areas on cells that receive hormones, causing the cell to perform a specific physiological action.
- Major glands are:
  - Pituitary:
    - Location: Base of the brain.
    - Posterior pituitary lobe stores and secretes:
      - Oxytocin: Promotes labor and delivery and stimulates the mammary glands to produce milk.
      - Antidiuretic hormone (ADH): Increases water absorption and decreases urine produced by the kidneys.
    - Anterior pituitary lobe secretes:
      - Growth hormone (GH) (somatotropin): Stimulates growth and cell production.
      - Thyroid-stimulating hormone (TSH) (thyrotropin): Stimulates the thyroid gland to produce thyroid hormones that regulate the basal metabolic rate.
      - Corticotropin: Stimulates the adrenal cortex to secrete aldosterone and cortisol.
      - Follicle-stimulating hormone (FSH): Stimulates maturation of ovarian follicles during the menstrual cycle.

- Luteinizing hormone (LH): Stimulates release of the egg from the mature follicle (ovulation).
- Prolactin: Stimulates the mammary glands to produce milk (lactation).

- Thyroid:
  - Location: Beneath the larynx and partly in front of the trachea.
  - Secretes:
    - Triiodothyronine (T3) and thyroxine (T4): Regulate metabolism.
    - Calcitonin: Inhibits calcium from being released from bone, leading to decreased calcium in the bloodstream.
- Parathyroid:
  - Location: Four parathyroid glands are located in the corners of the thyroid gland.
  - Secretes:
    - Parathyroid hormone (PTH): Increases calcium in the bloodstream by acting on bone, kidneys, and gastrointestinal tract.
- Adrenal:
  - Location: Above the kidneys.
  - Adrenal cortex (outer layer):
    - Secretes:
      - Cortisol: Reduces inflammation.
  - Adrenal medulla (core):
    - Secretes:
      - Epinephrine (adrenaline): Increases blood pressure and heart rate by narrowing blood vessels; also opens airways.
      - Norepinephrine: Increases blood pressure and heart rate by narrowing blood vessels.
- Pancreas:
  - Located: Behind the stomach.
  - Secretes:
    - Glucagon: Increases blood glucose.
    - Insulin: Decreases blood glucose.
  - Produces: Digestive enzymes.
- Thymus:
  - Located: Below the sternum.
  - Secretes:
    - Thymosin: Stimulates production of T cells.
    - Thymopoietin: Involved in cell structure.
  - Produces: T cells that are involved in cell-mediated immunity.
- Pineal:
  - Located: In the brain.
  - Secretes:
    - Melatonin: Regulates circadian rhythm.
- Gonads:
  - Ovaries:
    - Located: In the pelvis.

      - Secretes:
        - Estrogen: Causes secondary sex characteristics.
        - Progesterone: Promotes menstrual cycle.
    - Testes:
      - Located: In the scrotum.
      - Secretes:
        - Testosterone: Needed to support spermatogenesis.

7.1.2 Endocrine assessment

The endocrine critical care assessment:

- Look for clues for the underlying cause of the endocrine critical care issue:
  - Fatigue.
  - Weight changes.
  - Mental status changes.
  - Weakness.
  - Abnormal sexual function.
  - Frequent urination (polyuria).
  - Excessive thirst (polydipsia).
- Follow-up questions help probe further into the presenting endocrine problem.
  - Have you recently undergone any medical procedure?
    - What medical procedure?
    - When was the medical procedure performed?
  - Have you noticed recent bruises?
  - Have there been changes in your skin?
    - Increase/decrease in hair.
    - Increased dryness.
    - Increased moisture.
    - Tone.
  - Do you experience temperature intolerance?
- Inspect:
  - Appearance:
    - Distribution of body fat.
    - Posture.
    - Grooming.
    - General appearance.
    - Neck symmetry.
    - Nails:
      - Coloration.
      - Thickness.
      - Cracking.

- Clubbing.
- Separation from nail bed.

- Mental Status:
  - Level of consciousness.
  - Orientation.
  - Speech.
  - Facial expression.
  - Tremors.
- Skin:
  - Pigmentation (increased/decreased/absence).
  - Lesions.
  - Texture.
  - Hair distribution.
- Eye:
  - Conjunctiva.
  - Sclera.
  - Protrusion (exophthalamos).
  - Periorbital edema.

- Palpation:
  - Thyroid:
    - Abnormal:
      - Swelling.
      - Knot.
    - Chvostek's sign:
      - Tap facial nerve in front of the ear.
        - Hypocalcemia: Facial muscle contracts toward the ear.
    - Trousseau's sign:
      - Inflate the blood pressure cuff on the patient's arm.
        - Hypocalcemia: Thumb and digits contract within 3 minutes.
- Auscultation:
  - Thyroid:
    - Hyperthyroidism: Bruits heard over thyroid.

7.1.2.1 Signs and symptoms

Endocrine critical care assessment requires the nurse to recognize common signs and symptoms of underlying causes and then prepare for the anticipated treatment that the practitioner is likely to order. Commonly seen endocrine signs and symptoms are:

- Hypocalcemia (hypoparathyroidism).
- Increased urination (diabetes).
- Increased thirst (diabetes).
- Increased pigmentation (Addison's disease).
- Profound hypotension (Addison's disease).

- Intolerance to cold temperatures (hypothyroidism).
- Periorbital edema (myxedema coma).
- Thick dry tongue (myxedema coma).
- Irritability/restlessness (thyroid storm).
- Eye protrusion (exophthalamos) (thyroid storm).

7.2. Endocrine Tests

Endocrine critical care ocular tests are designed to assess the effectiveness and the capability of the endocrine system to function. Critical care practitioners order endocrine tests to collect objective data to further assess the patient and to assist in stabilizing the patient. The following are endocrine tests commonly ordered by critical care practitioners.

7.2.1 Endocrine computed tomography (CT) scan

An endocrine CT scan provides a three-dimensional image of endocrine glands using x-rays. It enables the practitioner to visualize normal and abnormal structures. CT can be performed with or without a contrast agent. A contrast agent is iodine based and enhances images of blood vessels and less dense areas. Common reasons the practitioner orders a CT scan is to assess for endocrine gland structural abnormalities.

The CT scan procedure:

- Assesses whether the patient is allergic to iodine or shellfish if the patient is undergoing a CT scan with contrast. Patients who are allergic to iodine or shellfish have a high likelihood of experiencing an allergic reaction to the contrast agent.
- Assesses whether the patient is claustrophobic. The patient will be placed in an enclosure during the test.
- Assesses whether the patient can remain still for 30 minutes during the CT scan.
- Administer diphenhydramine (Benadryl) and prednisone (Deltasone) before the CT scan to reduce the risk of an allergic reaction to the contrast agent if the contrast agent is ordered.
- Administer the contrast agent through an intravenous (IV) line. The patient may feel flushed and experience a salty or metallic taste in the mouth.
- The CT scanner encircles the patient for up to 30 minutes.
- Explain to the patient that the contrast material typically discolors the urine for up to 24 hours following the CT scan. The patient should increase fluid intake after the CT scan to flush the contrast agent from the patient's body if the contrast agent is used for the CT scan.

7.2.2 Radionuclide thyroid imaging

The radionuclide thyroid imaging study requires the administration of a radioisotope into the patient. Images of the thyroid gland are taken as the radioisotope enters the thyroid gland. Areas on the image are classified as:

- Hot spot: Black areas where excessive uptake of the radioisotope occurs (hyperfunctioning nodules).
- Cold spots: Light gray areas where little update of the radioisotope occurs (hypofunctioning nodules).

A common reason the practitioner orders radionuclide thyroid imaging is to assess an enlarged thyroid gland following palpation.

The radionuclide thyroid imaging procedure:

- Assesses whether the patient is allergic to iodine or shellfish if the patient is undergoing a CT scan with contrast. Patients who are allergic to iodine or shellfish have a high likelihood of experiencing an allergic reaction to the iodine.
- Administer diphenhydramine (Benadryl) and prednisone (Deltasone) before the CT scan to reduce the risk of an allergic reaction to the iodine.
- Administer the radioisotope orally or IV per practitioner's order.
- Several images are taken of the patient as the radioisotope enters the thyroid gland.
- Administer fluids orally or IV per practitioner's order, to flush the radioisotope from the patient.

7.2.3 Endocrine blood tests

Practitioners use blood studies to assist in diagnosing endocrine disorders. A practitioner may order one or multiple of the following blood studies. Common blood studies are:

- Calcium: Calcium levels assess parathyroid disorders:
  - Increase may indicate:
    - Parathyroid tumor.
    - Hyperparathyroidism.
  - Decrease may indicate:
    - Hypoparathyroidism.
- Catecholamine: Catecholamine levels are used to assess the function of the adrenal medulla.
  - Increase may indicate:
    - Pheochromocytoma.
- Cortisol: Cortisol levels are used to assess the function of the adrenal cortex.
  - Increase may indicate:
    - Cushing's disease.
    - Cushing's syndrome.
  - Decrease may indicate:
    - Addison's disease.
- Glucose tolerance test: A glucose tolerance test is used to assess for endocrine disorders.
  - Increase may indicate:
    - Cushing's disease.
    - Pheochromocytoma.
    - Diabetes.
  - Decrease may indicate:
    - Addison's disease.
    - Hypopituitarism.
    - Hypothyroidism.
    - Hypoglycemia.
- Glycosylated hemoglobin: The glycosylated hemoglobin test is used to assess the control of glucose in diabetes over a 3-month period.

  - Increase may indicate:
    - Uncontrolled diabetes.
- Gonadotropin: The gonadotropin test is used to assess the pituitary gland.
  - Increase may indicate:
    - Primary gonadal failure.
  - Decrease may indicate:
    - Pituitary insufficiency.
- GH: The GH test is used to assess secretion of GH.
  - Increase may indicate:
    - Pituitary tumor.
    - Hypothalamic tumor.
    - Diabetes.
  - Decrease may indicate:
    - Pituitary infarction.
- Insulin-induced hypoglycemia: The insulin-induced hypoglycemia test is used to assess for hypopituitarism.
  - Decrease may indicate:
    - Hypopituitarism.
- Parathyroid hormone: The parathyroid hormone test is used to assess the parathyroid gland.
  - Increase may indicate:
    - Hyperparathyroidism.
  - Decrease may indicate:
    - Hypoparathyroidism.
- Phosphorus: The phosphorus test is used to assess the parathyroid gland.
  - Increase may indicate:
    - Hypoparathyroidism.
    - Diabetic ketoacidosis.
  - Decrease may indicate:
    - Hyperparathyroidism.
- TSH: The TSH test is used to assess the thyroid gland.
  - Increase may indicate:
    - Hypothyroidism.
    - Thyroid cancer.
  - Decrease may indicate:
    - Hyperthyroidism .
- T4 radioimmunoassay: The T4 radioimmunoassay test is used to assess the thyroid gland.
  - Increase may indicate:
    - Hyperthyroidism.
  - Decrease may indicate:
    - Hypothyroidism.
- T3 radioimmunoassay: The T3 radioimmunoassay test is used to assess the thyroid gland.

- Increase may indicate:
  - Hyperthyroidism.
- Decrease may indicate:
  - Hypothyroidism.

7.2.4 Urine analysis

Practitioners use urine analysis to assist in diagnosing endocrine disorders. Common studies are:

- Cortisol: Cortisol is used to assess the adrenal cortex.
  - Increase may indicate:
    - Cushing's disease.
- The 17- hydroxycorticosteroid test: The 17- hydroxycorticosteroid test is used to assess the adrenal gland.
  - Increase may indicate:
    - Cushing's disease.
    - Pituitary tumor.
  - Decrease may indicate:
    - Hypothyroidism.
    - Addison's disease.
- The 17- ketosteroid test: The 17- ketosteroid test is used to assess the adrenal cortex.
  - Increase may indicate:
    - Congenital adrenal hyperplasia.
  - Decrease may indicate:
    - Adrenal insufficiency.

7.3 Endocrine Medication

Commonly used medications for endocrine disorders are thyroid hormone replacement and thyroid hormone antagonist, insulin, oral antidiabetes medications, and corticosteroids. These medications replace or block hormones produced by the endocrine system.

7.3.1 Thyroid hormone replacement

Thyroid replacement medication is administered to supplement production of the thyroid hormone for a patient diagnosed with hypothyroidism.

- Medications:
  - Levothyrozine (Synthroid):
  - Use: Hypothyroidism.
  - Considerations:
    - Administer medication early in the morning on an empty stomach.
    - Avoid antacids that contain aluminum and magnesium that can decrease absorption of the medication.

        - Blood level of medication must be monitored to avoid toxicity.
    - Adverse effects:
        - Thyrotoxicosis may occur, resulting in hypothyroidism.
            - Weight loss.
            - Palpitations.
            - Intolerance to heat.
            - Hair loss.
            - Hyperactivity.
            - Weakness.
            - Fatigue.
        - Tachycardia.
        - Hypertension.
        - Insomnia.
        - Tremors.

7.3.2 Antithyroid medication

Antithyroid medication is administered to reduce production of the thyroid hormone for a patient diagnosed with hyperthyroidism.

- Medications:
    - Propylthiouracil.
    - Use: Hyperthyroidism
    - Considerations:
        - Medication can affect cardiac medications.
        - Increased risk of bleeding when used with anticoagulants.
        - Blood level of medication must be monitored to avoid toxicity.
    - Adverse effects:
        - Myxedema coma may occur, resulting in hypothyroidism.
            - Altered mental status.
            - Hypothermia.
            - Hypoventilation.
            - Hypotension.
            - Hypoglycemia.
        - Drowsiness.
        - Nausea.
        - Vomiting.
        - Diarrhea.
        - Headache.
        - Loss of taste.
        - Joint pain.
        - Decreased white blood cells (leukopenia).
        - Dizziness (vertigo).

7.3.3 Corticosteroids

Corticosteroids are administered to a patient in acute adrenal crisis:

- Medications:
  - Glucocorticoid (hydrocortisone)
  - Use: Acute adrenal crisis.
  - Consideration:
    - Monitor blood pressure.
    - Monitor blood glucose.
    - Monitor for signs of infection.
    - Taper use. Adrenal gland is suppressed when medication is administered.
  - Adverse effects:
    - Diabetes.
    - Peptic ulcer.
    - Insomnia.
    - Increased hunger.
    - Hypertension.
    - Seizures.
    - Muscle wasting.
    - Delirium.
    - Delayed wound healing.
    - Masks infection symptoms.
    - Hirsutism.

7.3.4 Insulin

Insulin is administered when the pancreas no longer produces insulin for a patient diagnosed with diabetes.

- Medications:
  - Lispro (rapid-acting).
  - Regular (short-acting).
  - Neutral protamine Hagedorn (NPH) (intermediate-acting).
  - Ultralente (long-acting).
- Use: Insulin-dependent diabetes.
- Consideration:
  - Monitor blood glucose levels.
  - Alert patient to signs of hypoglycemia.
- Adverse effects:
  - Hypoglycemia may occur if too much insulin is administered:
    - Sweating.
    - Trembling.
    - Palpitations.
    - Clammy skin.
    - Increased hunger.

        - Irritability.
        - Confusion.
        - Headache.
        - Death.
    - Weight gain.

7.3.5 Oral antidiabetic medication

Oral antidiabetic medication is administered when the pancreas no longer produces sufficient quantity or quality insulin for a patient diagnosed with diabetes.

- Medications:
    - Metformin (glucophage).
    - Acarbose (Precose).
    - Glipizide (Glucotrol).
    - Glyburide (DiaBeta).
    - Pioglitazone (Actos).
    - Rosiglitazone (Avandia).
- Use: Non-insulin–dependent diabetes.
- Consideration:
    - Monitor blood glucose levels.
    - Alert patient to signs of hypoglycemia and hyperglycemia.
    - Administer medication with meals.
    - Monitor liver function.
    - Monitor kidney function.
    - Stop metformin (Glucophage) 24 hours before imaging test using contrast.
- Adverse effects:
    - Hypoglycemia may occur:
        - Sweating.
        - Trembling.
        - Palpitations.
        - Clammy skin.
        - Increased hunger.
        - Irritability.
        - Confusion.
        - Headache.
    - Hyperglycemia may occur:
        - Dry mouth.
        - Increased hunger (polyphagia).
        - Increased thirst (polydipsia).
        - Increased urination (polyuria).
        - Poor wound healing.
        - Weight loss.
        - Blurred vision.

- Diarrhea.
- Nausea.
- Flatulence (acarbose [Precose]).

7.4 Hypothyroidism (Myxedema)

Hypothyroidism is a lack of, or too little, thyroid hormone commonly caused by Hashimoto's thyroiditis. Hashimoto's thyroiditis is a chronic disorder caused by abnormal antibodies that attack the thyroid gland. Hypothyroidism can also be caused by decreased production of the TSH hormone from the pituitary gland, a side effect of surgery, inflammation of the thyroid gland, and treatment for hyperthyroidism.

7.4.1 Signs and symptoms

- Fatigue due to slow metabolism.
- Hypothermia due to slow metabolism.
- Brittle nails due to low levels of thyroid hormone, which helps growth and development.
- Thin, dry hair from lack of thyroid hormone.
- Dry skin from lack of thyroid hormone.
- Menstruation changes due to diminished levels of thyroid hormone.
- Slow cognitive function due to slow metabolism.
- Weight gain and low levels of thyroid hormone cause fatigue, sluggishness.

7.4.2 Medical tests

- Increased TSH unless the cause is a decreased production of TSH by the pituitary gland.
- Decreased T3, T4.
- Presence of thyroglobulin, indicating Hashimoto's thyroiditis.
- Presence of peroxidase autoantibodies appears in serum, indicating Hashimoto's thyroiditis.

7.4.3 Treatment

- Replacement hormone levothyroxine is the treatment of choice.
- Serum measurements of T3 and T4 will need to be performed after 6 to 8 weeks to determine whether the patient is taking the correct dose.
- The patient needs to be aware that this is lifetime replacement.

7.4.4 Intervention

- Monitor vital signs.
- Provide a warm environment.
- Low-calorie diet.
- Increase fluids and fiber to prevent constipation.

- Take thyroid replacement hormone each morning to avoid insomnia.
- Monitor for signs of thyrotoxcosis (an increase in T3) (nausea, vomiting, diarrhea, sweating, tachycardia).
- Instruct the patient:
  - Side effects of thyroid hormone replacement.
  - Review the signs of hyperthyroidism and hypothyroidism.

7.5 Hyperthyroidism (Graves' Disease)

In hyperthyroidism, there is an overproduction of T3 and T4 by the thyroid gland. This can be caused by an autoimmune disease in which the body's immune system attacks the thyroid gland. Other causes can be a benign tumor (adenoma), resulting in an enlarged thyroid gland (goiter) or an overproduction of TSH by the pituitary gland caused by a pituitary tumor.

7.5.1 Signs and symptoms

- Enlarged thyroid gland (goiter) caused by tumor .
- Protrusion of the eyeballs (exophthalmos) due to lymphocytic infiltration, which pushes out the eyeball.
- Sweating (diaphoresis): Excess thyroid hormone raises the metabolic rate.
- Increased appetite due to increased metabolism.
- Nervousness due to high levels of thyroid hormone.
- Weight loss due to increased metabolism.
- Menstrual changes due to elevated levels of thyroid hormone.

7.5.2 Medical tests

- Increased serum T3.
- Increased serum T4.
- Increased thyroid-releasing hormone (TRH) and TSH if pituitary gland is the cause of hyperthyroidism.
- Presence of antibodies if cause is Grave's disease.
- Thyroid scan reveals enlarged thyroid.

7.5.3 Treatment

- Radioactive iodine therapy to decrease production of thyroid hormones.
- Surgically reduce in size or remove the thyroid gland if the size of the thyroid gland interferes with swallowing or breathing.
- Administer:
  - Antithyroid medication to block synthesis of T3 and T4:
    - Propylthiouracil (PTU).
    - Methimazole (Tapazole).

- Beta blockers to decrease sympathetic activity and control tachycardia, tremors, and anxiety:
  - Propranolol (Inderal).

7.5.4 Intervention

- Monitor vital signs.
- Provide a cool environment.
- Protect the patient's eyes with dark glasses and artificial tears if the patient has exophthalmos.
- Provide a diet high in carbohydrates, protein, calories, vitamins, and minerals.
- Monitor for laryngeal edema following surgery:
  - Hoarseness.
  - Inability to speak clearly.
- Keep oxygen, suction, and a tracheotomy set near bed in case the neck swells and breathing is impaired.
- Keep calcium gluconate near the patient's bed following surgery to treat tetany and to maintain the serum calcium level.
- Place the patient in a semi-Fowler's position to decrease tension on the neck following surgery.
- Support the patient's head and neck with pillows.
- Monitor for muscle spasms and tremors (tetany).
- Check drainage and hemorrhage from incision line:
  - Frank hemorrhage.
  - Purulence.
  - Foul-smelling drainage.
- Monitor for signs of hypocalcemia (tingling of hands and fingers).
- Check for Chvostek's sign:
  - Tapping of the facial nerve causes twitching of the facial muscles.
  - Administer IV calcium quickly.
- Check for Trousseau's sign:
  - Inflate blood pressure cuff on the arm and muscles contract.

7.6 Addison's Disease

Addison's disease is inadequate secretion of corticosteroids from the adrenal cortex resulting from damage to the adrenal cortex. Autoimmune destruction of the adrenal gland and tuberculosis are two common causes of Addison's disease. A patient can experience Addisonian crisis when infection, surgery, or other stressful events result in a decrease in the production of cortisol and aldosterone. Addisonian crisis is a medical emergency. With ongoing treatment, patients can live a normal life span.

7.6.1 Signs and symptoms

- Weakness due to insufficient cortisol.
- Weight loss due to insufficient cortisol.

- Orthostatic hypotension due to poor fluid status from aldosterone deficiency.
- Bronzing of the skin due to hyperpigmentation from the autoimmune disease.

7.6.2 Medical tests

- Increased blood urea nitrogen (BUN) levels due to dehydration.
- Increased serum potassium from changes in aldosterone secretion.
- Decreased serum cortisol being secreted from the adrenal cortex.
- Decreased serum glucose from decreased corticosteroids.
- Positive 24-hour urine aldosterone level due to less aldosterone being secreted.
- Positive adrenocorticotropic hormone (ACTH) stimulation test. ACTH acts on the adrenal cortex to stimulate adrenal hormone secretion. An infusion of ACTH is given and the test is positive if the infusion fails to raise the cortisol level.
- Abnormal adrenal glands appear on CT.

7.6.3 Treatment

- Administer:
  - Cortisone or hydrocortisone to replace cortisol.
  - Fludrocortisone to regulate sodium and potassium balance.
- Maintain fluid balance.

7.6.4 Intervention

- Monitor fluids and electrolytes.
- Weigh the patient daily.
- Suggest bone density test for osteoporosis due to decrease in mineralocorticoids.
- Instruct the patient:
  - Medication must be taken every day.
  - Wear a medic alert bracelet.
  - Keep an emergency supply of medication available.

7.7 Syndrome of Inappropriate Antidiuretic Hormone Secretion (SIADH)

SIADH is caused by too much ADH being secreted by the posterior pituitary gland. ADH is responsible for controlling the amount of water reabsorbed by the kidney; it prevents loss of too much fluid. When too much water is detected, ADH production or secretion is halted. SIADH may be caused by damage to the hypothalamus or pituitary, inflammation of the brain, some medications such as selective serotonin receptor inhibitors (SSRIs), carbamazapine, cyclophosphamides, and chlorpropamide. Certain cancers, especially lung, may produce ADH.

If sodium (Na) levels are kept within normal limits, prognosis is excellent.

7.7.1 Signs and symptoms

- Headaches due to hyponatremia.
- Nausea and vomiting due to hyponatremia.
- Confusion due to hyponatremia.
- Personality changes due to hyponatremia.

7.7.2 Medical tests

- Hyponatremia (low serum sodium) due to the dilution.

7.7.3 Treatment

- Administer:
  - Saline IV to replenish sodium.
- Treat underlying cause.

7.7.4 Intervention

- Monitor electrolytes to monitor sodium levels.
- Restrict fluid because excess fluid dilutes sodium levels.
- Weigh the patient daily using the same scale, at the same time of day, with the patient wearing similar clothing.
- Monitor intake and output.

7.8 Cushing's Syndrome

The adrenal cortex secretes an excess of glucocorticoids or the pituitary gland secretes an excess of ACTH as a result of a pituitary tumor, adrenal tumor, or from ongoing glucocorticoid therapy. Patients can expect a normal life span once the tumor is removed; however, tumors may recur.

7.8.1 Signs and symptoms

- Moon face during excess cortisol production.
- Buffalo hump (fat pad located in the upper back) from excessive corticosteroids.
- Osteoporosis from an excess of corticosteroids, which weaken the bones.
- Absence of menstruation (amenorrhea) from the effects of excess steroids.
- Changes in mental status from excessive steroids.

7.8.2 Medical tests

- Dexamethasone suppression test: A dose of glucocorticoid is given to test the hypothalamus-pituitary-adrenal axis. If there is suppression with the dose, it indicates a pituitary origin of the excess cortisol. If no suppression occurs, the etiology is an adrenal or ectopic tumor.
- Increased cortisol in 24-hour urine collection from excess production.
- Presence of a pituitary tumor or adrenal tumor on a CT; the tumor will show on a CT scan.
- Increased blood glucose due to overproduction of steroids.
- Increased sodium due to excess fluid loss.
- Decreased potassium.

7.8.3 Treatment

- Surgical removal of the pituitary tumor or adrenal tumor.

7.8.4 Intervention

- Weigh daily to monitor fluid status.
- Monitor input and output to ensure adequate hydration.
- Monitor for glucose and acetone in urine as elevated levels of corticosteroids may produce hyperglycemia.
- Allow for adequate rest to allow the body to stabilize.
- Avoid skin because elevated levels of corticosteroids can delay wound healing.
- Bone densitometry to assess for osteoporosis as corticosteroids can leech calcium from the bone.
- Following surgery:
  - Assist in early ambulation, deep breathing, coughing to facilitate mucus mobilization, and decreased risk for emboli.
  - Monitor incision site for drainage, erythema, and signs of infection.
- Instruct the patient:
  - Maintain a high-calorie, high-calcium diet to aid in wound repair and replace calcium.
  - Administer pain medication as needed.

7.9 Diabetes Insipidus

Either a decrease in ADH production by the hypothalamus or the increase of ADH by the pituitary causes a decreased ability of the kidneys to concentrate urine, resulting in the excretion of large amounts of diluted urine. The patient then drinks large amounts of fluid to replace the increased urine output. Treatment will eliminate the symptoms of diabetes insipidus, and the patient can expect a normal life span.

7.9.1 Signs and symptoms

- Increased urination as the kidneys fail to concentrate urine.
- Increased thirst as the body attempts to replace lost fluid.

7.9.2 Medical tests

- Normal blood glucose, indicating that diabetes insipidus is not a complication of diabetes mellitus.
- Low specific gravity in urine due to increased fluid in the urine.
- Increased BUN, indicating dehydration because the concentration of solutes to fluid is rising.
- Electrolytes indicate dehydration; Na and Cl will rise as the concentration increases.
- Desmopressin stimulation test:
  - If urine output decreases and urine specific gravity increases, the problem is with the pituitary gland and the kidneys are normal.
  - If urine output remains unchanged and urine specific gravity remains low, the pituitary gland is normal and the kidneys are the problem.
- Presence of a pituitary tumor or hypothalamus tumor appear on magnetic resonance imaging (MRI).

7.9.3 Treatment

- Administer:
  - Replacement ADH hormone to return normal urination:
    - Desmopressin.
  - Diuretic to decrease urination:
    - Hyrdrochlorothiazide (Dyazide).
- Place the patient on a low-salt diet to reduce urine production by the kidneys.
- Increase fluid intake until urination returns to normal.

7.9.4 Intervention

- Maintain fluid and electrolyte balance.
- Monitor intake and output.
- Weigh the patient each day using the same scale, at the same time of day, with the patient wearing similar clothing.
- Instruct the patient:
  - Medication must be taken every day.
  - Wear a MedicAlert alert necklace/bracelet to alert healthcare providers that you have diabetes insipidus.

7.10 Primary Aldosteronism (Conn's Syndrome)

In primary aldosteronism, the adrenal cortex is secreting an excessive amount of aldosterone caused by an adrenal tumor, malfunctioning adrenal cortex, or sources outside the adrenal gland producing aldosterone. Some medications, such as calcium channel blockers, can lower aldosterone levels, which can confuse the diagnosis. The patient can expect a normal life span if diagnosed and treated early.

7.10.1 Signs and symptoms

- Increased blood pressure caused by the excess aldosterone.
- Headache caused by increased blood pressure.
- Muscle weakness from decreased serum potassium.
- Increased thirst (polydipsia) due to high levels of aldosterone.
- Increased urination (polyuria) due to high levels of aldosterone.

7.10.2 Medical tests

- Decreased serum potassium.
- A 24-hour urine test for aldosterone, creatinine, and cortisol levels.
- Increased urinary aldosterone.
- Presence of an adrenal tumor on a CT.

7.10.3 Treatment

- Administer:
  - Diuretics to control hypertension and raise potassium levels.
    - Spironolactone (Aldactone).
  - Mineralocorticoid receptor antagonists to block the effect of aldosterone.
    - Eplerenone (Inspra).
- Surgically remove the adrenal tumor if present.

7.10.4 Intervention

- Restrict sodium intake.
- Monitor intake and output.
- Weigh the patient daily.
- Instruct the patient:
  - Thirst and dry mucous membranes are caused by low sodium. Swallow sips of water, ice chips.

7.11 Pheochromocytoma

In pheochromocytoma, a tumor on the adrenal medulla secretes excessive amounts of epinephrine and norepinephrine. Patients who are diagnosed and treated early can expect a normal life with close follow-up if the tumor is benign. Patients can expect a limited prognosis if the tumor is malignant. Metastasis may develop at any time. The patient's hypertension often resolves with removal of the tumor but may recur later in life.

7.11.1 Signs and symptoms

- Uncontrollable hypertension as a result from increased epinephrine and norepinephrine.
- Headaches as a result of hypertension.
- Palpitations and tachycardia due to increased production of catecholamines.
- Dilated pupils from increased production of epinephrine and norepinephrine.

7.11.2 Medical tests

- Presence of catecholamines in serum.
- Increased catecholamines, metanephrines, and vanillylmandelic acid (VMA) in 24-hour urine collection.
- Presence of an adrenal tumor shown in CT scan.

7.11.3 Treatment

- Surgical removal of the adrenal tumor.
- Administer:
    - Antihypertensive medication to help lower blood pressure.
    - Beta blockers to diminish effects of epinephrine and norepinephrine.
        - Nifedipine (Procardia).
        - Nicardipine (Cardene).
        - Propranolol (Inderal).

7.11.4 Intervention

- Monitor blood pressure.
- Decrease stress.
- Instruct the patient:
    - No smoking, which helps lower blood pressure.
    - Reduce caffeine consumption to help lower blood pressure.

7.12 Hyperparathyroidism

In hyperparathyroidism, overactivity of the parathyroid glands caused by a tumor produces too much PTH, resulting in hypercalcemia and hypophosphatemia. Excess calcium is reabsorbed by the kidneys and may result in kidney stones. However, malfunction in the feedback mechanism prevents detection of excessive calcium levels in the blood, failing to adjust to the secretion of PTH. Parathyroid tumors are usually benign. Patients can expect a normal life span once the parathyroid tumor is removed.

7.12.1 Signs and symptoms

- Hyperparathyroidism is asymptomatic.
- Increased serum calcium level.
- Bone pain or fracture as a result of excreting calcium from bone.
- Kidney stones.
- Frequent urination as a result of increased calcium in the urine (hypercalciuria).

7.12.2 Medical Tests

- Increased serum calcium.
- Increased serum PTH.
- Decreased serum phosphate.
- Increased urine calcium.
- Presence of parathyroid tumor in ultrasound.
- Fine-needle biopsy of the parathyroid tumor.

7.12.3 Treatment

- Surgical removal of the parathyroid tumor.
- Administer:
  - Bisphosphanates to lower serum calcium by increasing calcium absorption in the bone.
  - Ibandronate sodium (Bonviva).
  - Risedronate (Actonel).
  - Alendronate sodium (Fosamax).
- IV normal saline to dilute serum calcium.
- Diuretic to excrete excess calcium in the urine.
  - Furosemide (Lasix).

7.12.4 Intervention

- Monitor intake and output.
- Monitor for fluid overload.
- Monitor electrolyte balance.
- Force fluids.
- Give the patient acidic juices such as cranberry juice.
- Strain urine for kidney stones.
- Place the patient on a low-calcium and high-phosphorus diet.

- Instruct the patient:
  - Avoid over-the-counter calcium supplements.
  - Maintain daily activities.

7.13 Diabetes Mellitus

Diabetes mellitus occurs when beta cells in the pancreas either are unable to produce insulin (type I diabetes mellitus) or produce an insufficient amount of insulin (type II diabetes mellitus). As a result, glucose does not enter cells and remains in the blood. Glucose levels in the blood increase, signaling the patient to increase intake of fluid in an effort to flush glucose out of the body in urine. Patients then experience increased thirst and increased urination. Cells become starved for energy because of the lack of glucose and signal the patient to eat, causing the patient to experience an increase in hunger. There are three types of diabetes mellitus:

- Type I, known as insulin-dependent (IDDM): Beta cells are destroyed by an autoimmune process.
- Type II known as non-insulin–dependent (NIDDM): Beta cells produce insufficient insulin.
- Gestational diabetes mellitus that occurs during pregnancy.

Patients with type I and type II diabetes mellitus are at risk for complications such as vision loss (diabetic retinopathy), damaged blood vessels and nerves (diabetic neuropathy), and kidney damage (nephropathy). However, complications can be minimized by maintaining a normal blood glucose level through consistent monitoring, administering insulin, and dieting. Patients with gestational diabetes mellitus will recover following pregnancy; however, they are at risk for developing type II diabetes mellitus later in life.

7.13.1 Signs and symptoms

- Type I:
  - Fast onset because no insulin is being produced.
  - Increased appetite (polyphagia) because cells are starved for energy, signaling a need for more food.
  - Increased thirst (polydipsia) from the body attempting to rid itself of glucose.
  - Increased urination (polyuria) from the body attempting to rid itself of glucose.
  - Weight loss because glucose is unable to enter cells.
  - Frequent infections as bacteria feed on the excess glucose.
  - Delayed healing because elevated glucose levels in the blood hinders the healing process.
- Type II:
  - Slow onset because some insulin is being produced.
  - Increased thirst (polydipsia) from the body attempting to rid itself of glucose.
  - Increased urination (polyuria) from the body attempting to rid itself of glucose.
  - Candidal infections as bacteria feed on the excess glucose.
  - Delayed healing because elevated glucose levels in the blood hinder the healing process.
- Gestational:
  - Asymptomatic.
  - Some patients may experience increased thirst (polydipsia) from the body attempting to rid itself of glucose.

7.13.2 Medical tests

- Increased glucose in urine (glucosuria).
- Fasting plasma blood glucose test with a serum glucose level of 126 mg/dl (7.0 mmol/L) on three different tests.
- Oral glucose tolerance test (OGTT) with plasma glucose of 200 mg/dl or 11.1 mmol/L 2 hours after ingesting 75 g oral glucose.
- Random plasma glucose at or above 200 mg/dl or 11.1 mmol/L.
- Glycosylated hemoglobin A1C 6.0% or higher.

7.13.3 Treatment

- Type I:
  - Regular monitoring of blood glucose.
  - Maintain a diabetic diet.
  - Administer:
    - Insulin to maintain normal blood glucose levels (see table 7.1).

TABLE 7.1 Insulin Guide

Drug	Synonym	Appearance	Onset	Peak	Duration	Compatibility
Rapid acting	Regular	Clear	1/2 to 1 hr	2 to 4 hr	6 to 8 hr	All insulin except ulralente
Intermediate acting	NPH	Cloudy	1 to 1.5 hr	8 to 12 hr	18 to 24 hr	Regular insulin
Long acting	Ultralente	Cloudy	4 to 6 hr	16 to 20 hr	30 to 36 hr	Regular

- Type II
  - Maintain ideal body weight through diet and exercise.
  - Regular monitoring of blood glucose.
  - Administer:
    - Oral sulfonylureas to stimulate secretion of insulin from the pancreas (see table 7.2).

TABLE 7.2 Oral Hypoglycemic Agents

Drug	Onset	Peak	Duration	Comments
Oral sulfonylureas				
Dymelor	1 hr	4 to 6 hr	12 to 24 hr	
Diabinase	1 hr	4 to 6 hr	40 to 60 hr	
Micronase, DiaBeta	15 min to 1 hr	2 to 8 hr	10 to 24 hr	
Oral biguanides				Decreases glucose production in liver,
Glucophage	2 to 2.5 hr		10 to 16 hr	decreases intestinal absorption of glucose, and improves insulin sensitivity
Oral alpha-glucosidose inhibitor		1 hr		Delays glucose absorption and digestion of carbohydrates, lowers blood sugar, reduces plasma glucose and insulin
Precose		2 to 3 hr		
Glyset	Rapid	2 to 3 hr		

- Gestational
  - Maintain weight through diet and exercise.
  - No oral diabetes medication; most are contraindicated in pregnancy.
  - Administer insulin if diet and exercise fail to control blood glucose levels.

7.13.4 Intervention

- Educate the patient about the disease and the importance of maintaining normal glucose levels.
- Demonstrate blood glucose monitoring.
- Review diet and food choices, including portion sizes.
- Encourage exercise.
- Discuss coping skills to reduce stress.
- Teach self-injection of insulin (type I).
- Urge smoking cessation.
- Instruct the patient:
  - Self-care.
  - Acute management.
  - Prevention of complications.
  - Importance of daily medications.
  - Hypoglycemia signs, symptoms, and interventions:
    - Sweating.
    - Lethargy.
    - Confusion.
    - Hunger.
    - Dizziness.
    - Weakness (type I).
  - Management of hypoglycemia:
    - Glucose tablets.
    - Four (4) oz fruit juice.
    - Several hard candies.
    - Small amount of a carbohydrate.
  - Signs and symptoms of hyperglycemia:
    - Fatigue.
    - Headache.
    - Blurry vision.
    - Dry, itchy skin.
  - Management of hyperglycemia:
    - Change in medication or dosage.
    - Increase in regular exercise.
    - More careful food intake and meal planning.

    - Increase in the number of finger sticks.
    - Discussion with the practitioner.
    - Glucagon injection for hypoglycemic events.

7.14 Metabolic Syndrome (Syndrome X/Dysmetabolic Syndrome)

In metabolic syndrome, patients have a collection of symptoms that include high blood glucose, obesity, high blood pressure, and high triglycerides based on family history. Beta cells in the pancreas are unable to produce sufficient insulin, and the liver produces a higher level of glucose. The patient is also insulin resistant. This syndrome leads to cardiovascular disease. A diagnosis of metabolic syndrome puts one at high risk for the development of diabetes and heart disease. Changes in lifestyle must be made to decrease the chance of incurring these diseases.

7.14.1 Signs and symptoms

- Hypertension.
- Abdominal obesity.

7.14.2 Medical tests

- Decreased high-density lipoprotein (HDL) level.
- Increased low-density lipoprotein (LDL) level.
- Increased triglycerides.
- Elevated fasting glucose.

7.14.3 Treatment

- Administer:
  - Statin to lower LDL:
    - Atorvastatin (Lipitor).
    - Simvastatin (Zocor).
    - Rosuvastatin (Crestor).
  - Antihyperlipidemic agent to raise HDL:
    - Niacin (Niaspan).
    - Fibrates to lower triglycerides.
  - Ace inhibitors to lower blood pressure:
    - Lisinopril (Prinivil).
    - Captopril (Capoten).
    - Enalapril (Vasotec).

- Angiotensin receptor blockers to lower blood pressure.
  - Losartan (Cozaar).
  - Candesartan (Atacand).
  - Irbesartan (Avapro).
- Insulin sensitizers to increase the effectiveness of insulin (see table 7.2).

- Manage weight through diet and exercise.

7.14.4 Intervention

- Monitor blood glucose.
- Encourage weight loss.
- Instruct the patient:
  - Continue medication even if symptoms are not present.

Solved Problems

7.1 What are signs of myxedema?

- Fatigue due to slow metabolism.
- Hypothermia due to slow metabolism.
- Brittle nails due to low levels of thyroid hormone, which helps growth and development.
- Thin, dry hair from lack of thyroid hormone.
- Dry skin from lack of thyroid hormone.
- Menstruation changes due to diminished levels of thyroid hormone.

7.2 What is a common rationale for a radionuclide thyroid imaging study?

To assess an enlarged thyroid gland following palpation.

7.3 Why is serum calcium assessed?

To assess parathyroid disorders.

7.4 What would a decreased calcium level indicate?

Hypoparathyroidism.

7.5 Why are serum catecholamine levels assessed?

Catecholamine levels are used to assess the function of the adrenal medulla.

7.6 Why would a practitioner order a glucose tolerance test?

A glucose tolerance test is used to assess for endocrine disorders.

7.7 What might be indicated by an increase in serum cortisol levels?

- Cushing's disease.
- Cushing's syndrome.

7.8 What would a decreased value resulting from the thyroid stimulating hormone test indicate?

Hyperthyroidism.

7.9 Why would a practitioner order antithyroid medication?

Antithyroid medication is administered to reduce production of the thyroid hormone for a patient diagnosed with hyperthyroidism.

7.10 What interventions are used to treat myxedema?

- Monitor vital signs.
- Provide a warm environment.
- Low-calorie diet.
- Increase fluids and fiber to prevent constipation.
- Take thyroid replacement hormone each morning to avoid insomnia.
- Monitor for signs of thyrotoxicosis (an increase in T3) (nausea, vomiting, diarrhea, sweating, tachycardia).

7.11 What medication is administered to a patient experiencing acute adrenal crisis?

Corticosteroids.

7.12 What is diabetes insipidus?

Either a decrease in antidiuretic hormone (ADH) production by the hypothalamus or the increase of ADH by the pituitary causes a decreased ability of the kidneys to concentrate urine. This results in the excretion of large amounts of diluted urine. The patient then drinks large amounts of fluid to replace the increased urine output.

7.13 What is Cushing's syndrome?

The adrenal cortex secretes an excess of glucocorticoids or the pituitary gland secretes an excess of ACTH as a result of a pituitary tumor, adrenal tumor, or ongoing glucocorticoid therapy.

7.14 What is SIADH?

Syndrome of inappropriate antidiuretic hormone secretion (SIADH) is caused by too much ADH being secreted by the posterior pituitary gland.

7.15 What might you suspect if a patient experiences uncontrollable hypertension, headaches, palpitations, and tachycardia?

Pheochromocytoma.

7.16 What are common instructions for patients who undergo thyroid hormone replacement?

- Administer medication early in the morning on an empty stomach.
- Avoid antacids that contain aluminum and magnesium that can decrease absorption of the medication.
- Blood level of medication must be monitored to avoid toxicity.

7.17 Why would you monitor signs of infection if the patient is receiving corticosteroids?

Corticosteroids decrease the inflammation response and may hide some common signs of infection.

7.18 Why would Benadryl and prednisone be administered to the patient before a radionuclide thyroid imaging study?

To reduce the risk of an allergic reaction to the iodine.

7.19 What is a hormone?

Hormones are chemical transmitters that stimulate organs to perform a specific physiological action.

7.20 What are causes of myxedema?

Hypothyroidism or myxedema can be caused by decreased production of the TSH hormone from the pituitary gland, a side effect of surgery, inflammation of the thyroid gland, and treatment for hyperthyroidism.

7.21 Why is it important to provide a cool environment for a patient diagnosed with Graves' disease?

The patient experiences an increased metabolic rate, which causes the patient to become sensitive to heat.

7.22 Why is calcium gluconate kept near the patient's bed if the patient underwent thyroid surgery?

The patient is at risk for decreased calcium levels, and calcium gluconate is administered to restore calcium levels.

7.23 What would you suspect if a patient who underwent thyroid surgery reports tingling of the hands and fingers?

Hypocalcemia.

7.24 What would you suspect if the patient who underwent thyroid surgery could not speak clearly and appeared hoarse?

Laryngeal edema.

7.25 What would you suspect if a patient appeared to have bronzing of the skin?

Addison's disease.

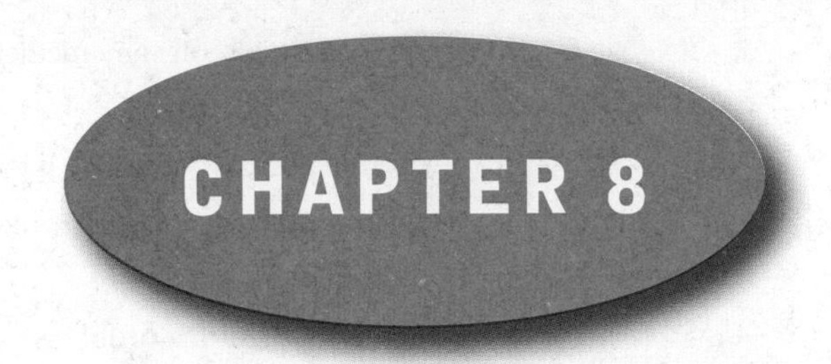

Environmental Critical Care

8.1 Definitions

- An environmental critical condition is a condition caused by environmental factors, such as temperature and exposure to materials, that can cause burns that alter any part of the body. This results in the patient becoming unstable.
- The patient's physiology can be disrupted by an inflammation, infection, or trauma.
- An environmental critical condition can be life threatening if the injury compromises the airway.
- An environmental critical condition can result in pain, discomfort, and disfigurement.
- Focus on the environmental critical symptoms after the patient's airway, breathing, circulation, and cervical spine are stabilized.
- An environmental critical condition requires immediate care.

8.1.1 Goal of treating environmental critical conditions

- The goal is to supplement the patient's systems until the patient's systems can maintain functionality during the healing process.
- Thoroughly assess the patient before beginning treatment.
- Diagnose acute problems.
- Stabilize the patient by relieving pain and treat acute problems.
- Refer the patient to a step-down unit.

8.1.2 Environmental assessment

- The environmental assessment interview:
  - Look for clues for underlying cause of the environmental emergency.
    - What happened prior to you noticing this problem?

    - Have you recently undergone any medical procedure?
        - What medical procedure?
        - When was the medical procedure performed?
  - Follow up questions help probe further into the presenting environmental problem.
    - When did this problem start?
    - How long have you had this problem?
    - Can you describe the problem?
    - How badly does the problem bother you?
    - Where do you feel uncomfortable?
    - Is the problem spreading or is the problem remaining in one place?
    - Does anything make the problem worse?
    - Does anything make the problem better?
    - Did you have this problem or a similar problem in the past?
        - Explain.
    - Have you been diagnosed with any medical condition?
        - What medical condition?
        - Are you being treated for the medical condition?
        - What is your treatment?
        - Who is treating you?
    - What medications do you use?
        - Prescribed.
        - Over the counter.
        - Cultural.
        - Herbal.
- Perform a physical assessment as described in Chapter 1 (1.4 Critical Care Thinking)
  - Inspect:
    - Ask the patient to show you the site of the injury or confirm the site if the injury is visible.
    - Remove the patient's clothes and inspect the patient beginning with the head. Look for other sites of injury besides those presented by the patient.
  - Percussion.
  - Palpation.
  - Auscultation:
    - In a fire, a patient's lungs may be burned without obvious signs and symptoms, resulting in pulmonary inflammation that can place the patient in respiratory distress.
    - Pulmonary inflammation can occur at any time.

8.1.2.1 Signs and symptoms

Environmental assessment in a critical care situation requires the nurse to recognize common signs and symptoms of underlying causes and then prepare for the anticipated treatment that the practitioner is likely to order. Commonly seen environmental signs and symptoms are:

- Disruption of skin (burns).
- Abnormal lung sounds (rhonchi, stridor, crackles).
- Discoloration of skin (reddened, cyanotic).

- Pain (burn).
- Burning sensation.
- Lack of pain in presence of severe burn (nerves are damaged).
- Change in voice (inflammation).
- Unusual breath odor (chemical ingestion).
- High or low temperature.
- Loss of consciousness.

8.2 Environmental Tests and Procedures

Environmental tests are designed to assess the effectiveness and capability of the cardiovascular and respiratory systems to function. Critical care practitioners order tests to collect objective data to further assess and to supplement that patient's systems. Once stabilized, the patient is transferred to a step-down care unit to treat the underlying cause of the current episode, which may require additional tests and procedures. The following environmental tests and procedures are commonly ordered by critical care practitioners.

8.2.1 Bronchoscopy

Bronchoscopy is a procedure that enables the healthcare provider to view the patient's larynx, trachea, and bronchi using a bronchoscope. The bronchoscope is a flexible tube that uses fiber optics to display images of the respiratory structure. The healthcare provider uses the bronchoscope to remove airway obstructions, including mucus, tumors, and foreign bodies. The bronchoscope is also used to obtain specimens for further testing. The bronchoscopy procedure:

- Administer atropine to decrease secretions.
- Administer midazolam (Versed) or other sedative and antianxiety medication to help relax the patient.
- Administer a topical anesthetic to the nasopharynx, vocal cords, and trachea to suppress the gagging reflex.
- Administer oxygen.
- Monitor vital signs.
- Insert the bronchoscope through the mouth or nose.
- Suction as necessary.
- Remove the obstruction or sample.
- After the bronchoscope is removed, raise the head of the bed 30 degrees or place the patient on his or her side.
- The patient must not receive anything by mouth until the gag response returns.
- Test for the return of the gag response.
- Monitor the patient's vital signs until the gag response returns.

8.2.2 Arterial blood gas (ABG)

The ABG test is a blood test in which an arterial blood sample is taken from the patient and assessed for oxygen (Pao_2), carbon dioxide ($Paco_2$), bicarbonate (HCO_3-), saturation oxygen (Sao_2), and pH levels in the blood. Normal ranges are:

- Pao_2: 80 to 100 mmHg.
- $Paco_2$: 35 to 45 mmHg.
- HCO_3-: 22 to 26 mEq/L.

- Sao_2: 95% to 100% of hemoglobin.
- pH: 7.35 to 7.45.

The pH value measures the concentration of hydrogen ions in arterial blood. A value greater than 7.45 indicates alkalosis, and a value lower than 7.35 indicates acidosis. The patient's blood must be within normal limits to be considered stabilized. Abnormal values indicate that the patient's body is trying to reestablish the acid-base (alkalosis) balance by having the metabolic system work together with the respiratory system to compensate for the acid-base imbalance.

The imbalance can be caused by a problem with the respiratory system. This is referred to as respiratory acidosis or respiratory alkalosis. The imbalance can be caused by a problem with the metabolic system. This is referred to as metabolic acidosis or metabolic alkalosis. The results of the ABG test can help you identify the underlying cause, as shown in table 8.1.

TABLE 8.1 Acid-Base Values

	pH	Pco_2	HCO3-	Signs	Causes
Respiratory acidosis (too much carbon dioxide retained)	<7.35	>45 mmHg	>26 mEq/L (metabolic system compensating)	Flushed face Sweating Restlessness Tachycardia Headache	Hypoventilation Asphyxia Decreased central nervous system function
Respiratory alkalosis (too little carbon dioxide retained)	>7.45	<35 mmHg	<22 mEq/L	Anxiety Rapid deep breathing Light-headedness	Hyperventilation Gram-negative bacteria infection Increased respiratory function related to medication
Metabolic acidosis (too little bicarbonate retained)	<7.35	<35 mmHg (respiratory system compensating)	<22 mEq/L (metabolic system compensating)	Drowsiness Vomiting Nausea Rapid deep breathing Fruity breath Headache	Diarrhea Renal disease Hepatic disease Medication intoxication Shock Endocrine disorder
Metabolic alkalosis (too much bicarbonate retained)	>7.45	>45 mmHg (respiratory system compensating)	>26 mEq/L	Ringing in the ear Confusion Slow, shallow breathing Irritability	Vomiting Gastric suctioning Steroid administration Diuretic therapy Decreased potassium levels

It is important that any supplemental oxygen or ventilation assistance administered to the patient shortly before or when the sample is taken is noted on the sample documentation. This enables the lab to adjust the results accordingly.

Because the sample is taken from an artery, you must apply pressure to the puncture site for 5 minutes and apply a pressure dressing for 30 minutes once the bleeding stops. The site then needs to be monitored regularly to ensure there is no residual bleeding.

8.2.3 Electrocardiograph (ECG)

The ECG shows a graphic representation of the electrical activity of the heart in a three-dimensional perspective. An electrical signal is generated each time the heart contracts. Small pads containing electrodes are placed on the surface of the skin to detect the electrical signal. Six electrodes are placed on the chest and six on the arms and legs. Each electrode is connected with wires to an ECG machine that draws up to 12 different graphical representations of the electrical signal. *Schaum's Outline of ECG Interpretation* provides details on how to administer an ECG and how to interpret the results.

- P wave: The first deflection is recorded as the P wave and starts when there is electrical activity at the SA node of the heart, indicating atrial contraction (depolarization).
- PR interval: The period between the end of the P wave and the beginning of the QRS complex is called the PR interval (PRI). This is the time the electrical impulse takes to travel to the ventricles after atrial relaxation (repolarization).
- QRS complex: This represents ventricle contraction (depolarization).
- ST segment: The S wave represents the end of ventricle contraction. The T wave represents ventricle relaxation.
- QT interval (QTI): This represents the complete cycle of ventricle contraction and ventricle relaxation.

8.2.4 Blood chemistry

Blood chemistry is a laboratory test of venous blood. It examines levels of enzymes and other elements in blood to develop a profile of the patient's health. This test is usually performed routinely for critical care patients because results provide the healthcare provider with objective information about how well the patient's systems are functioning.

Blood chemistry results typically include:

- Electrolyte balance (sodium, potassium, bicarbonate, magnesium, calcium, phosphorus).
- Kidney function (blood urea nitrogen [BUN], creatinine).
- Liver function (aspartate aminotransferase [AST]/alanine aminotransferase [ALT]).
- Diabetes: (serum glucose).
- Cholesterol level: cholesterol, LDL, HDL, triglycerides).

Enzymes are normally inside the cell. As cells rupture during normal events, enzymes leave the cell and enter the bloodstream. The laboratory determines the normal level of a particular enzyme in the blood. A level greater than the normal level indicates more than the normal number of cells was injured, indicating something unusual is happening with the patient.

Enzyme levels might increase gradually and then return to normal level. This might occur with a myocardial infarction, when blood supply to a port of cardiac tissue is interrupted, leading to the death of some cardiac tissue. Several hours may pass before the enzyme levels are abnormal, and then they decrease hours later when no more cardiac tissue is injured.

It is important to look for obvious reasons why enzyme levels or other values are abnormal before assuming that the patient is unstable related to the test results. For example, a patient who exercised before coming to the emergency department will have elevated muscle cell enzymes because exercising injures muscles. Likewise, a patient who ate a normal breakfast before visiting the emergency department will have high blood glucose levels.

8.2.5 Hematologic studies

Hematologic studies profile the patient's blood and include:

- Red blood cell (RBC) count.
- White blood cell (WBC) count, indicating inflammation.
- Erythrocyte sedimentation rate (ESR).
- Bleeding (prothrombin time [PT], international normalized ratio [INR], partial thromboplastin time, platelet count).
- Hemoglobin and hematocrit (Hgb, Hct).

8.2.6 Gastric lavage

Gastric lavage is a procedure used to flush the stomach of ingested material using a lavage tube that is inserted into the patient's esophagus and stomach. Gastric lavage is typically used following poisoning, resulting in decreased gag reflex and as directed by poison control. Gastric lavage is only effective within a half hour following ingestion of the toxin material. Activated charcoal (see 8.3.5 Activated charcoal) is administered following gastric lavage and if more than a half-hour has passed since the patient ingested the toxin. Gastric lavage can be:

- Intermittent: Flushing occurs as needed and is specified in the practitioner's order.
- Continuous: Flushing occurs without interruption.

Do not use gastric lavage if you suspect that the following material was ingested because the material may compromise the integrity of the gastric lavage tube, resulting in the material injuring the esophagus:

- Ammonia.
- Mineral acids.
- Petroleum products.
- Alkalis.
- Corrosive material.

The material may remain corrosive once removed from the patient, and therefore the material must be disposed of appropriately, based on hospital policy.

8.2.7 Dialysis

Dialysis is mechanical/chemical process that is used to assist the kidney remove toxins from the blood when an antidote is unavailable and gastric lavage and activated charcoal are ineffective or not appropriate. In dialysis, the patient's vascular system is attached to the dialysis device that filters the blood, replacing the function of the kidneys.

During dialysis:

- Monitor vital signs constantly or at least every 15 minutes per practitioner's order.
- Perform an INR/PT/PTT blood test periodically to assess for clotting.

8.3 Environmental Medication

Commonly used medications in environmental critical care are nonsteroidal anti-inflammatory drugs (NSAIDs), corticosteroids, analgesics, and antibiotics. These medications reduce pain and discomfort by reducing pressure on nerves caused by inflammation and by blocking neurologic transmission. Antibiotics assist the immune system with combatting bacterial infection.

8.3.1 Nonsteroidal Anti-inflammatory Drugs (NSAIDs)

NSAIDs are medications that reduce swelling, pain, and stiffness without exposing the patient to the adverse side effects that occur when using corticosteroid medication.

- Aspirin (ASA).
- Ibuprofen (Motrin, Advil, Nuprin).
- Naproxen (Naprosyn, Aleve).
- Oxaprozin (Daypro).
- Ketoprofen (Orudis).
- Diclofenac sodium (Voltaren).
- Ketorolac (Toradol).
- Celecoxib (Celebrex).

8.3.2 Corticosteroids

Corticosteroids are used to reduce inflammation and cerebral edema. Corticosteroids may increase the risk of pancreatitis, heart failure, and thromboembolism.

- Dexamethasone (Dexone).
- Methylprednisolone (Solu-Medrol).
- Dexamethasone (Decadron).

8.3.3 Analgesics

Analgesics are used to reduce pain.

- Oxycodone (OxyContin).
- Morphine (Duramorph).

8.3.4 Antibiotics

Antibiotics are used to treat bacterial infections such as sinus infection and conjunctivitis.

- Bacitracin (Baciguent).
- Cefuroxime (Ceftin).
- Cephalexin (Keflex).
- Ceftibuten (Cedax).
- Erythromycin (Ilotycin).
- Gentamicin (Garamycin).
- Neosporin (Bactrim).
- Tobramycin (Tobrex).

8.3.5 Activated charcoal

Activated charcoal is used to treat ingestion of toxic chemicals or drugs by absorbing the toxin in the gastrointestinal tract. The patient ingests the fine, black powder activated charcoal, which absorbs up to 60% of the toxin using the process called adsorption. Adsorption occurs when the toxin attaches to the activated charcoal. Activated charcoal is not absorbed by the body and therefore passes through the gastrointestinal tract and is eliminated through a bowel movement. Activated charcoal is administered in conjunction with sorbitol (see 8.3.6 Sorbitol).

- Activated charcoal is administered:
  - Awake and alert: Drinking a black liquid drink.
  - Patient vomiting: Through a nasogastric or orogastric tube.
- Activated charcoal does not bind well with:
  - Sodium.
  - Iron.
  - Lithium.
  - Iodine.
  - Boric acid.
  - Fluorine.
  - Lead.
  - Iron.
  - Alcohol.
  - Acetone.
  - Petroleum products.
  - Plant oils.
- Do not administer activated charcoal if:
  - There is an intestinal obstruction.
  - A corrosive (acid/alkali) toxin was ingested.
  - An antidote was administered.

8.3.6 Sorbitol

Sorbitol is a sugar substitute that stimulates the bowels and is used in conjunction with activated charcoal to move the activated charcoal through the gastrointestinal tract quickly, reducing the risk of constipation, which is a side effect of activated charcoal. Monitor the patient for dehydration and chemical imbalance because frequent doses of sorbitol can cause diarrhea.

Do not administer sorbitol if:

- The patient is less than one year old because doing so can result in excessive fluid losses.
- The patient is fructose intolerant.

8.4 Hyperthermia

Hyperthermia is a condition in which body temperature is greater than 99°F, resulting from the body's inability to dissipate heat sufficiently to maintain normal body temperature. Heat is generated by ambient temperature such as being exposed to very hot temperature. Heat can also increase when the body's temperature-regulating mechanism has malfunctioned. The hypothalamus coordinates changes in the neurological and cardiovascular systems to regulate body temperature. Veins dilate with hot temperatures to help cool blood. Sweat glands excrete fluids to cool the skin. Veins contract in cold temperatures to help warm the blood. Disorders such as cardiovascular disorders and dehydration can lead to malfunction of the temperature-regulating system, leading to hyperthermia and the risk of hypovolemic shock.

There are three classifications of hyperthermia. These are:

- Mild: Heat cramps. Excessive perspiration. Temperatures 99°F to 102°F.
- Moderate: Heat exhaustion. Blood accumulates in the skin, decreasing the amount of circulating blood. Temperatures 104°F to 106°F.
- Critical: Heatstroke. Internal organs are affected. Temperatures greater than 106°F.

8.4.1 Signs and symptoms

- Skin: Moist, cool (mild).
- Skin: Pale, moist (moderate).
- Skin: Hot, dry, reddened (critical).
- Hypertension (mild).
- Hypotension (moderate).
- Agitation (mild).
- Confusion (moderate).
- Combativeness (critical).
- Nausea (mild).
- Vomiting (moderate).
- Tachycardia (mild, moderate, critical).
- Loss of consciousness (critical).
- Muscle spasms (mild).
- Syncope (moderate).
- Dizziness (moderate).
- Low urine output (oliguria) (moderate).
- Fixed, dilated pupils (critical).
- Weakness (moderate).
- Seizures (critical).
- Tachypnea (critical).

8.4.2 Medical tests

- Urinalysis: Increases in:
  - Protein.
  - Concentration.
  - Myoglobin.
  - Tubular casts.

- Complete blood count: Increases in:
  - Hematocrit.
  - WBCs.
  - BUN.

8.4.3 Treatment

- Remove patient's clothes.
- Apply cooling blankets.
- Apply ice packs to groin area.
- Avoid cooling too quickly, which might result in shivering, leading to decreased circulation and increased oxygen demand.
- Administer:
  - Chlorpromazine (Thorazine) or diazepam (Valium) to reduce shivering.
  - Oxygen.

8.4.4 Intervention

- Monitor vital signs.
- Classify the degree of hyperthermia.
- Monitor renal functions.
- Monitor fluids and electrolytes.
- Monitor cardiac function using an ECG.
- Instruct the patient:
  - How to avoid hyperthermia.
  - How to recognize signs of hyperthermia.
  - To hydrate with water.
  - To avoid outdoor exercise in hot weather.

8.5 Hypothermia

Hypothermia is a condition in which body temperature is less than 95°F, resulting from the body's inability to retain heat sufficiently to maintain normal body temperature. Heat is lost by exposure to very cold temperatures. Heat can also be lost when the body's temperature-regulating mechanism has malfunctioned. Veins contract in cold temperatures to help warm the blood. The body shivers to stay warm, resulting in decreased circulation and increased oxygen demand.

There are three classifications of hypothermia. These are:

- Mild: Shivering, slurred speech, loss of coordination, and amnesia. Temperatures 88.6°F to 95°F.
- Moderate: Cyanosis, rigidity, and unresponsive. Temperatures 86°F to 88.6°F.
- Critical: No pulse, absence of deep tendon reflexes, pupils dilated, ventricular fibrillation. Temperature below 86°F.

Caution:

- Do not use tympanic thermometer to measure temperature.
- Surface warming is ineffective in critical hypothermia.
- Lidocaine is ineffective in ventricular dysrhythmias related to hypothermia.
- Do not perform chest compressions if the patient's chest is frozen.
- Do not defibrillate when patient's temperature is below 86ºF.

8.5.1 Signs and symptoms

- Slurred Speech (mild).
- Shivering (mild).
- Cyanosis (moderate).
- Amnesia (mild).
- Atrial fibrillation (critical).
- Ventricular fibrillation (critical).
- Pupils dilated (critical).
- Absence of deep tendon reflex (critical).
- Rigidity (moderate).
- Unresponsive (critical).
- No pulse (critical).

8.5.2 Medical tests

- Doppler: Used to locate pulse.
- Plethysmography: Used to assess the impact of frostbite.
- Pertechnetate scan: Shows perfusion and assesses damage to deep tissue.

8.5.3 Treatment

- Remove patient's wet clothes and replace with dry clothes.
- Provide external warming with heated blankets and radiant heat lamps.
- Extracorporeal rewarming to rewarm core blood.
- Full-body immersion in warm water (Hubbard tank technique).
- Administer:
  - Heated normal saline administered intravenously.
  - Oxygen.

8.5.4 Intervention

- Monitor vital signs.
- Monitor cardiac rhythms with an ECG.

- Measure core temperatures with rectal, esophageal, or bladder thermometer.
  - Make sure that the thermometer can measure very low temperatures.
  - Do not insert rectal thermometer into stool.
- Classify the degree of hypothermia.
- Be alert for a sudden drop in blood pressure (warming shock).
- Carefully handle the patient in moderate to critical hypothermia to prevent cardiac degeneration.
- Instruct the patient:
  - To avoid exposure to cold temperatures.
  - To remove wet clothes immediately.

8.6 Burns

A burn is damage to the skin as a result of exposure to an external heat source such as fire, electricity, or chemicals. Cells die directly from the trauma or as a result of decreased circulation to the affected area. Collagen in the skin is destroyed, leading to intravascular fluid moving into interstitial spaces. There is increased capillary permeability as the inflammation process mediates the burn site.

Burns are described by the depth of the burn:

- Superficial burn (first-degree): Affects the surface of the epidermis. There is pain and redness. No blisters.
- Superficial partial-thickness (first-degree): Affects the epidermis. The injury is painful. The skin remains a barrier between the environment and internal structures.
- Deep partial-thickness (second-degree): Affects the epidermis and dermis. Blisters form. There is swelling (edema) and pain. Hair follicles remain functional. There is less pain because of neurologic damage at the site. The skin no longer remains a barrier between the environment and internal structures.
- Full-thickness (third-degree): Affects the epidermis, dermis, subcutaneous tissues, and muscle. There is swelling but little pain related to neurologic damage at the site.

Measure the burn size using the body surface area (BSA) charts, the rule of nines, and Lund and Browder Classification to estimate the amount of fluids that need to be replaced. There are two BSA charts used to estimate the size of the burn. These are the adult BSA chart (fig. 8.1) and the infant BSA chart (fig. 8.2).

The rule of nines is used estimate the burn size of an adult. Each area of the body is assigned a percentage based on the number 9 except for the groin area, which is 1%. This enables you to quickly assess the size of the burn.

The Lund and Browder Classification is used to estimate the burn size for infants and children because of their different body shapes. Table 8.2 lists the burn percentage by age to determine the Lund and Browder Classification of the patient.

TABLE 8.2 Lund and Browder Classification

At Birth	0 to 1 yr	1 to 4 yr	5 to 9 yr	10 to 15 yr	Adult
A: Half of head					
8.5%	8.5%	6.5%	5.5%	4.5%	4.3%
B. Half of one thigh					
2.75%	3.25%	4%	4.25%	4.25%	4.75%
C. Half of one leg					
2.5%	2.5%	2.75%	3%	3.25%	3.5%

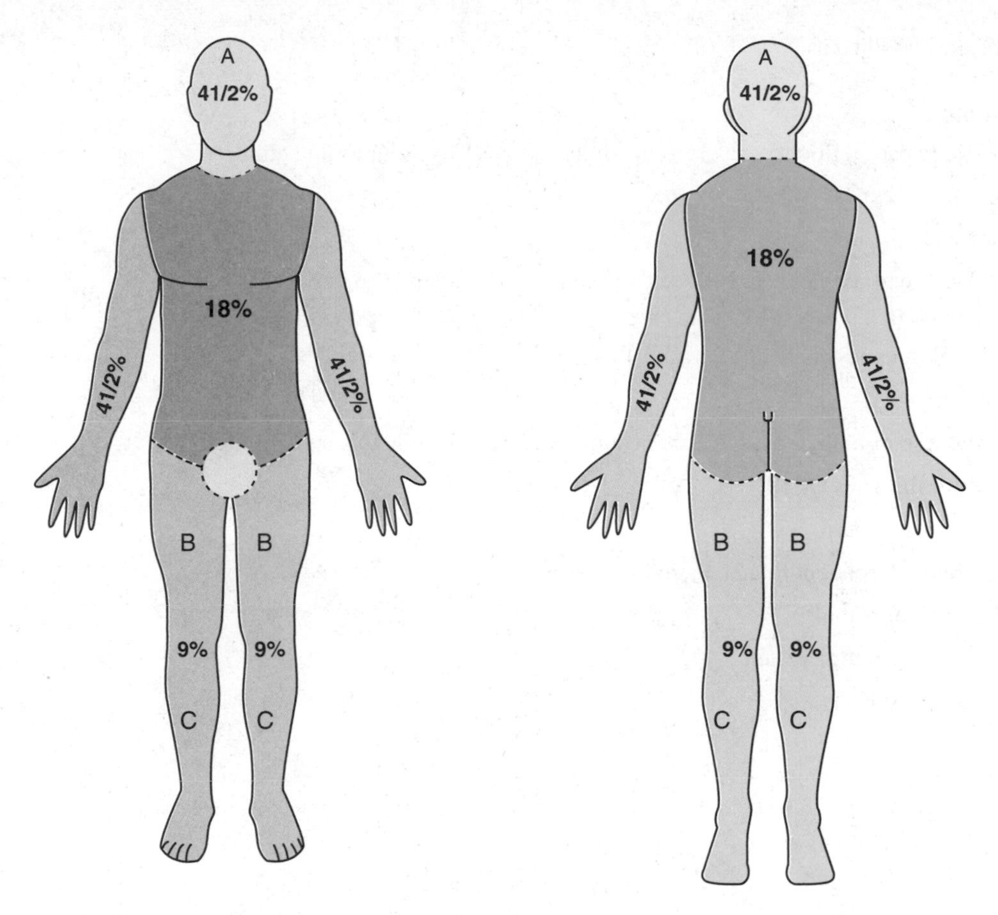

Figure 8.1 Apply the rule of nines to calculate the size of the burn for adults.

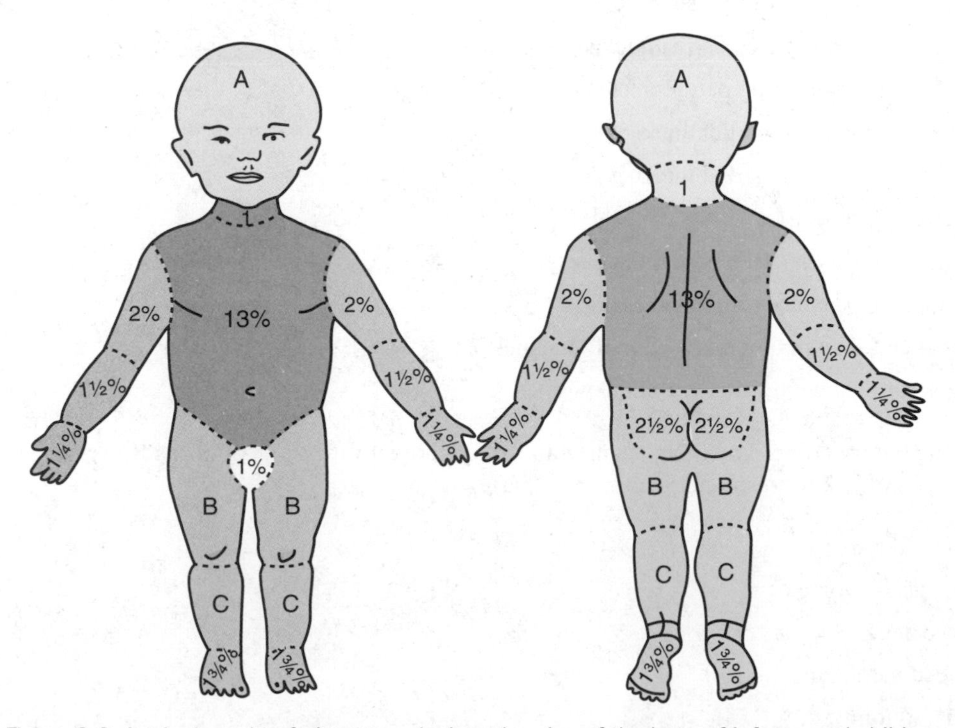

Figure 8.2 Apply the rule of nines to calculate the size of the burn of infants and children.

Burns are classified as:

- Minor:
  - Deep partial thickness <15% in adults and <10% in infants and children.
  - Full thickness <2%.
- Moderate:
  - Deep partial thickness between 15% and 25% in adults and between 10% and 20% in infants and children.
  - Full thickness between 2% and 10%.
- Major:
  - Deep partial thickness >25% in adults and <20% in infants and children.
  - Full thickness <10%.
  - Electrical burn.
  - High-risk patient related to codiagnosis.
  - Involvement of:
    - Respiratory system.
    - Fractures.
    - Face.
    - Hands.
    - Genitalia.
    - Feet.

8.6.1 Signs and symptoms

- Reddened skin (erythema) (superficial).
- Swelling (edema) (deep partial thickness).
- Nausea/vomiting (deep partial thickness).
- Shivers (superficial partial thickness).
- Blisters (superficial partial thickness).
- Charred site (electrical).
- Waxy, white color (deep partial thickness).
- Leathery appearance (full thickness).
- Blood clot seen in blood vessels (full thickness).
- Black, brown, white color (full thickness).

Caution: Respiratory compromise can occur with little or no outward signs of burns if respiratory tissues are damaged. Signs of risk for respiratory compromise are:

- Mucosal burns.
- Changes in voice.
- Wheezing.
- Singed nasal hairs.
- Dark sputum.

- Coughing.
- Darkened nose and mouth.
- Burns on the neck or chest.

8.6.2 Medical tests

- Urine tests:
  - Myoglobin: Presence indicates renal involvement.
- Blood tests:
  - Creatine kinase (CK): Elevated indicates muscle damage.
  - Myoglobin: Elevated indicates muscle damage.
  - Carboxyhemoglobin: Elevated indicates smoke inhalation.
  - BUN: Elevated relates to increased protein breakdown and fluid loss.
  - Total protein: Decrease indicates protein breakdown.
  - Albumin: Decrease indicates fluid switch to interstitial space.
  - Hct: Increase relates to decrease in fluid.
  - WBCs: Increase relates to inflammation or infection.
  - Hgb: Decrease relates to the breakdown of red blood cells.
  - Sodium: Decrease relates to fluid shift.
  - Potassium: Increase relates to the destruction of cells and fluid shift.

8.6.3 Treatment

- Irrigate chemical burns with saline solution.
- Insert nasogastric tube to suction or aspirate stomach contents.
- Insert indwelling urinary catheter to monitor urinary output.
- Fluid replacement:
  - Lactated Ringer's solution: Use the Parkland formula to calculate the amount of lactated Ringer's solution to administer over the first 24 hours.
    - Amount to infuse = 4 ml × weight in kilograms × BSA percentage of affected area.
  - Administer the total amount to infuse:
    - Fifty percent (50%) in the first 8 hours of time of injury, not the time of arrival.
    - Fifty percent (50%) over the next 16 hours.
- Administer:
  - Humidified oxygen.
  - Nonsteroidal anti-inflammatory:
    - Ibuprofen (Motrin, Advil).
    - Naproxen (Naprosyn, Aleve).
    - Flurbiprofen (Ansaid).

- Topical antibiotic:
  - Neosporin (superficial).
  - Bacitracin (superficial and ocular burns).
  - Silvadene (severe dermal burns).
- Analgesics:
  - Morphine sulfate.
  - Meperidine (Demerol).
  - Vicodin.
- Diuretics:
  - Mannitol (Osmitrol) (restores urinary output).

8.6.4 Intervention

- Monitor airway, breathing, and circulation.
- Nothing by mouth (NPO).
- Position patient in semi-Fowler's position.
- Intubate if airway is compromised.
- Remove patient's clothes. Clothes may contain the material that caused the burn.
- Cover burn site with sterile, dry bed sheets.
- Monitor for signs of overreplacement of fluid:
  - Pulmonary edema.
  - Cardiac failure.
- Monitor for signs of underreplacement of fluid:
  - Hypovolemic shock.
- Administer medication intravenously and not intramuscularly due to impaired absorptions of damaged muscle tissue.
- Monitor for signs of compartment syndrome in full-thickness burns. As tissue rehydrates from infusion of fluids, the inelasticity of burnt tissue can decrease circulation, resulting in decreased pulse in the affected area. The practitioner may perform an escharotomy, a surgical procedure to expose fatty tissue below the site, resulting in reducing the constriction.
- Instruct the patient:
  - Drink 3 L of fluid per day to avoid crystallization of uric acid.
  - Eat a low-fat, low-cholesterol diet.
  - Avoid foods that are high in purine proteins such as turkey, organ meats, sardines, smelts, mackerel, anchovies, herring, and bacon.
  - Avoid alcohol, which inhibits renal excretion of uric acid.

8.7 Poisoning

A poison is a material that results in a chemical reaction that disrupts bodily functions, resulting in nausea, vomiting, changes in heart rate, changes in breathing, confusion, or seizures. Symptoms reflect the type of poison and can occur immediately or hours, days, or months following exposure. The goal is to identify the poison and to prevent or reduce the absorption of the poison by administering an antidote or eliminating the poison from the body.

A poison enters the body through:

- Ingestion.
- The skin.
- Inhalation.
- Injection.
- Animal bite.

8.7.1 Signs and symptoms

- Delayed symptoms.
- Increase or decrease in heart rate.
- Increase or decrease in respiration.
- Dilated or constricted pupils.
- Low level of consciousness or hyperactivity.
- Sweating or excessive dryness.

8.7.2 Medical tests

- Toxicology screen: Tests for common poisons.
- ECG: Assesses for abnormal cardiac activity related to a poison.
- Brain CT scan: Assesses structural changes in the brain related to a poison.

8.7.3 Treatment

- Intubation if the patient is unconscious.
- Call poison control (1-800-222-1222) and follow their advice.
- Gastric lavage, if not caustic material and material has not passed the stomach.
- Administer:
  - Poison-specific antidote provided by poison control.
  - Activated charcoal, if caustic material and if material has passed the stomach.
  - Whole bowel irrigant to flush the gastrointestinal tract to prevent absorption:
    - Golytely.
  - Sedative, if patient is agitated:
    - Clonazepam (Klonopin).
    - Diazepam (Valium).
  - Antiseizure, if patient has a seizure.
    - Lorazepam (Ativan).

8.7.4 Intervention

- Monitor airway, breathing, and circulation.
- Ask the patient, friends, or relatives for information that may lead you to identify the poison.
- Make sure everyone knows that telling the truth may save the patient's life. Some patients, friends, and relatives may conceal the truth to avoid undesirable consequence related to the poisoning.
- Determine medication that is available to the patient, either prescribed to the patient or to friends and family.
- Determine whether the patient uses street drugs.
- Assess what poisonous materials may be around the patient's house or workplace.
- Ask whether the patient was bitten or was in the outdoors any time prior to when the signs and symptoms of the poisoning began.
- Estimate the time that the poison was introduced into the patient's body.
- Assume that the material is caustic until proven otherwise.
- Assume that the patient has been poisoned even if no signs and symptoms are present. The patient, friends, or family have reason to believe that a poisoning may have occurred. Signs and symptoms of poisoning can be delayed.
- Assess the patient's general medical condition. Signs and symptoms of poisoning may actually be signs and symptoms of an underlying medical condition rather than a poison.
- Instruct the patient:
  - That treatment will minimize the impact of the poison on the patient's body.
  - How to avoid accidental poisoning.
  - What to do if an accidental poisoning occurs again and the importance of getting medical help immediately.

Solved Problems

8.1 What is the goal of treating a patient who is in an environmental critical condition?

The goal is to supplement the patient's systems until the patient's systems can maintain functionality during the healing process.

8.2 When should you focus on the patient's environmental critical symptoms?

Focus on the environmental critical symptoms after the patient's airway, breathing, circulation, and cervical spine are stabilized.

8.3 What are the common signs and symptoms of an environmental critical condition?

- Disruption of skin (burns).
- Abnormal lung sounds (rhonchi, stridor, crackles).
- Discoloration of skin (reddened, cyanotic).
- Pain (burn).
- Burning sensation.
- Lack of pain in the presence of severe burn (nerves are damaged).
- Change in voice (inflammation).

- Unusual breath odor (chemical ingestion).
- High or low temperature.
- Loss of consciousness.

8.4 Why is atropine administered when the patient undergoes bronchoscopy?

To decrease secretions.

8.5 When can the patient receive fluids by mouth after bronchoscopy?

The patient must not receive anything by mouth until the gag response returns.

8.6 What is the purpose of testing arterial blood gas?

A primary reason to test arterial blood gas is to determine whether the body is compensating for failure of a system that results in acidosis or alkalosis.

8.7 What would a low platelet count indicate?

Risk of bleeding.

8.8 Why would a critical care patient receive dialysis?

Dialysis compensates for the patient's kidneys when the kidneys are unable to fully remove toxins from the blood.

8.9 What internal abnormality might cause hyperthermia?

Malfunctioning of the hypothalamus may result in hyperthermia.

8.10 Why would a patient receive sorbitol on a critical care unit?

Sorbitol is a sugar substitute that stimulates the bowels and is used in conjunction with activated charcoal to move the activated charcoal through the gastrointestinal tract quickly, reducing the risk of constipation, which is a side effect of activated charcoal. The patient would receive sorbitol on the critical care unit if the patient received activated charcoal in the emergency department.

8.11 What symptoms would you suspect in a patient who has heatstroke?

- Temperature greater than 106°F.
- Skin is hot, dry, reddened.
- Patient is combative.
- Tachycardia.
- Pupils are fixed and dilated.
- Loss of consciousness.
- Seizure.
- Tachypnea.

8.12 What medication would you expect to administer to a patient diagnosed with hyperthermia who is shivering?

Chlorpromazine (Thorazine) or diazepam (Valium) to reduce shivering.

8.13 How would you respond if you were ordered to surface warm a patient whose temperature is less than 86°F?

Ask for clarification, because surface warming is ineffective in critical hypothermia.

8.14 What is warming shock?

Warming shock is a sudden drop in blood pressure as the patient is warmed.

8.15 What are two factors to avoid when measuring a patient's temperature who has hypothermia or hyperthermia?

- Make sure that the thermometer can measure very low and very high temperatures.
- Make sure not to insert the rectal thermometer into stool.

8.16 How would you determine the amount of lactated Ringer's solution to administer to a burn patient?

Use the Parkland formula.

8.17 What would you use to irrigate a chemical burn?

Saline solution.

8.18 Why would mannitol be administered to a burn patient?

To restore urinary output.

8.19 What is a sign of replacement fluid overload in a burn patient?

Pulmonary edema.

8.20 What can result if too little fluid is administered to a burn patient?

Hypovolemic shock.

8.21 What is the best method of administering medication to a burn patient?

Large-bore IV.

8.22 What would you do if a medication order stated to administer the medication intramuscularly to a burn patient?

Ask for clarification. Intramuscular medication is not administered to a burn patient because of impaired absorption of damaged muscle tissue.

8.23 What must be considered when assessing signs and symptoms of a patient who is reported to have been poisoned?

Signs and symptoms of poisoning may actually be signs and symptoms of an underlying medical condition rather than a poison.

8.24 Why would a brain CT scan be ordered for a patient who has been poisoned?

Assesses structural changes in the brain related to a poison.

8.25 What would you do if a burn patient's voice changes?

Assess for respiratory compromise. A change in voice may indicate edema that may lead to respiratory distress.

Neurologic Critical Care

9.1 Definitions

- A neurologic critical condition is a condition that alters the neurologic system, resulting in a temporary or permanent disability that may be life threatening to the patient.
- A neurologic critical condition is considered life threatening until proven otherwise.
- Subtle changes in the patient's presentation can indicate deterioration of the patient's neurologic system.
- Focus on neurologic problems after the patient's airway, breathing, circulation, and cervical spine are stabilized.
- The first sign of a neurologic critical condition is the patient's altered mental status (AMS). Level of conscience (LOC) is the most important indicator of neurologic function.
- Neurologic critical care requires immediate intervention.

9.1.1 Goals of treating neurologic critical conditions

- The goal of the critical care staff is to identify the neurologic critical condition and supplement the patient's systems until the patient is stabilized.
- Stabilize the airway, breathing, and circulation before focusing on the underlying neurologic problem.
- Diagnose and treat the acute problem.
- Establish a baseline of the patient's mental status on arrival. Reassess the patient's mental status during the patient's stay, comparing the results to the baseline to determine whether the patient's mental status has changed.
- Assess the patient completely before beginning treatment.
- Refer the patient to a step-down unit once the patient stabilizes.

9.1.2 Neurologic assessment

- Begin with a head-to-toe examination.
- Assess for causes of altered mental status.
    - AEIOU:
        - Alcohol, arrhythmia.
        - Endocrine/exocrine, electrolytes, encephalopathy.
        - Insulin.
        - Oxygen, opiates.
        - Uremia.
    - TIPS:
        - Trauma, temperature disorders.
        - Infection.
        - Psychiatric, porphyria, poisons.
        - Shock, seizures, stroke, subarachnoid hemorrhage, space-occupying lesion.
- A patient who has a neurologic impairment may present as:
    - Alert and oriented, reporting signs of neurologic impairment.
        - Focus your interview on the patient.
    - Disoriented and in an altered mental state and unable to report signs of neurologic impairment.
        - Focus your interview on family and friends who accompanied the patient to the hospital or who can provide information about the patient's condition via phone.
- The neurologic assessment interview begins with open-ended questions:
    - Why did you come to the hospital today?
    - What makes you feel that something is wrong?
- Next gather more information about each sign reported by the patient:
    - Describe what you are feeling.
    - When did you first notice it?
    - What were you doing when you first noticed it?
    - Did this ever happen before today?
- Next ask about the patient's health history:
    - Are you being treated for any illness?
    - Were you treated for any illness in the past?
    - Were your injured recently or in the past?
    - Do you have any allergies?
    - Have you had any surgeries?
- Next ask about the patient's lifestyle:
    - What is your occupation?
    - Were you ever exposed to toxic chemicals?
    - Do you or people around you use recreational drugs?

    - Do you smoke?
    - Do you drink alcohol?
    - Do you have any hobbies that may have exposed you to toxic chemicals?
- Assess the patient's altered mental status.
    - Alert: The patient responds to stimuli with little or no delay.
    - Oriented: The patient is oriented to time, person, and place.
        - What day is this?
        - What is your name?
        - Where are you?
- Sleepy: The patient is arousable to a normal level of awareness.
- Lethargic: The patient has a global depressed awareness of the environment and of the patient himself or herself.
- Stupor: The patient is sleepy and can be aroused to a seminormal level of awareness using noxious stimuli.
- Coma: The patient cannot be aroused.
- Delirium: The patient is acutely confused, showing psychomotor excitement and impaired memory and perception. The patient may experience hallucination.
- Dementia: A gradual deterioration of mental function.
- Assess for mental impairment using the Abbreviated Mental Test Score (AMTS). Each question is valued at 1 point. A score of 6 or less suggests mental impairment that requires further testing.
    - What is your age?
    - What is the time to the nearest hour?
    - What year is this?
    - What is the name of this hospital?
    - Do you know who I am? Do you know who this person is? The patient is expected to recognize two people who are in the room by name or title.
    - When was Pearl Harbor attacked? Any important historical event can be asked.
    - Who is the president of the United States?
    - Count backwards from 20 to 1.
    - Mention an address to the patient then ask the patient to repeat the address.
- Develop the patient's baseline mental status using the Glasgow Coma Scale (see Chapter 1, 1.4.3 Assessment).
- Assess breath odor.
    - Alcohol: Might indicate alcohol intoxication as a cause of neural impairment. However, do not assume that alcohol is the underlying cause of neural impairment because the patient's breath smells of alcohol. Rule out other possible causes.
    - Acetone: Might indicate diabetic ketoacidosis as a cause for neural impairment that can be reversed by administering insulin and fluids.
- Assess cardiac effectiveness.
    - Cardiac arrhythmia results in decreased circulatory function, leading to decreased oxygenation and neural impairment.

- Assess respiratory effectiveness.
    - Respiratory disorder may result in ineffective gas exchange, leading to decreased oxygenation and neural impairment.

9.1.2.1 Signs and symptoms

Neurologic assessment in a critical care situation requires the nurse to recognize common signs and symptoms of underlying causes and then prepare for the anticipated treatment that the practitioner is likely to order.

Commonly seen signs and symptoms:

- Changes in pupils:
    - Pinpoint bilateral nonreactive to light indicates:
        - Lesion in the pons resulting from a hemorrhage.
        - Drug intoxication (heroin, opiates).
    - Dilated bilateral fixed nonreactive to light indicates:
        - Cerebral ischemia.
        - Anticholinergic toxicity.
        - Severe brain damage.
        - Hypoxia.
        - Drug (sympathomimetic) intoxication (cocaine, methamphetamine, amphetamines, ecstasy, bath salts, stimulants).
    - Small unilateral nonreactive to light indicates:
        - Spinal cord lesion.
    - Dilated, unilateral fixed nonreactive to light indicates:
        - Normal if patient has a history of severe eye injury.
        - Increased intracranial pressure.
        - Subdural hematoma or epidural hematoma.
        - Brainstem compression.
        - Brain herniation, leading to oculomotor nerve damage.
    - Midsize, bilateral, fixed, nonreactive indicates:
        - Contusion.
        - Brain edema.
        - Brain hemorrhage.
        - Laceration of the brain.
        - Infarction in the brain.
- Abnormal cranial nerve function:
    - There are 12 cranial nerves responsible for motor and sensory pathways to the brain.
    - Assess cranial nerves (see table 9.1).

TABLE 9.1 How to Assess the Cranial Nerves

Cranial Nerve	Function	Examine
I Olfactory	Smell	Test each nostril with scents such as peppermint, coffee, and vanilla.
II Optic	Vision	Eyes with Snellen eye chart.
III Oculomotor	Eye movement Constricting pupils Raising eyelid	Pupil size. Pupil shape. Pupil response to light.
IV Trochlear	Moving eyes down and in	Ask the patient to move eyes down and in.
V Trigeminal	Sensation for face and scalp Chewing Corneal reflex	Ask the patient to look up and out. Touch a piece of cotton to the other side of the eye. Both eyes should blink. Ask patient to close both eyes. Randomly press a sharp and blunt object on the patient's forehead, jaw, and cheek. Ask the patient whether he or she feels anything and if so, to describe the feeling as sharp or dull. Ask the patient to open his or her mouth and clench the teeth.
VI Abducens	Moving eyes laterally	Ask the patient to move eyes laterally.
VII Facial	Taste Moving mouth, eyes, and forehead to show expression. Tears (lacrimation), salivation	Raise and lower eyebrows. Smile showing teeth. Puff cheeks. Wrinkle forehead.
VIII Acoustic	Balance Hearing	Stand an arm's length away from the patient's ear and rub two fingers. Ask whether the patient hears anything. Repeat the test on the other ear. Conduct the Weber's test by placing the vibrant fork on top of the patient's head, asking, "Where do you hear the sound coming from? The response should be midline. Conduct the Rinne's test. Place a vibrating fork on the mastoid bone behind the ear. Ask the patient when he or she stops hearing it. Then move the fork to the patient's ear so the patient can hear the tone. The patient should hear better with the fork by the ear rather than on the mastoid bone.
IX Glossopharyngeal	Taste Swallowing Gag reflex Salivating	Ask patient to swallow.
X Vagus	Gag reflex Swallowing Heart rate Peristalsis Talking Abdominal function Thoracic functions	Ask the patient to talk. Check the gag reflex by touching the back of the tongue with the tongue blade. Ask the patient to open his or her mouth and say "Ah." Uvula should be midline and soft palate should be upward symmetrically.

(*Continued*)

TABLE 9.1 How to Assess the Cranial Nerves (Continued)

Cranial Nerve	Function	Examine
XI Accessory	Rotation of head Moving shoulder	Ask patient to shrug the shoulders while you press down on the shoulders. The shrug should be bilaterally equal. Apply resistance to the side of the patient's head while the patient rotates his head against the resistance. Repeat on the other side of the head. Ask the patient to stick out his tongue. The tongue should be midline.
XII Hypoglossal	Moving tongue	Ask the patient to say, "Round the rugged rock that ragged rascal ran." The patient should show little problem articulating. Results are dependent on the patient's cognitive ability. Ask the patient to push his tongue against his cheek. Apply resistance to the cheek. The tongue should be symmetrical.

- Motor function:
  - Ask the patient to push against your hands. There should be equal pressure from both arms.
  - Ask the patient to close his eyes then extend both arms palms up for 20 seconds. Both arms should remain in position without any drift.
  - Ask the patient to sit at the edge of the bed and raise both legs against your hands. There should be equal pressure from both legs.
  - Ask the patient to push his feet against your hands. There should be equal pressure from both legs.
  - Ask the patient to stand. The patient should stand without assistance or support.
  - Ask the patient to sit. The patient should sit without assistance or support.
  - Ask the patient to walk. The patient's gait should be steady.
    - Bias toward one side may indicate a cerebellar lesion on that side.
    - Unsteady gait may indicate abnormal cerebellar functioning.
  - Ask the patient to touch his nose with an extended finger one hand at a time. The patient should be able to perform this action without hesitation.
  - Ask the patient to touch your extended finger as you move your finger. The patient should be able to perform this action without hesitation.
  - Ask the patient to touch each finger with the thumb on his same hand. Perform the test on the other hand. The patient should be able to perform this action without hesitation.
  - Inability to perform this exercise quickly may indicate alcohol toxicity, cerebellar disorder, or stroke.
- Reflexes:
  - Tactile stimulation: Stroke the patient's skin. The more you stroke, the less of a reflex response should be noticed.
  - Plantar reflex: Use a tongue blade and slowly stroke from the patient's heel to the great toe. Toes should flex. The Babinski's reflex (fanning of the smaller toes and upward movement of the great toe) is abnormal unless the patient is 2 years of age or younger.
  - Abdominal reflex: Stroke one side of the abdomen with the handle of the reflex hammer. Abdominal muscles contract and the umbilicus should deviate toward the same side. Repeat this on the opposite side.

9.2 Neurologic Tests and Procedures

Neurologic tests are designed to assess the effectiveness and the capability of the nervous system to function. Critical care practitioners order neurologic tests to collect objective data to further assess the patient and to assist in stabilizing him or her. Neurologic procedures are performed to stabilize the patient. The following are neurologic tests and procedures commonly ordered by critical care practitioners.

9.2.1 Spinal x-ray

During a spinal x-ray, x-ray particles are beamed through the front, back, and side of the patient onto a photographic film or to a computer. Dense structures such as bone block x-ray particles, causing those structures to appear white. Less dense structures such as lesions and deteriorated bone block some x-ray particles, causing those structures to appear gray. Spinal tissue that does not block x-ray particles appears dark.

Common reasons for the practitioner to order a spinal x-ray are to assess for:

- Fractures.
- Displacements.
- Lesions.
- Tumors.

The spinal x-ray procedure:

- Be sure that the patient's spine is stabilized. Immobilize the spine, if necessary.
- Be sure that the patient is not pregnant.
- Remove all jewelry in the area because jewelry may appear on the x-ray image.
- Assess whether the patient has scars in the spinal area. If so, note the location of the scar because it may appear on the x-ray image.
- The patient removes clothes. Provide the patient with a gown.
- The patient lies on the x-ray table and the x-ray plate is positioned below the table.
- The initial result, called a wet read, provides a relatively superficial assessment of the image. A more thorough reading is taken hours or days later.

9.2.2 Brain and spinal computed tomography (CT) scan

A brain CT scan provides a three-dimensional image of the brain using x-rays. It enables the practitioner to visualize normal and abnormal structures within the brain. A spinal CT scan provides a three-dimensional image of the spine. A CT can be performed with or without a contrast agent. A contrast agent is iodine based and enhances images of blood vessels and less dense areas of the brain and spine.

Common reasons for the practitioner to order a brain CT scan are to assess for:

- Inflammation.
- Lesions.
- Contusion.
- Vascular anomalies.
- Cerebral atrophy.

- Blood clots.
- Aneurysms.
- Infarctions.
- Calcifications.
- Hydrocephalus.
- Foreign bodies.

Common reasons for the practitioner to order a spinal CT scan are to assess for:

- Fractures.
- Dislocation.
- Herniated disk.
- Tumors.
- Spinal stenosis.

The CT scan procedure:

- Assesses whether the patient is allergic to iodine or shellfish if the patient is undergoing a CT scan with contrast. Patients who are allergic to iodine or shellfish have a high likelihood of experiencing an allergic reaction to the contrast agent.
- Assesses whether the patient is claustrophobic. The patient will be placed in an enclosure during the test.
- Assesses whether the patient can remain still for 30 minutes during the CT scan.
- Administer diphenhydramine (Benadryl) and prednisone (Deltasone) before the CT scan to reduce the risk of an allergic reaction to the contrast agent if the contrast agent is ordered.
- Administer the contrast agent through an intravenous (IV) line. The patient may feel flushed and experience a salty or metallic taste in the mouth.
- The CT scanner encircles the patient for up to 30 minutes.
- Explain to the patient that the contrast material typically discolors the urine for up to 24 hours following the CT scan. The patient should increase fluid intake after the CT scan to flush the contrast agent from the patient's body if the contrast agent was used for the CT scan.

9.2.3 Central nervous system (CNS) magnetic resonance imaging (MRI)

A CNS MRI provides a three-dimensional view of the central nervous system, using radio waves, a strong magnet, and a computer. An MRI is used particularly to assess fluid-filled soft tissue and to identify tumors from other structures within the central nervous system.

The MRI procedure:

- All metal must be removed from the patient.
- No metal must enter the room containing the MRI scanner. The MRI scanner's magnet is always activated.
- Assesses whether the patient is claustrophobic. If so, then ask the healthcare provider if an open MRI scanner should be used for the test or the patient should be sedated before the scan begins.
- The MRI scan takes about 30 minutes.
- The MRI scan is noninvasive. The patient will not feel any discomfort.

9.2.4 Cerebral angiograph

A cerebral angiograph is a test that enables the practitioner to examine blood vessels in the brain. Radiopaque contrast medium is injected into the brachial artery or femoral artery. The contrast medium highlights blood vessels on the image.

Common reasons for the practitioner to order a cerebral angiograph are to assess for:

- Hematoma.
- Cerebral edema.
- Displaced vessels.
- Aneurysms.
- Stenosis.
- Occlusion.
- Arteriovenous malformations.
- Circulation.

The cerebral angiograph procedure:

- Assessed whether the patient is allergic to iodine or shellfish. Patients who are allergic to iodine or shellfish have a high likelihood of experiencing an allergic reaction to the contrast agent.
- Administer diphenhydramine (Benadryl) and prednisone (Deltasone) before the cerebral angiograph to reduce the risk of an allergic reaction to the contrast agent.
- Explain to the patient that the contrast material typically discolors the urine for up to 24 hours following the cerebral angiograph. The patient should increase fluid intake after the cerebral angiograph to flush the contrast agent from the patient's body.
- Assesses renal function (serum creatinine and BUN) before the procedure, to ensure that the patient is able to void the contrast medium.
- Assesses coagulation (prothrombin time [PT], partial thromboplastin time [PTT], international normalized ratio [INR], platelet count) before the procedure to ensure that there will not be excessive bleeding following the procedure.
- Use a Femstop device on the injection site to maintain pressure on the site following the procedure.
- Monitor the patient for neurologic changes during and after the procedure.

9.2.5 Lumbar puncture

A lumbar puncture is a procedure in which the practitioner samples the patient's spinal fluid. A sterile needle is inserted into a subarachnoid space between the third and fourth lumbar vertebrae while the patient lies on his or her side held by staff. The sample is then sent to the laboratory for analysis.

Common reasons for the practitioner to order a lumbar puncture are to assess for:

- Bacteria.
- Blood.
- Relative intracranial pressure.

The lumbar puncture procedure:

- Is not performed if the patient has a lumbar spine deformity.
- Explain that the patient may feel discomfort.
- A local anesthetic is administered at the injection site.
- Assess the patient for back spasms, headache, or seizures following the procedure.

9.3 Neurologic Medication

Several categories of medication are commonly used for neurologic critical conditions. These are used to counter conditions that make the patient's neurologic system unstable. Each medication can cause adverse side effects. Therefore, the patient must be monitored carefully following administration of these medications.

9.3.1 Anticonvulsants

Anticonvulsant medication is used to treat seizures, which are episodes of disturbed brain activity that can affect muscular capability and behavior. Seizures can be caused by epilepsy or head trauma. Anticonvulsant medications can increase intracranial pressure and cause cerebral edema in addition to causing bradycardia.

- Fosphenytoin (Cerebyx).
- Phenytoin (Dilantin).

9.3.2 Anticoagulants

Anticoagulant medication is used to prevent an embolism following a cerebral vascular accident (CVA). Anticoagulant medication increases the risk of bleeding.

- Heparin.

9.3.3 Antiplatelet medication

Antiplatelet medication is used to reduce coagulants following a CVA or a transient ischemic attack (TIA). Antiplatelet medication increases the risk of low platelet count (thrombocytopenia) and low white blood cell count (agranulocytosis).

- Aspirin.
- Ticlopidine (Ticlid).

9.3.4 Barbiturates

Barbiturates are used to reduce patient irritability and agitation. In addition, barbiturates are used to treat seizures, except febrile seizures and absence seizures. Barbiturates increase the risk of respiratory depression and bradycardia.

- Phenobarbital (Luminal).

9.3.5 Benzodiazepines

Benzodiazepines are used to reduce patient anxiety and agitation. In addition, barbiturates are used to treat seizures and muscle spasm. Benzodiazepines increase the risk of respiratory depression and bradycardia and can cause the patient to experience withdrawal symptoms.

- Diazepam (Valium).
- Lorazepam (Ativan).

9.3.6 Calcium channel blockers

Calcium channel blockers are used to reduce vasoconstriction caused by vasospasm, which occurs after the rupture of an aneurysm. Calcium channel blockers increase the risk of edema and tachycardia related to hypotension.

- Nisoldipine (Sular).

9.3.7 Corticosteroids

Corticosteroids are used to reduce inflammation and cerebral edema. Corticosteroids increase the risk of pancreatitis, heart failure, and thromboembolism.

- Dexamethasone (Dexone).
- Methylprednisolone (Solu-Medrol).

9.3.8 Diuretics

Diuretics are used to reduce cerebral edema and reduce intracranial pressure. Diuretics increase the risk of seizures, electrolyte imbalance, renal failure, heart failure, and dehydration.

- Furosemide (Lasiz).
- Mannitol (Osmitroil).

9.3.9 Opioid analgesics

Opioid analgesics are used to reduce pain. Diuretics increase the risk of respiratory depression, bradycardia, sedation, and constipation.

- Oxycodone (OxyContin).
- Morphine (Duramorph).

9.3.10 Thrombolytics

Thrombolytics are used to remove a blood clot following an acute ischemic CVA. Thrombolytic medication increases the risk of bleeding.

- Alteplase (Activase).

9.3.11 Serotonin inhibitors

Serotonin inhibitors are used to treat migraine headaches. Serotonin inhibitors increase the risk of unstable blood pressure.

- Sumatriptan (Imitrex).

9.4 Cerebral Hemorrhage

Cerebral hemorrhage is bleeding within the brain, the layers covering the brain, or between the skull and the dura mater. It can occur at the time of an injury or hours or days later. Types of cerebral hemorrhages are:

- Epidural hematoma: Bleeding from an artery with blood accumulating between the dura and skull.
- Subdural hematoma: Bleeding from a vein in the area between the dura mater and the arachnoid mater, resulting in slow, chronic bleeding.
- Subarachnoid hemorrhage: Bleeding between the arachnoid mater and the pia mater, the location of cerebrospinal fluid.
- Intracerebral hemorrhage: Bleeding within brain tissue caused by shearing or tearing of small vessels within the brain and between the cerebrum and brainstem.
- Concussion: Blunt force trauma thrusts the brain against the inside of the skull, resulting in bruising.
- Cerebral contusion: Blunt force trauma thrusts the brain against the inside of the skull, resulting in cerebral edema, cerebral hemorrhage, and loss of consciousness longer than that in a concussion.
- Coup injury: Blunt force trauma thrusts the brain against the inside of the skull at the point of the blunt force trauma.
- Countrecoup injury: Blunt force trauma causes the head to recoil, thrusting the brain against the inside of the skull at a point opposite the blunt force trauma.
- Cerebral edema: Fluid within the skull moves to the third space, resulting in increased cranial pressure.

9.4.1 Signs and symptoms

- Nausea.
- Vomiting.
- Disorientation.
- Headache.
- Unequal pupil size.
- Diminished or absent pupil reaction.
- Cognitive changes.
- Speech changes.
- Motor movement changes.
- Decreased level of consciousness or loss of consciousness.
- Amnesia.
- Unilateral paralysis.
- Facial weakness or droop.

9.4.2 Medical tests

- CT scan: Shows cerebral edema and hemorrhage.
- MRI: Shows edema and hemorrhage.

9.4.3 Treatment

- Craniotomy:
  - Stop bleeding surgically.
  - Debridement of wound and tissue necrosis.
  - Decompress cerebral pressure by drilling burr holes to relieve pressure.
  - Remove hematoma surgically.
- Intubation to open airway.
- Supplemental oxygen.
- Mechanical ventilation to assess breathing.
- Administer:
  - Osmotic diuretics to decrease cerebral edema.
    - Mannitol.
  - Loop diuretics to decrease edema and circulating blood volume.
    - Furosemide (Lasix).
  - Analgesics.
    - Acetaminophen (Tylenol).
  - Antibiotics (open head wound) to prevent infection.
  - Antihypertensives.
    - Nitroprusside (Nitropress).
  - Opioids (low dose) for restlessness agitation and pain (if on ventilator).
    - Morphine sulfate.
    - Fentanyl citrate.

9.4.4 Intervention

- Supplemental oxygen.
- Seizure precautions.
- Monitor vital signs.
- Monitor signs of increased intracranial pressure: Widening pulse pressure, increased blood pressure, and slow pulse.
- High-protein, high-calorie, high-vitamin diet.
- Monitor intake and output.
- Monitor for diabetes insipidus due to injury to the pituitary gland.
- Monitor neurologic status (Glasgow Coma Scale).
- Instruct the patient:
  - To call the healthcare provider if the patient becomes lethargic, experiences a change in personality, or is drowsy.
  - About seizure precautions.

9.5 Bell's Palsy

Bell's palsy is facial paralysis of the seventh cranial nerve affecting one side of the face. It is related to inflammation and common in diabetics. It leads to the patient being unable to close the eyelid, smile, or raise the eyebrow. Patient may experience a change in taste and pain around the ear. This disorder is self-resolving in most patients.

9.5.1 Signs and symptoms

- Unilateral facial paralysis.
- Change in taste.
- Ear and jaw pain.

9.5.2 Medical tests

- Electromyogram (EMG) used to assess recovery time.

9.5.3 Treatment

- Administer:
  - Corticosteroids to decrease inflammation.
    - Prednisone.
  - Artificial tears to moisten eyes.

9.5.4 Intervention

- Monitor for eye irritation.
- Provide meals in private.
- Instruct the patient:
  - How to properly apply artificial tears.

9.6 Brain Abscess

With a brain abscess, pus collects within the brain as a result of infection from the ear, sinuses, systemic circulation, or from within the brain. It leads to cerebral edema. The cause is streptococci, staphylococci, anaerobes, or mixed organism infections.

9.6.1 Signs and symptoms

- Seizures.
- Headache.

- Drowsiness.
- Confusion.
- Ataxia (loss of coordination).
- Widened pulse pressure.
- Nystagmus (involuntary eye movement).
- Aphasia (inability to use or understand language).

9.6.2 Medical tests

- Elevated white blood cell (WBC) count.
- MRI shows abscess.
- CT shows abscess.
- Biopsy to identify organism.

9.6.3 Treatment

- Drain the abscess.
- Administer:
    - Antibiotics.
        - Nafcillin sodium (penicillinase-resistant penicillin).
        - Penicillin G benzathine.
        - Chloramphenicol.
        - Metronidazole (Flagyl).
        - Vancomycin (Vancocin).
    - Corticosteroids.
        - Dexamethasone (Decadron).
    - Anticonvulsants.
        - Phenytoin (Dilantin).
        - Phenobarbital (Solfoton).
    - Osmotic diuretics to decrease cerebral edema.
        - Mannitol (Osmitrol).

9.6.4 Intervention

- Monitor vital signs.
- Monitor mental status.
- Monitor fluid intake and output.
- Monitor movement.
- Monitor senses.
- Instruct the patient:
    - To continue antibiotic treatments.

9.7 Brain Tumor

A brain tumor is a growth of abnormal cells within the brain, leading to increased intracranial pressure. Abnormal cells may be metastasized cancer cells from a site outside the brain (secondary).

- Meningiomas: Benign tumor generated from the meninges.
- Gliomas: Malignant rapid growing tumor generated from neuroglial cells.
- Astrocytoma: Type of glioma.
- Oligodendroglioma: Slower growing glioma.
- Glioblastoma: Differentiated glioma.

9.7.1 Signs and symptoms

- Parietal lobe:
  - Visual-field defect.
  - Sensory loss.
    - Seizures.
- Frontal lobe:
  - Anosmia (loss of sense of smell).
  - Personality changes.
  - Expressive aphasia.
  - Slowing of mental activity.
- Occipital lobe:
  - Prosopagnosia.
  - Impaired vision.
- Cerebellum or brainstem:
  - Ataxia.
  - Lack of coordination.
  - Hypotonia of limbs.
- Temporal lobe:
  - Receptive aphasia.
  - Auditory hallucinations.
  - Depersonalization.
  - Seizures.
  - Smell hallucinations.
  - Emotional changes.
  - Visual-field defects.

9.7.2 Medical tests

- CT: Shows meningioma.
- MRI with contrast: Shows tumor.

9.7.3 Treatment

- Craniotomy to remove the tumor.
- Radiation to decrease tumor size.
- Administer:
    - Glucocorticoid to decrease inflammatory:
        - Dexamethasone (Decadron).
    - Anticonvulsant to decrease seizure activity.
        - Phenytoin (Dilantin), phenobarbital, carbamazepine (Tegretol), divalproex sodium (Depakote), valproic acid (Depakene), levetiracetam (Keppra), lamotrigine (Lamictal), clonazepam (Klonopin), topiramate (Topamax), ethosuximide (Zarontin).
    - Osmotic diuretic to reduce cerebral edema.
        - Mannitol (Osmitrol).
    - Proton pump inhibitors to decrease gastric irritation.
        - Lansoprazole (Prevacid), omeprazole (Prilosec), esomeprazole (Nexium), rabeprazole (Aciphex), pantoprazole (Protonix).
    - Histamine 2 (H_2) receptor antagonists: to decrease gastric irritation.
        - Ranitidine (Zantac), famotidine (Pepcid), nizatidine (Axid), cimetidine (Tagamet).
    - Mucosal barrier fortifier to decrease gastric irritation.
        - Sucralfate.
    - Chemotherapeutic agents based on cell type.
        - Carmustine, lomustine, procarbazine, vincristine, temozolomide, erlotinib, and gefitinib.

9.7.4 Intervention

- Monitor neurologic function.
- Seizure precautions.
- Instruct the patient:
    - On seizure precautions.

9.8 Cerebral Aneurysm

Weakening of a blood vessel wall in the brain resulting in ballooning of the vessel wall that might lead to a rupture and intracranial bleeding. This can be caused by congenital malformation, infection, lesion on the blood vessel wall, trauma, or atherosclerosis.

9.8.1 Signs and symptoms

- Asymptomatic unless rupture occurs.
- Decreased LOC.
- Headache due to hemorrhage and increased intracranial pressure.

9.8.2 Medical tests

- CT shows the aneurysm.
- Single-photon emission computed tomography (SPECT) shows the aneurysm.
- Angiogram shows the aneurysm.
- Digital subtraction angiography shows the aneurysm.
- Diffusion/perfusion magnetic resonance angiography (MRA) shows the aneurysm.

9.8.3 Treatment

- Surgical resection of the aneurysm is commonly replaced with endovascular procedures.
- Administer:
  - Glucocorticoid to decrease inflammation.
    - Dexamethasone (Decadron).
  - Anticonvulsant to decrease seizure activity.
    - Phenytoin (Dilantin), phenobarbital, carbamazepine (Tegretol), divalproex sodium (Depakote), valproic acid (Depakene), levetiracetam (Keppra), lamotrigine (Lamictal), clonazepam (Klonopin), topiramate (Topamax), ethosuximide (Zarontin).
  - Stool softener to decrease the need to strain.
    - Docusate sodium (Colace).

9.8.4 Intervention

- Elevate the head of the bed 30 degrees.
- Bed rest.
- Monitor LOC.
- Monitor vital signs for indication of increased intracranial pressure (widened pulse pressure and bradycardia).
- Instruct the patient:
  - To report any headache to the healthcare provider immediately.

9.9 Encephalitis

Encephalitis is inflammation of the brain in response to an infection by a virus (common), bacteria, fungus, or protozoa.

9.9.1 Signs and symptoms

- Fever.
- Stiff neck.

- Headache.
- Nausea and vomiting.
- Drowsiness.
- Lethargy.
- Seizure.

9.9.2 Medical tests

- Blood cultures and sensitivity.

9.9.3 Treatment

- Administer:
  - Glucocorticoid to decrease inflammation.
    - Dexamethasone (Decadron).
  - Anticonvulsant to decrease seizure activity.
    - Phenytoin (Dilantin), phenobarbital, carbamazepine (Tegretol), divalproex sodium (Depakote), valproic acid (Depakene), levetiracetam (Keppra), lamotrigine (Lamictal), clonazepam (Klonopin), topiramate (Topamax), ethosuximide (Zarontin).
  - Diuretic to reduce cerebral edema.
    - Mannitol, Lasix (furosemide).
  - Antipyretics to reduce fever.
    - Acetaminophen (Tylenol).

9.9.4 Intervention

- Monitor vital signs for indication of increased intracranial pressure (widened pulse pressure and bradycardia).
- Monitor neurologic changes.
- Monitor fluid input and output.
- Monitor electrolyte levels.
- Provide a quiet environment.
- Range-of-motion exercises, active or passive.
- Turn and position patient.
- Instruct the patient:
  - That the patient will be turned every 2 hours by staff.

9.10 Guillain-Barré Syndrome

Guillain-Barré syndrome is an autoimmune reaction that damages the myelin surrounding the axon on the peripheral nerves resulting in an acute, progressive weakness and paralysis of muscles. This occurs a few weeks following a viral infection, acute illness, or surgery. Damage may be permanent if nerve cells are damaged. Damage may be temporary if axons are damaged.

- Ascending Guillain-Barré: The damage begins at the distal lower extremities and moves upward.
- Descending Guillain-Barré: The damage begins in the muscles in the face and throat and moves downward, resulting in paralysis of the diaphragm and intercostal muscles. This leads to respiratory compromise.

9.10.1 Signs and symptoms

- Acute illness or infection within the past several weeks.
- Absence of deep tendon reflexes.
- Burning or pricking feeling.
- Symmetrical weakness.
- Flaccid paralysis.
- Fluctuating blood pressure.
- Cardiac dysrhythmias.
- Facial weakness.
- Difficulty swallowing (dysphagia).

9.10.2 Medical tests

- Nerve conduction studies: Show slowed velocity.
- Pulmonary function tests: Show diminished tidal volume and vital capacity.
- Lumbar puncture: Shows increased protein in cerebrospinal fluid.

9.10.3 Treatment

- Plasmapheresis to remove antibodies from blood.
- Endotracheal intubation if necessary.
- Monitor respirations and support ventilation if necessary.
- Administer:
    - Immunoglobulin IV.

9.10.4 Intervention

- Monitor airway, breathing, and circulation.
- Monitor vital signs.

- Monitor for progression of change.
- Monitor gag reflex.
- Insert nasogastric tube if dysphagia present.
- Develop nonverbal communication method (e.g., call bell).
- Instruct the patient:
    - That the patient will be turned every 2 hours by staff.

9.11 Meningitis

Meningitis is an infection of the meningeal coverings of the brain and spinal cord commonly caused by bacteria (*Streptococcus pneumoniae* (pneumococcal), *Neisseria meningitidis* (meningococcal), or *Haemophilus influenza*). It can also be caused by a virus, fungus, protozoa, or toxic exposure. Bacterial meningitis is transmitted when people live in close quarters. Viral meningitis may follow a viral infection and is self-limiting. Fungal meningitis may occur in patients who are immunocompromised.

9.11.1 Signs and symptoms

- Fever.
- Nuchal rigidity (pain when flexing chin toward chest).
- Stiff neck.
- Petechial rash on skin and mucous membranes.
- Photophobia (sensitivity to light).
- Headache.
- Malaise and fatigue.
- Seizures.
- Nausea and vomiting.
- Myalgia (muscle aches).
- Chills.
- Altered LOC.

9.11.2 Medical tests

- Lumbar puncture to sample cerebrospinal fluid.
- Polymerase chain reaction (PCR) test of cerebrospinal fluid for organisms.
- Culture and sensitivity of cerebrospinal fluid and blood.
- CT brain to rule out a lesion.

9.11.3 Treatment

- Administer:
  - Glucocorticoid to decrease inflammation.
    - Dexamethasone (Decadron).
  - Anticonvulsant to decrease seizure activity.
    - Phenytoin (Dilantin), phenobarbital, carbamazepine (Tegretol), divalproex sodium (Depakote), valproic acid (Depakene), levetiracetam (Keppra), lamotrigine (Lamictal), clonazepam (Klonopin), topiramate (Topamax), ethosuximide (Zarontin).
  - Diuretic to reduce cerebral edema.
    - Mannitol, Lasix (furosemide).
  - Antipyretics to reduce fever.
    - Acetaminophen (Tylenol).
  - Antibiotics for bacterial meningitis.
    - Penicillin G, cefotaxime (Rocephin), vancomycin plus ceftriaxone, cefotaxime (Claforan), ceftazidime (Fortaz).
  - Antifungal medication for fungal infection.
    - Amphotericin B (Fungizone), fluconazole (Diflucan), flucytosine (Ancobon).

9.11.4 Intervention

- Isolation.
- Darken room.
- Seizure precautions.
- Bed rest.
- Monitor fluid intake and output.
- Monitor neurologic function every 2 hours.
- Instruct the patient:
  - Explain restrictions.

9.12 Spinal Cord Injury

Pulling, twisting, compressing, or severing the spinal cord may result in damage to partial (incomplete) or entire thickness (complete) of the spinal cord. Damage is assessed after inflammation related to trauma subsides. Spinal cord tissue does not regenerate. The level of damage to the spinal cord determines the degree of disability.

9.12.1 Signs and symptoms

- Tingling (paresthesia).
- Reduced sensation (hypoesthesia).

- Increased sensation (hyperesthesia).
- Weakness (flaccid paralysis).
- Absence of reflexes.
- Lack of bowel control.
- Loss of bladder control.
- Hypotension.
- Hypothermia.
- Bradycardia.
- Loss of motor control below the level of the injury.

9.12.2 Medical tests

- CT scan: Shows injury.
- MRI: Shows injury.

9.12.3 Treatment

- Administer:
  - Corticosteroid to decrease inflammation.
    - Methylprednisolone (Medrol), prednisone (Deltasone), dexamethasone (Decadron).
  - Plasma expander to increase circulation and oxygen to injured tissues.
    - Dextran (Infed).
  - H_2 receptor antagonists to prevent formation of stress ulcer.
    - Cimetidine (Tagamet), ranitidine (Zantac), famotidine (Pepcid), nizatidine (Axid).
  - Gastric mucosal protective agent to prevent formation of stress ulcer.
    - Sucralfate (Carafate).
  - Surgical decompression or repair of fracture.

9.12.4 Intervention

- Position flat on rotating bed to prevent pressure ulcers.
- No flexion.
- Immobilize spinal cord with traction to decrease irritation.
- Monitor traction to prevent skin irritation.
- Monitor for spinal shock (reflex loss below injury, bradycardia, hypotension, paralytic ileus, flaccid paralysis).
- Monitor vital signs.
- Monitor intake and output.
- Monitor mental status.

- Monitor neurologic status.
- Monitor skin for pressure ulcers.
- Care of cervical traction pin sites.
- Instruct the patient:
  - Proper transferring from wheelchair to bed.
  - Need for regular bowel movement and urination.
  - Need to use the incentive spirometer.
  - Turning and positioning.

9.13 Cerebrovascular Accident (CVA)

A CVA is an interruption of blood supply to the brain resulting in infarction (necrosis) in the affected tissue. Patients with high cholesterol, diabetes mellitus, smoking, obesity, oral contraceptive use, or atrial fibrillation have a high risk for CVA. There are three types of CVA:

- Ischemic stroke (common in 88% of all strokes) is an interruption of arterial blood flow by an obstruction (clot) by the thrombus or embolus.
- Hemorrhagic stroke is an interruption of blood flow by rupture or leakage of a blood vessel into brain tissues and ventricles.
- TIA is a temporary interruption of blood flow that resolves in a few hours with no permanent neurologic deficit.

9.13.1 Signs and symptoms

- Difficulty speaking (aphasia).
- Personality changes.
- Confusion.
- Sensory changes.
- Numbness.
- Weakness.
- Severe headache.
- Seizure.
- Difficulty with gait and coordination.
- Facial droop.
- Altered vision.

9.13.2 Medical tests

- Single photon emission computed tomography (SPECT): Shows decreased perfusion.
- Magnetic resonance angiography (MRA): Shows abnormal vessels.

- CT scan: Shows bleeding.
- MRI: Shows ischemic vessels.

9.13.3 Treatment

- Carotid artery endarterectomy to remove plaque from carotid artery (ischemic).
- Surgical implantation of a stent in the carotid artery (ischemic).
- Surgical correction of bleeding (hemorrhagic).
- Administer:
  - Thromoblytic agent (tissue plasminogen activator [t-PA]) within 3 hours of onset of symptoms (ischemic).
    - Alteplase (Activase).
  - Anticoagulants after t-PA (ischemic).
    - Heparin, warfarin (Coumadin), enoxaparin (Lovenox), aspirin.
  - Antiplatelet medications to decrease platelet adhesiveness (ischemic).
    - Clopidogrel (Plavix), ticlopidine hydrochloride (Ticlid), dipyridamole (Persantine).
  - Corticosteroid to decrease inflammation.
    - Dexamethasone (Decadron).

9.13.4 Intervention

- Bed rest.
- Monitor vital signs.
- Monitor neurologic status.
- Monitor for increased intracranial pressure (decreased LOC, restlessness, confusion, headaches, nausea, and vomiting).
- Develop nonverbal communication method (call bell).
- Physical therapy to maintain muscle tone.
- Speech therapy to assist with swallowing and speech.
- Occupational therapy to regain independent living.
- Instruct the patient:
  - Proper transferring from wheelchair to bed.
  - Effects of CVA on activities of daily living.

9.14 Seizure Disorder

Seizure disorder is a sudden, uncontrolled discharge of neurons in the brain resulting in abnormal behavior caused by metabolic disorder, intracranial pressure, tumor, CVA, medication, or seizure disorder. Prior to the seizure (preictal stage), the patient may experience alterations in sight, sound, or smell. After the seizure (postictal stage), the patient is fatigued, confused, and may not recall the seizure.

9.14.1 Signs and symptoms

- General seizures:
  - Tonic/clonic: First tonic (limbs rigid), loss of consciousness, and then clonic (rhythmic jerking).
  - Tonic: Limbs rigid, loss of consciousness.
  - Clonic: Rhythmic jerking.
  - Absence: Staring and brief loss of consciousness.
  - Myoclonic: Brief rhythmic jerking.
  - Atonic: Loss of muscle tone.
- Partial seizures:
  - Simple partial: No loss of consciousness, unusual sensation, unusual movement, begins with aura.
  - Complex partial: Lip smacking, patting, picking, loss of consciousness.

9.14.2 Medical tests

- CT scan of brain to rule out tumor or bleed.
- MRI of brain to rule out tumor or bleed.
- Electroencephalogram (EEG): Shows abnormal electrical activity in brain.

9.14.3 Treatment

- Treat underlying cause.
- Surgically remove seizure focal area.
- Implantation of vagal nerve stimulator to decrease frequency of seizures.
- Administer:
  - Antiepileptic.
    - Phenytoin (Dilantin), phenobarbital, carbamazepine (Tegretol), divalproex sodium (Depakote), valproic acid (Depakene), levetiracetam (Keppra), lamotrigine (Lamictal), clonazepam (Klonopin), topiramate (Topamax), ethosuximide (Zarontin), gabapentin (Neurontin), levetiracetam (Keppra), oxcarbazepine (Trileptal), primidone (Mysoline), tiagabine (Gabitril).

9.14.4 Intervention

- Seizure precautions.
- During seizure:
  - Place patient on side to decrease risk of aspiration.
  - Remove objects from around patient to prevent injury.
  - Note duration and patient's actions during seizure.
  - Monitor for status epilepticus (prolonged seizures or repeated seizures).
  - Do not insert anything in patient's mouth during seizure.

- Instruct the patient:
  - Explain seizure precautions to family and friends.
  - Instruct family and friends what to do during a seizure.
  - Importance of taking medications as prescribed.

9.15 Concussion

Head trauma causes the brain to move within the skull, resulting in neural dysfunction. There is no bruising of brain tissue. The patient typically loses consciousness for a few minutes but no more than 6 hours. The patient experiences a headache for months. Full recovery occurs within 48 hours of the head trauma.

9.15.1 Signs and symptoms

- Vomiting.
- Lethargy.
- Unusual behavior.
- Headache.
- Temporary amnesia related to traumatic event.
- Dizziness.
- Blurry vision.
- Not thinking clearly.

9.15.2 Medical tests

- CT scan: Shows absence of bruising of brain tissue.
- MRI shows: Absence of bruising of brain tissue and evidence of head trauma.

9.15.3 Treatment

- Bed rest.
- Apply cold pack wrapped in thin cloths for up to 20 minutes on any swelling.
- Administer:
  - Analgesic.
    - Acetaminophen (Tylenol).
    - Ibuprofen (Advil, Motrin).

9.15.4 Intervention

- Monitor vital signs.
- Monitor neurologic status.

- Monitor for increased intracranial pressure (decreased LOC, restlessness, confusion, headaches, nausea, and vomiting).
- Instruct the patient:
  - No activities that are physically or mentally demanding.
  - No alcohol or illegal drugs.

9.16 Contusion

A contusion is a bruise of the brain as a result of acceleration-deceleration brain trauma, a coup injury in which bruising occurs at the site of the impact, such as in a force blow to the head, or a contrecoup injury, in which bruising occurs at the opposite side of the impact, such as when the head hits the windshield in a motor vehicle accident.

9.16.1 Signs and symptoms

- Difficulty breathing.
- Disorientation.
- Confusion.
- Loss of consciousness.
- Visible wound may or may not exist.
- Agitated.
- Unequal pupils.
- Drowsiness.
- Violent.
- Weakness on one side (hemiparesis).
- Abnormal posturing.
- Nausea and/or vomiting.
- Visual disturbance.
- Difficulty speaking.

9.16.2 Medical tests

- CT scan: Shows bruising of brain tissue and evidence of head trauma.
- MRI: Shows bruising of brain tissue and evidence of head trauma.

9.16.3 Treatment

- Administer:
  - Diuretic to reduce cerebral edema.
    - Mannitol, furosemide (Lasix).

- Antiepileptic.
  - Phenytoin (Dilantin), phenobarbital, carbamazepine (Tegretol), divalproex sodium (Depakote), valproic acid (Depakene), levetiracetam (Keppra), lamotrigine (Lamictal), clonazepam (Klonopin), topiramate (Topamax), ethosuximide (Zarontin), gabapentin (Neurontin), levetiracetam (Keppra), oxcarbazepine (Trileptal), primidone (Mysoline), tiagabine (Gabitril).

9.16.4 Intervention

- Elevate the head of the bed.
- Monitor vital signs.
- Monitor neurologic status.
- Monitor for increased intracranial pressure (decreased LOC, restlessness, confusion, headaches, nausea, and vomiting).
- Instruct the patient:
  - No activities that are physically or mentally demanding.
  - No alcohol or illegal drugs.

9.17 Subdural Hematoma

A subdural hematoma is blood (blood clot) that accumulates between the dura mater and arachnoid, called the subdural space, and has the highest mortality and morbidity rate of all hematomas. Subdural hematoma can be caused by head trauma as the result of a lumbar puncture or other procedures, administration of anticoagulants, or spontaneously. Bleeding is typically from veins in the venous sinus and cerebral cortex. There are three classifications of subdural hematomas, each of which can be bilateral or unilateral:

- Acute: Less than 72 hours old and considered a medical emergency requiring surgical intervention to prevent increased intracranial pressure from occurring.
- Subacute: 48 hours to 2 weeks following the acute injury.
- Chronic: 21 days or older following the acute injury.

9.17.1 Signs and symptoms

- Unequal pupils indicate increased intracranial pressure.
- Severe headache that is worsening related to increased bleedings.
- Decreased LOC (acute).
- Confusion.
- Weakness on one side of the body (hemiparesis) (acute).
- Fixed/dilated pupils (acute).

9.17.2 Medical tests

- CT scan: Shows hematoma.
- MRI: Shows hematoma.

- Arteriography: Shows altered blood flow.
- Lumbar puncture: Cerebrospinal fluid yellow and low protein if chronic subdural hematoma.

9.17.3 Treatment

- Small subdural hematomas are monitored and typically are self-resolving.
- Surgical removal of the hematoma.
- Administer:
    - Antiemetic for nausea and vomiting.
        - Metoclopramide (Reglan).
        - Ondansetron (Zofran).
        - Prochlorperazine (Compazine).
    - Diuretic to reduce cerebral edema.
        - Mannitol, furosemide (Lasix).

9.17.4 Intervention

- Bed rest.
- Monitor vital signs.
- Monitor neurologic status.
- Monitor for increased intracranial pressure (decreased LOC, restlessness, confusion, headaches, nausea, and vomiting).
- Instruct the patient:
    - No aspirin.
    - No anticoagulants (heparin, Coumadin, Plavix).

9.18 Diffuse Axonal Injury

A diffuse axonal injury is a traumatic injury to the brain resulting in damage to axons (white matter) in the brain stem, cerebral hemispheres, and corpus callosum, leading to axon disconnection and swelling. Diffuse axonal injuries are classified as:

- Mild: Returns to baseline neurologic function within 24 hours of the injury.
- Moderate: Patient is in a coma for a few days.
- Severe: Patient is in a coma for weeks.

9.18.1 Signs and symptoms

- Loss of consciousness.
- Abnormal posturing.

- Coma.
- Dysautonomia (dysfunction of the autonomic nervous system).

9.18.2 Medical tests

- CT scan: Shows cerebral edema and cerebral tissue damage.
- MRI (more sensitive than a CT scan): Shows cerebral edema and cerebral tissue damage.

9.18.3 Treatment

- Administer:
  - Polyethylene glycol to seal the membrane and prevent severe calcium influx.
  - Diuretic to reduce cerebral edema.
    - Mannitol, furosemide (Lasix).
  - Corticosteroid to decrease inflammation.
    - Dexamethasone (Decadron).

9.18.4 Intervention

- Bed rest.
- Total care. The patient is typically in a coma.
- Monitor vital signs.
- Monitor neurologic status.
- Instruct the patient:
  - The patient may experience amnesia when the patient returns to baseline neurologic function.
  - The patient may require rehabilitation therapy.

9.19 Skull Fracture

A skull fracture is breakage of bones in the skull caused by blunt force head trauma. Common skull fractures are:

- Linear: Breakage transverses the thickness of the skull. No bone displacement occurs.
- Comminuted: Bone is crushed, broken, and splintered.
- Depressed: Breakage causes bone to be displaced inward, leading to increased intracranial pressure.
- Basilar: Breakage occurs at the base of the skull.
- Diastatic: Breakage occurs at a suture line.
- Compound: Breakage causes the bone to tear the epidermis, meninges, paranasal sinuses, or the middle ear.

9.19.1 Signs and symptoms

- Asymptomatic.
- Bleeding from nose, ears, eyes, or site of wound.
- Pupils unequal and not reactive to light.
- Visual disturbances.
- Drainage of clear fluid (cerebrospinal fluid) from the ears or nose.
- Bruising behind the ears (Battle sign) or under the eyes (raccoon eyes).
- Loss of smell.
- Confusion.
- Irritability.
- Nausea/vomiting.
- Confusion.
- Restlessness.
- Headache.
- Seizure.

9.19.2 Medical tests

- CT scan: Shows fracture, hemorrhage, and swelling.
- MRI: Shows fracture, hemorrhage, and swelling.

9.19.3 Treatment

- Linear fractures: No treatment.
- Overnight observation.
- Do not probe wound.
- Stabilize head and neck.
- Surgical repair (nonlinear fractures).
- Administer:
  - Antibiotic (compound fracture).
  - Diuretic to reduce cerebral edema.
    - Mannitol, furosemide (Lasix).
  - Corticosteroid to decrease inflammation.
    - Dexamethasone (Decadron).
  - Antiepileptic.
    - Phenytoin (Dilantin), phenobarbital, carbamazepine (Tegretol), divalproex sodium (Depakote), valproic acid (Depakene), levetiracetam (Keppra), lamotrigine (Lamictal), clonazepam (Klonopin), topiramate (Topamax), ethosuximide (Zarontin), gabapentin (Neurontin), levetiracetam (Keppra), oxcarbazepine (Trileptal), primidone (Mysoline), tiagabine (Gabitril).

9.19.4 Intervention

- Bed rest.
- Monitor vital signs.
- Monitor neurologic status.
- Monitor for increased intracranial pressure (decreased LOC, restlessness, confusion, headaches, nausea, and vomiting).
- Instruct the patient:
  - No aspirin.
  - No anticoagulants (heparin, Coumadin, Plavix).

9.20 Intracerebral Hematoma

An intracerebral hematoma is blood (a blood clot) that accumulates in the cerebrum related to shear force brain trauma, leading to movement of the brain and surrounding nerve tissue. This also can be caused by hypertension. Bleeding is typically from veins, resulting in slower bleeding.

9.20.1 Signs and symptoms

- Unequal pupils indicate increased intracranial pressure.
- Severe headache that is worsening related to increased bleedings.
- Decreased LOC.
- Confusion.
- Nausea/vomiting.
- Memory loss.
- Impaired language ability (aphasia).

9.20.2 Medical tests

- CT scan: Shows hematoma.
- MRI: Shows hematoma.

9.20.3 Treatment

- Surgical removal of the hematoma.
- Administer:
  - Antiemetic for nausea and vomiting.
    - Metoclopramide (Reglan).

        - Ondansetron (Zofran).
        - Prochlorperazine (Compazine).
    - Diuretic to reduce cerebral edema.
        - Mannitol, furosemide (Lasix).
    - Antiepileptic
        - Phenytoin (Dilantin), phenobarbital, carbamazepine (Tegretol), divalproex sodium (Depakote), valproic acid (Depakene), levetiracetam (Keppra), lamotrigine (Lamictal), clonazepam (Klonopin), topiramate (Topamax), ethosuximide (Zarontin), gabapentin (Neurontin), levetiracetam (Keppra), oxcarbazepine (Trileptal), primidone (Mysoline), tiagabine (Gabitril).

9.20.4 Intervention

- Bed rest.
- Monitor vital signs.
- Monitor neurologic status.
- Monitor for increased intracranial pressure (decreased LOC, restlessness, confusion, headaches, nausea, and vomiting).
- Instruct the patient:
    - No aspirin.
    - No anticoagulants.

9.21 Subarachnoid Hemorrhage

A subarachnoid hemorrhage is bleeding into the area between the arachnoid membrane and the pia mater surrounding the brain called the subarachnoid space. It is commonly caused by the rupture of a cerebral aneurysm and often seen in elderly who have fallen and hit their head.

9.21.1 Signs and symptoms

- Asymptomatic.
- Thunderclap headache.
- Low LOC.
- Vomiting.
- Seizures.
- Neck stiffness.
- Drowsy.
- Coma.
- Confusion.
- Bleeding into the eyeball (Terson syndrome) (intraocular hemorrhage).

9.21.2 Medical tests

- CT scan: Shows bleeding.
- MRI scan: Shows bleeding.
- Cerebral angiography: Shows altered blood flow.
- Arteriography: Shows altered blood flow.
- Lumbar puncture: Cerebrospinal fluid contains elevated number of red blood cells.

9.21.3 Treatment

- Surgical repair of bleeding.
- Administer:
  - Antiemetic for nausea and vomiting.
    - Metoclopramide (Reglan).
    - Ondansetron (Zofran).
    - Prochlorperazine (Compazine).
  - Diuretic to reduce cerebral edema.
    - Mannitol, furosemide (Lasix).
  - Antiepileptic.
    - Phenytoin (Dilantin), phenobarbital, carbamazepine (Tegretol), divalproex sodium (Depakote), valproic acid (Depakene), levetiracetam (Keppra), lamotrigine (Lamictal), clonazepam (Klonopin), topiramate (Topamax), ethosuximide (Zarontin), gabapentin (Neurontin), levetiracetam (Keppra), oxcarbazepine (Trileptal), primidone (Mysoline), tiagabine (Gabitril).

9.21.4 Intervention

- Bed rest.
- Monitor vital signs.
- Monitor neurologic status.
- Monitor for increased intracranial pressure (decreased LOC, restlessness, confusion, headaches, nausea, and vomiting).
- Instruct the patient:
  - No aspirin.
  - No anticoagulants.

Solved Problems

9.1 What would you suspect had occurred if your patient suddenly appeared confused, angry, and experienced aphasia?

Cerebrovascular accident.

9.2 Why would a prescriber order dexamethasone for a patient diagnosed with meningitis?

To decrease inflammation.

9.3 Why would a prescriber order Lasix for a patient diagnosed with encephalitis?

To reduce cerebral edema.

9.4 What is a coup injury?

Blunt force trauma thrust the brain against the inside of the skull at the point of the blunt force trauma.

9.5 What are the signs of a cerebral hemorrhage?

- Nausea.
- Vomiting.
- Disorientation.
- Headache.
- Unequal pupil size.
- Diminished or absent pupil reaction.
- Cognitive changes.
- Speech changes.
- Motor movement changes.
- Decreased LOC or loss of consciousness.
- Amnesia.
- Unilateral paralysis.
- Facial weakness or droop.

9.6 What is a cerebral angiograph?

A cerebral angiograph is a test that enables the practitioner to examine blood vessels in the brain. Radiopaque contrast medium is injected into the brachial artery or femoral artery. The contrast medium highlights blood vessels on the image.

9.7 When is damage assessed in a spinal cord injury?

Damaged is assessed when inflammation related to trauma subsides.

9.8 What is an intracerebral hematoma?

An intracerebral hematoma is blood (a blood clot) that accumulates in the cerebrum related to shear force brain trauma. It leads to movement of the brain and surrounding nerve tissue. This may also be caused by hypertension. Bleeding is typically from veins, resulting in slower bleeding.

9.9 What is a concussion?

Head trauma causes the brain to move within the skull, resulting in neural dysfunction. There is no bruising of brain tissue. The patient typically loses consciousness for a few minutes but no more than

6 hours. The patient experiences a headache for months. Full recovery occurs within 48 hours of the head trauma.

9.10 What is a contusion?

A contusion is a bruise of the brain as a result of acceleration-deceleration brain trauma; a coup injury, in which bruising occurs at the site of the impact, such as in a force blow to the head; or a contrecoup injury, in which bruising occurs at the opposite side of the impact, such as when the head hits the windshield in a motor vehicle accident.

9.11 Why would you place a patient who is experiencing a seizure on his or her side?

To decrease the risk of aspiration.

9.12 What would you suspect if a patient suddenly stared and had a brief loss of consciousness?

The patient is experiencing an absence seizure.

9.13 What would you suspect if the patient reported progressive weakness and paralysis beginning in the lower extremities and moving upward?

Ascending Guillain-Barré.

9.14 What is a common cause of encephalitis?

Viral infection.

9.15 What is a meningioma?

A benign tumor generated from the meninges.

9.16 What is the risk of prescribing antiplatelet medication?

Antiplatelet medication increases the risk of low platelet count (thrombocytopenia) and low white blood cell count (agranulocytosis).

9.17 What test may be ordered if the practitioner suspects inflammation in the brain?

CT scan.

9.18 Why would a calcium channel blocker be prescribed to a patient diagnosed with an aneurysm?

To reduce vasospasm, which increases pressure on the aneurysm.

9.19 What are common risks in the use of opioid analgesic?

Respiratory depression, bradycardia, sedation, and constipation.

9.20 Why would you expect a prescriber to order alteplase?

Alteplase is a thrombolytic used to remove a blood clot following an acute ischemic cerebral vascular accident.

9.21 Why would a prescriber order sumatriptan?

For migraine headaches.

9.22 Why would a prescriber order docusate sodium for a patient diagnosed with an aneurysm?

To decrease the need to strain during a bowl movement.

9.23 Why would a prescriber assess the level of Dilantin in a patient who has a history of seizures?

Dilantin is prescribed to reduce seizure activity. The level of Dilantin in blood will determine whether the patient has a therapeutic level of Dilantin to reduce seizure activity.

9.24 Why would a prescriber order plasma expander in a spinal injury?

Plasma expander increases circulation and oxygen to injured tissues.

9.25 What medications would you expect to be prescribed after the patient receives t-PA?

Heparin, warfarin (Coumadin), enoxaparin (Lovenox), and aspirin to reduce coagulation.

Hematologic and Immune Critical Care

10.1 Definitions

- Hematologic and immune critical care focuses on conditions that alter bone marrow, blood, and elements of the immune system that result in the patient becoming unstable.
- Hematologic and immune physiology can be disrupted by an inflammation, infection, or trauma, leading to life-threatening conditions that compromise other systems.
- The hematologic and immune critical care condition requires immediate, quick assessment and intervention.

10.1.1 Hematologic cycle

- Bone marrow produces stem cells that differentiate into blood cells.
- Red blood cells (RBCs, erythrocytes):
    - RBCs leave bone marrow as recticulocytes (immature cells) and mature in 24 hours.
    - RBCs contain hemoglobin (Hgb) and antigens.
    - Hgb carries oxygen from the lungs throughout the body and carbon dioxide from cells to the lungs.
    - Antigen is a substance on the surface of RBCs that triggers an immune response and determines the blood type.
    - RBC function for 120 days.
    - The spleen removes old RBC.
    - Recticulocyte production rate equals removal rate by the spleen.
- White blood cells (WBCs, leukocytes):
    - WBCs leave bone marrow as one of five types of cells, each playing a role in the immune process.

      - Neutrophils:
        - Immature neutrophils (bands) are produced by bone marrow in response to infection and mature in blood.
        - Neutrophils engulf, ingest, and digest foreign substances in tissue at the infection site.
        - Old neutrophils form pus.
      - Eosinophils:
        - Eosinophils are produced by bone marrow in response to an allergic reaction.
        - Eosinophils ingest antigen-antibody units at the site of the allergic reaction.
      - Basophils:
        - Basophils secrete histamine, heparin, and bradykinin to increase permeability of blood vessels so fluid passes freely into tissues.
      - Monocytes:
        - Monocytes dispose of remnants of cells as part of wound healing.
        - Monocytes are found in the spleen, lymph nodes, and the liver, where monocytes engulf, ingest, and digest microorganisms.
      - Lymphocytes:
        - Lymphocytes form one of two types of cells:
          - T lymphocytes attack nonspecific invading microorganisms.
          - B lymphocytes (antibodies) attack specific invading microorganisms.
- Platelets:
  - Platelets leave bone marrow as megakaryocytes.
  - Platelets form clots:
    - Platelets group together at the site of a rupture in a blood vessel wall to form a plug (clot).
    - Platelets also release substances that constrict blood vessels at the rupture site.

10.1.2 Immune cycle

- The immune system protects the body from microorganisms (bacteria, viruses, toxins, and parasites) by attacking these microorganisms before they can impede physiological activity of the cells within the body. Microorganisms include:
  - Bacteria are single-cell organisms that are able to reproduce and frequently release toxins that interrupt the physiological activity of cells.
  - A virus is a fragment of DNA in a protective shell that attaches to a cell and injects its DNA into the cell, in a sense taking over the cell. As the cell ruptures, the viral DNA attacks other cells.
  - A toxin is a substance that is poisonous to cells. The substance might be man-made or produced by a cell.
  - A parasite is an organism that lives on or in another organism.
- The immune system creates a barrier that prevents the microorganism from entering the body or cell and has a specialized cell (see 10.1.1 Hematologic cycle) to attack and kill the microorganism. In addition, the immune system destroys the body's imperfect cells (i.e., cancer).
- The immune system consists of:
  - Skin: The skin provides a barrier between microorganisms and cells within the body. The epidermis contains antibacterial substances that kill many microorganisms. Saliva, tears, and mucus contain enzymes that kill bacteria.

- Thymus: The thymus is a gland where T cells mature (see 10.1.1 Hematologic cycle) into one of five T cells:
  - Memory cells: Respond to second exposure to an antigen during which the antigen is attacked.
  - Lymphokine-producing cells: Delay hypersensitivity reactions.
  - Cytotoxic cells: Kill antigen-carrying cells and the antigen.
  - Helper cells (T4): Facilitate the cell-mediated response necessary to recognize foreign antigens.
  - Suppressor cells (T8): Inhibit the cell-mediated response.
- Spleen: The spleen is a blood filter where foreign cells and mature RBCs are removed from blood.
- Lymph system: The lymph system consists of lymph vessels, lymph nodes, and lymph. Lymph is blood plasma that receives nutrients and water from blood and carries nutrients and water to cells. Lymph surrounds cells. Protein and waste from cells enter the lymph. Lymph vessels drain and filter these byproducts of physiological activity of cells and remove bacteria. Lymph is collected in lymph nodes. Lymph nodes filter lymph. The filtered lymph is then returned into blood. The lymph nodes swell with bacteria and antibodies when the body has a bacterial infection. The swelling subsides as the antibodies destroy the bacteria.
- Bone marrow: Bone marrow produces WBCs, some of which are transformed into antibodies that attack microorganisms (see 10.1.1 Hematologic cycle).
- Complement system: The complement system consists of protein produced by the liver that freely floats in blood. It is activated by antibodies. These proteins cause invading cells to rupture (lysing) and signal the phagocytes to remove cell parts.
- Hormones: Hormones are chemical messengers that signal. Immune system hormones care called lymphokines:
  - Corticosteroids: Corticosteroids are hormones that suppress the immune system.
  - Tymosin: Tymosin is a hormone that causes production of WBCs.
  - Interleukin: Interleukin is a hormone produced by macrophages once the macrophage destroys the invading cell. Interleukin causes the hypothalamus to increase body temperature to a degree that bacteria die.
  - Tumor necrosis factor (TNF): TNF is a hormone produced by macrophages that causes tumor cells to be killed and helps to create new blood vessels.
  - Interferon: Interferon is a hormone produced by many cells when a virus is detected. Interferon causes cells to produce a protein that prevents the virus from replicating in other cells.

- Infection and inflammation:
  - Inflammation is a response to cell damage caused by injury or by a microorganism. Inflammation is different from an infection. An infection is the invasion of a microorganism into the body, which causes an inflammation response. However, the inflammation response can also occur in reaction to the cell damage caused by injury, not by a microorganism.
  - The inflammation response begins with damage to cells. The pattern recognition receptors (PRRs) at the injury site cause blood vessels at the site to dilate (vasodilation), resulting in increased blood flow to the site. PRRs also release bradykinin, which stimulates nerves at the site, causing the patient to focus on the injury.
  - Increased blood flow causes the site to become warm, swollen, and reddened (RBCs are closer to the surface of the skin). Blood vessels also become more permeable, enabling plasma and WBCs to enter the injured tissue. WBCs remove damaged cells. Plasma contains nutrients that promote new cell growth at the site. As damaged cells are removed and new cells grow, PRRs decrease and eventually stop the inflammation response at the site, resulting in contraction of blood vessels to their normal size (no swelling), and stopping the release of bradykinin (no pain).

- There are two categories of inflammation:
  - Acute inflammation: Acute inflammation occurs in response to an injury or invasion by a microorganism. Once damaged cells are removed and replaced by new cells, the inflammation process stops.
  - Chronic inflammation: Chronic inflammation is persistent inflammation caused by continued injury (e.g., osteoarthritis) or a malfunction to the immune system, preventing the inflammation response from shutting off once new cells replace damaged cells.
- Infection occurs as a result of invasion of a microorganism. The presence of the microorganism causes the immune response, which includes the inflammation response.
- Infection occurs when the chain of infection is in place:
  - Etiologic agent: There is a microorganism.
  - Reservoir: A place where the microorganism can grow (i.e., the body).
  - Portal of exit: A method of leaving the reservoir (airborne [sneeze, cough], contact [touch], ingestion).
  - Transmission: The microorganism moves to the patient.
  - Portal of entry: The microorganism enters the patient (i.e., through the nose, mouth, eyes, or a break in the skin).
  - Susceptible host: Barriers to infection are compromised. The patient's immune system (i.e., antibodies, WBCs) is unable to quickly kill the microorganism.

10.1.3 Hematologic and immune system assessment

The hematologic and immune critical care assessment:

- Look for clues of underlying cause of the hematologic and immune critical care issue:
  - Fatigue.
  - Fever.
  - Chills.
  - Frequent infections.
  - Slow wound healing.
  - Bruising (ecchymoses).
  - Enlarged lymph nodes.
  - Broken capillary (petechiae).
  - Bone pain.
  - Bleeding.
- Follow-up questions help probe further into the presenting hematologic and immune problem.
  - Have you recently undergone any medical procedure?
    - What medical procedure?
    - When was the medical procedure performed?
  - Have you noticed recent bruises?
  - Do you experience frequent fevers?
  - How long does it take for cuts to heal?
  - Do you experience shortness of breath?
  - Do you feel tried frequently?

- Inspect:
  - Skin:
    - Wounds.
    - Bruises.
    - Broken capillaries (decrease platelets [thrombocytopenia]).
    - Pallor (iron deficiency anemia).
    - Ruddy coloring (inflammation).
    - Dryness (iron deficiency anemia).
  - Nails:
    - Spoon-shaped (iron deficiency anemia).
    - Longitudinal striations (anemia).
  - Eyes:
    - Retinal hemorrhage (anemia, decreased platelets).
    - Signs of infection or inflammation.
  - Mouth:
    - White patches (candidiasis).
  - Abdomen:
    - Enlarged liver.
    - Enlarged spleen (overdestruction or production of RBCs).
- Palpation:
  - Lymph nodes.
    - Normal: Lymph nodes cannot be seen and should not be enlarged.

10.1.3.1 Signs and symptoms

The hematologic and immune critical care assessment requires the nurse to recognize common signs and symptoms of underlying causes and then prepare for the anticipated the treatment that the practitioner is likely to order. Commonly seen hematologic and immune signs and symptoms are:

- Fever (infection).
- Chills (infection).
- Frequent bleeding (decreased platelets).
- Fatigue (anemia).
- Shortness of breath (anemia).
- Swollen glands (infection).
- Increased WBC count without fever (leukemia).
- Frequent infection (immunodeficiency).
- Fatigue, muscle aches, low-grade fever (autoimmune disease).

10.2 Hematologic and Immune Tests

Hematologic and immune critical care tests are designed to assess the effectiveness and capability of the function of blood and the immune system. Critical care practitioners order hematologic and immune tests to collect objective data to further assess the patient and to assist in the stabilization of the patient. The following are commonly ordered hematologic and immune tests by the critical care practitioners.

10.2.1 Blood type test

Blood is identified by an antigen on the surface of RBCs. Major types of these antigens are blood group antigens and the Rh antigen. There are four types of blood group antigens that are determined by performing the ABO test:

- Type A: Has the A antigen and antibodies in plasma against B antigen.
- Type B: Has the B antigen and antibodies in plasma against the A antigen.
- Type O: Has neither the A antigen nor the B antigen, and antibodies in plasma against A antigen and B antigen.
- Type AB: Has the A antigen and the B antigen and no antibodies in plasma against the A antigen and B antigen.
- RBCs may have attached to it the Rh antigen, sometimes called the Rh factor. It is determined by the Rh test:
  - Rh positive (+): The Rh antigen is present on the RBCs.
  - Rh negative (−): The Rh antigen is not present on the RBCs.
- A patient's blood type is described as a combination of the blood group antigen and Rh antigen by using the blood type letter(s) followed by a plus (+) or minus (−) sign, indicating whether the Rh antigen is present. For example, type A− means that the patient has the A antigen but does not have the Rh antigen attached to the RBCs.
- Table 10.1 lists compatibility of blood for transfusion.
- Assess the patient for conditions that might affect the test results:
  - The patient has taken methyldopa, levodopa, or cephalexin. These medications can cause a false Rh+ test result
  - Recent x-ray with contrast.
  - Bone marrow transplant.
  - A blood transfusion in the previous 3 months.
  - Has or has had cancer or leukemia.

TABLE 10.1 Blood Transfusion Capability Chart

Recipient	Donor
A–	A– O–
A+	A– A+ O– O+
B–	B– O–
B+	B– B+ O– O+
AB–	AB– O–
AB+	AB– AB+ A– A+ B– B+ O– O+
O–	O–
O+	O– O+

10.2.2 Partial thromboplastin time (PTT)

PTT test measures clotting time of blood. This test is performed prior to any invasive procedure and to assess the effectiveness dose of heparin. Aspirin and antihistamines may affect the results of the test. A patient with a high PTT value is at risk for bleeding and bruising. Patients who have inherited bleeding disorders may have normal PTT values.

- Normal range is:
  - PTT: 30 to 40 seconds.
  - Proper heparin dose: The PTT is 1.5 to 2.5 greater than the normal value.
- Longer times may indicate:
  - Hemophilia.
  - Von Willebrand's disease.
  - A blood clotting factor is low or absent.
  - Nephrotic syndrome.
  - Cirrhosis.
  - Antiphospholipid antibody syndrome.
  - Lupus anticoagulant syndrome.
  - Factor XII deficiency.
  - Disseminated intravascular coagulation (DIC).
  - The patient has been administered heparin.
  - Hypofibrinogenemia.

10.2.3 Total serum protein

The total serum protein test assesses the levels of albumin, globulin, and total protein in a blood sample. The result compares the ratio of albumin to globulin. Protein is not stored. It is continuously metabolized into amino acids, which are used to make enzymes, hormones, and new proteins. Liver damage reduces the protein level in blood, but this level may not be reduced for 2 weeks after the damage because protein stays in blood for up to 18 days.

- Albumin is a protein produced by the liver that keeps blood from leaking from blood vessels. Albumin is also important for tissue growth and healing because it carries medicine to tissues.
- Globulin is a group of proteins made by the liver and the immune system that binds with Hgb and transports iron and metals in the blood to help fight infection. Globulin is composed of three different proteins: alpha, beta, and gamma.
- The total serum protein test reports separate values for total protein, albumin, and globulin. The amounts of albumin and globulin also are compared (albumin to globulin ratio).
- Test results can be affected by:
  - Taking androgens (male sex hormones), estrogen, corticosteroids, insulin, growth hormone, which can affect the test results
  - A chronic illness that interferes with nutrition.
  - Any recent injuries or infections.
  - Pregnancy.
  - Extended bed rest.

- Normal range is:
  - Total protein: 5.5 to 9.0 g/dl.
  - Albumin: 3.5 to 5.5 g/dl.
  - Globulin: 2.0 to 3.5 g/dl.
  - Albumin to globulin ratio: Greater than 1.0.
- High albumin levels may indicate:
  - Severe dehydration.
- High globulin levels may indicate:
  - Liver disease.
  - Kidney disease.
  - Hodgkin's lymphoma.
  - Leukemia.
  - Hemolytic anemia.
  - Macroglobulinemia.
  - Rheumatoid arthritis.
  - Lupus.
  - Sarcoidosis.
  - Autoimmune hepatitis.
  - Tuberculosis.
- Low albumin levels may indicate:
  - Malnutrition.
  - Kidney disease.
  - Liver disease.
  - Uncontrolled diabetes.
  - Hodgkin's lymphoma.
  - Severe burns.
  - Systemic lupus erythematosus (SLE).
  - Rheumatoid arthritis.
  - Heart failure.
  - Hyperthroidism.
  - Crohn's disease.
  - Celiac disease.
- Albumin to globulin ratio:
  - A ratio less than 1 indicates abnormal function in the body.

10.2.4 C-reactive protein (CRP)

CRP is produced as part of the inflammatory process and attaches to the invading microorganism or damaged cells, enhancing phagocytosis in the destruction of the microorganism or damaged cell. The CRP test measures the CRP level in the blood. A high level indicates inflammation, but not the source of the inflammation. The health-care provider will order other tests to identify the source of the inflammation. The CRP level peaks 6 hours following surgery and decreases by the third day. Infection as a result of surgery is suspected if the CRP level remains high after the third day. Elevated CRP level prior to surgery increases the risk of infection following surgery.

- Normal CRP range is: 0 to 1 mg/ml.
- High CRP values may indicate:
  - Inflammation.
  - Infection.
  - Risk of a heart attack.

10.2.5 Complete blood count (CBC)

The CBC test measures several components of blood to assess the patient for various disorders and is part of a routine blood screening. Components measured are:

- Leukocyte count (WBC): Leukocytes normally increase when infection is present but can also increase in the absence of infection if the patient has leukemia.
- Leukocyte cell type (WBC differential): There are five major types of leukocyte cells, each having a role in the immune process. These are neutrophils, lymphocytes, monocytes, eosinophils, and basophils. The quantity of each leukocyte cell type provides important information in diagnosing the patient's condition.
- Erythrocyte count (RBC): Erythrocyte cells carry oxygen and carbon dioxide.
- Erythrocyte indices:
  - Mean corpuscular volume (MCV): This is the size of erythrocytes.
  - Mean corpuscular Hgb (MCH): This is the amount of Hgb in an erythrocyte cells.
  - Mean corpuscular Hgb concentration (MCHC): This is the concentration of Hgb in an erythrocyte cell.
  - Red cell distribution width (RDW): This shows the different sizes of erythrocyte cells.
- Hematocrit (Hct, packed cell volume): The test measures the volume in percentage taken up by erythrocytes in the patient's blood.
- Hgb: The Hgb test measures the amount of Hgb in blood. Hgb is the part of the erythrocyte that carries oxygen.
- Thrombocyte count (platelet): Platelets form blood clots.
- Test results can be affected by:
  - Taking antibiotics, steroids, Equanil, thiazide diuretics, Miltown, quinidine, Meprospan, or chemotherapy.
  - High levels of triglycerides, which can affect the Hgb test.
  - An enlarged spleen, which can reduce the platelet count.
  - Pregnancy.
  - Smoking.
  - Stress.
  - Exercising before the test is administered.
- Normal leukocyte (WBC) count range is:
  - Men: 5000 to 10,000 μl^3.
  - Nonpregnant women: 4500 to 11,000 μl^3.

- Pregnant women:
  - First trimester: 6600 to 14,100 μl^3.
  - Second trimester: 6900 to 17,100 μl^3.
  - Third trimester: 5900 to 14,700 μl^3.
  - Postpartum: 9700 to 25,700 μl^3.
- Normal leukocyte cell type range is:
  - Neutrophils: 55% to 70%.
  - Band neutrophils: 0% to 3%.
  - Lymphocytes: 20% to 40%.
  - Monocytes: 2% to 8%.
  - Eosinophils: 1% to 4%.
  - Basophils: 0.5% to 1%.
- Normal erythrocyte (RBC) count range is:
  - Men: 4.7 to 6.1 million µl.
  - Women: 4.2 to 5.4 million µl.
  - Children: 4.0 to 5.5 million µl.
  - Newborns: 4.8 to 7.1 million µl.
- Normal Hct range is:
  - Men: 42% to 52%.
  - Women: 37% to 47%.
  - Pregnant women:
    - First trimester: 35% to 46%.
    - Second trimester: 30% to 42%.
    - Third trimester: 34% to 44%.
    - Postpartum: 30% to 44%.
  - Children: 32% to 44%.
  - Newborns: 44% to 64%.
- Normal Hgb range is:
  - Men: 14 to 18 g/dl.
  - Women: 12 to 16 g/dl.
  - Pregnant women:
    - First trimester: 11.4 to 15 g/dl.
    - Second trimester: 10 to 14.3 g/dl.
    - Third trimester: 10.2 to 14.4 g/dl.
    - Postpartum: 10.4 to 18 g/dl.
  - Children: 9.5 to 15.5 g/dl.
  - Newborns: 14 to 24 g/dl.
- Normal erythrocyte indices range is:
  - Mean corpuscular volume: 80 to 95 fl.
  - Mean corpuscular Hgb: 27 pg to 31 pg.
  - Mean corpuscular Hgb concentration: 32 to 36 g/dl.

- Normal red cell distribution width range is: 11% to 14.5%.
- Normal thrombocyte count range is:
  - Adults and children: 150,000 to 400,000 mm^3.
  - Babies: 200,000 to 475,000 mm^3.
  - Newborns: 150,000 to 300,000 mm^3.
- High leukocyte (WBC) count might indicate:
  - Inflammation.
  - Infection.
  - Leukemia.
  - Tissue damage.
  - Stress.
  - Malnutrition.
  - Lupus.
  - Kidney failure.
  - Rheumatoid arthritis.
  - Thyroid gland problems.
- High erythrocyte (RBC) counts might indicate:
  - Lung disease.
  - Alcoholism.
  - Polycythemia vera.
  - Smoking.
  - The patient is using diuretics.
- High thrombocyte counts might indicate:
  - Bleeding.
  - Bone marrow problems.
  - Iron deficiency.
- High MCV might indicate:
  - Folate deficiency.
  - Vitamin B12 deficiency.
- Low leukocyte (WBC) count might indicate:
  - Alcoholism.
  - Lupus.
  - Cushing's syndrome.
  - Aplastic anemia.
  - Enlarged spleen.
  - Viral infection.
- Low erythrocyte counts might indicate:
  - Anemia.
  - Addison's disease.
  - Sickle cell disease
  - Inflammatory bowel disease.

        - Peptic ulcer.
        - Removal of the spleen.
        - Pernicious anemia.
    - Low thrombocyte counts might indicate:
        - Risk of bleeding.
        - Idiopathic thrombocytopenic purpura.
        - Pregnancy.
        - Enlarged spleen.
    - Low MCV might indicate:
        - Iron deficiency.
        - Thalassemia deficiency.

10.2.6 Cold agglutinins

Agglutinins are antibodies that cause RBCs to aggregate, forming a clump called Rouleaux formation at low temperatures as an immune reaction to an infection. High levels of agglutinins can impede blood flow to the extremities when exposed to cold, resulting in tissue damage unless the extremity is warmed. High levels of agglutinins can cause hemolytic anemia. The cold agglutinin test measures the level of agglutinins in a blood sample.

- The test is affected by:
    - Taking penicillin or cephalosporins.
    - Measles, malaria, congenital syphilis, pneumonia, chickenpox, anemia, infectious mononucleosis, cirrhosis, or multiple myeloma.
- Normal cold agglutinins titer range is below 1 to 40 (1:40).
- High cold agglutinins titer may indicate:
    - Pneumonia.
    - Hepatitis C.
    - Cirrhosis.
    - Infectious mononucleosis.
    - Rheumatoid arthritis.
    - Malaria.

10.2.7 Prothrombin time

There are 12 factors that must be present to coagulate (clot) blood. Prothrombin is clotting factor II synthesized by the liver with the assistance of vitamin K. When a blood vessel is injured, prothrombin is converted to thrombin, a protein, which forms a blood clot with other proteins to stop the bleeding. The PT test determines the time necessary for plasma to clot. The healthcare provider orders the PT test to assess the patient's risk of bleeding and to assess the therapeutic effect of anticoagulation medication.

- The test is affected by:
    - Vomiting or diarrhea.
    - Alcohol.
    - Taking vitamin K, Tagamet, birth control pills, aspirin, antibiotics, hormone replacement therapy, or Coumadin.

- Normal test results:
  - PT: 10 to 13 seconds.
  - INR: 1 to 1.4 seconds.
  - Coumadin PT: 1.5 to 2.5 times normal PT.
  - Coumadin INR time: 2 to 3 times normal PT.
- Longer PT may indicate:
  - Cirrhosis.
  - Risk of bleeding.
  - Vitamin K deficiency.
  - DIC.
  - Too much Coumadin or heparin.
- Low Coumadin PT may indicate:
  - Not enough Coumadin.

10.2.8 Reticulocyte count

Reticulocyte is an immature RBC that is released by bone marrow and develops into a mature RBC in 2 days. The reticulocyte count test determines the amount of reticulocyte in a blood sample.

- The test may be affected by:
  - Radiation therapy.
  - Pregnancy.
  - Blood transfusion in the previous week.
  - A prostate biopsy in the past 8 weeks.
  - Taking Bactrim, Septra, corticotrophin, Imuran, levodopa, Chloromycetin, methotrexate, or Cosmegen.
- Normal test results: 0.5% to 2.5%.
- Higher levels may indicate:
  - Hemolysis.
  - Anemia.
  - Hemorrhaging.
- Low levels may indicate:
  - Aplastic anemia.
  - Iron deficiency anemia.
  - Folic acid deficiency.
  - Vitamin B12 deficiency.

10.2.9 Sedimentation Rate

An increase in fibrinogen in blood during the inflammatory process causes erythrocytes (RBCs) to adhere to each other, forming a stack called rouleaux. The sedimentation rate test measures how many millimeters per hour erythrocytes settle to the bottom of a test tube. Rouleaux settles quicker than erythrocytes. Therefore, the increased sedimentation rate indicates that the patient has inflammation. Not all inflammation increases the sedimentation rate. Therefore, a normal sedimentation rate does not rule out inflammation.

- Test results can be affected by:
  - Pregnancy.
  - Menstrual period.
  - Anemia.
- Normal test results:
  - Men: 0 to 15 mm/hr.
  - Women: 0 to 20 mm/hr.
  - Children: 0 to 10 mm/hr.
  - Newborn: 0 to 2 mm/hr.
- Higher levels may indicate:
  - Inflammation.
  - Rheumatoid arthritis.
  - SLE.
- Lower levels may indicate:
  - Sickle cell disease.
  - Hyperglycemia.
  - Polycythemia.

10.2.10 Iron

Iron is a mineral in food that is needed for cell growth. Once metabolized, iron binds to the transferrin protein, which transports iron to bone marrow and other tissues. Iron tests measure the amount of iron that is bound to transferrin. There are three iron tests:

- Total iron-binding capacity (TIBC) test: This test measures the capacity of the blood to carry iron by determining the amount of iron needed to bind to all the available transferring proteins.
- Serum iron test: This test measures the amount of circulated iron in the blood.
- Transferrin saturation test: This is the percentage of serum iron of total iron-binding capacity.
- Test results may be affected by:
  - Taking iron supplements 12 hours before the test is administered.
  - Taking vitamin B12 supplements 2 days before the test.
  - Sleep deprivation.
  - Stress.
  - A blood transfusion 4 months prior to the test.
- Normal test results:
  - Serum iron:
    - Men: 80 to 180 μg/dl.
    - Women: 60 to 160 μg/dl.
    - Children: 50 to 120 μg/dl.

  - TIBC: 250 to 450 μg/dl.
  - Transferrin saturation:
    - Men: 20% to 50%.
    - Women: 15% to 50%.
- High levels may indicate:
  - Hemochromatosis.
  - Kidney disease.
  - Cirrhosis.
  - Lead poisoning.
- Low levels may indicate:
  - Iron deficiency anemia.
  - Iron deficient diet.
  - Bleeding.
  - Pregnancy.
  - Rapid growth.

10.2.11 Blood culture

Blood can be infected by bacteria or fungi. A blood culture identifies the bacteria or fungi by allowing the microorganism to grow in a controlled environment and then examining the microorganism under a microscope.

- Test results are affected by:
  - Taking antibiotics.
- Normal is negative: No bacteria or fungi found in the blood sample.
- Normal false-negative: Improper processing or improper sampling results in bacteria or fungi not found in the blood sample, but the patient's blood is infected.
- Abnormal is positive: Bacteria or fungi found in the blood sample.
- Abnormal false-positive: Contaminated sample or improper processing results in bacteria or fungi found in the blood sample but not in the patient's blood.

10.2.12 Mononucleosis tests

The Epstein-Barr virus EBV causes mononucleosis. Mononucleosis tests identify antibodies for EBV in the blood sample. There are two kinds of mononucleosis tests:

- Monospot test: This test identifies heterophil antibodies that form between 2 weeks and 9 weeks after the patient becomes infected.
- EBV antibody test: This test is ordered when the patient shows symptoms of mononucleosis and the monospot test is negative.
- Test results can be affected by:
  - A false-negative result can occur if the test is administered within 2 weeks of the patient being infected.
- Normal (negative) heterophil antibody range is 0.

- High (positive) heterophil antibody levels greater than 0 may indicate:
  - Mononucleosis.
  - Rheumatoid arthritis.
  - Leukemia.
  - Hepatitis.
  - Lymphoma.

10.2.13 *Helicobacter pylori* tests

Helicobacter pylori (*H. pylori*) is a type of bacteria that infects the stomach and duodenum. It may result in a peptic ulcer. Many patients have *H. pylori* but few develop peptic ulcer disease. Four tests are used to detect *H. pylori*:

- *H. pylori* blood antibody test: This test determines whether the blood sample has *H. pylori* antibodies.
- Urea breath test: This test determines the presence of *H. pylori* in the stomach.
- *H. pylori* stool antigen test: This test determines the presence of *H. pylori* antigens in feces.
- Stomach biopsy: This is endoscopic removal of the lining of the stomach and small intestine, which is examined for the presence of *H. pylori*.
- Test results can be affected by:
  - Pregnancy or breastfeeding.
  - Taking antibiotics.
  - Taking Prilosec, Carafate, Pepcid, Aciphex, Zantac, or Pepto-Bismol.
- Blood test:
  - Normal result is: No *H. pylori* antibodies.
  - Abnormal blood test result is: Presence of *H. pylori* antibodies.
- Urea breath test:
  - Normal result is: No tagged hydrocarbon.
  - Abnormal blood test result is: Tagged hydrocarbon present.
- Stool antigen test:
  - Normal result is: No *H. pylori* antigens.
  - Abnormal blood test result is: Presence of *H. pylori* antigens.
- Stomach biopsy:
  - Normal result is: No *H. pylori*.
  - Abnormal blood test result is: Presence of *H. pylori*.

10.2.14 Immunoglobulins

Immunoglobulins are antibodies made by the immune system in response to microorganisms that enter the body, an allergen, and abnormal cells such as cancer cells. An antibody is specific to an antigen. The immunoglobulin test measures the level of an immunoglobulin in the patient's blood. A low level of a specific immunoglobulin increases the risk of repeated infections from an antigen. There are five major types of immunoglobulins. These are:

- IgA: This is found in tears and saliva and protects the ears, eyes, breathing passages, digestive tract, and vagina that are exposed to outside antigens; 10% of immunoglobulins.

- IgG: This is found in all body fluids and defends the body against viruses and bacteria. This immunoglobulin crosses the placenta; 80% of immunoglobulins.
- IgM: This is found in blood and lymph fluid and is the first response to infection; 5% of immunoglobulins. Forms when an infection occurs for the first time.
- IgE: This is found on mucous membranes, lungs, and skin and defends against allergens. A high level of IgE immunoglobulins is common in patients who are hyperallegenic. Less than 5% of immunoglobulins.
- IgD: This is found in abdominal and chest tissues; less than 5% of immunoglobulins.
- Test results can be affected by:
  - Taking hydralazine (Apresoline), phenylbutazone, birth control pills, anticonvulsants (phenytoin), methotrexate, aminophenazone, asparaginase, and corticosteroids.
  - Receiving a blood transfusion within 6 months before the test.
  - Using alcohol or illegal medication.
- Normal ranges are:
  - IgA = 85 to 385 mg/dl.
  - IgG = 565 to 1,765 mg/dl.
  - IgM = 55 to 375 mg/dl.
  - IgD = less than 8 or 5 to 30 μg/l.
  - IgE = 10 to 1,421 μg/l.
- Abnormally high values and low values are not used to diagnose a condition.

10.2.15 Antinuclear antibodies (ANA)

In autoimmune diseases, the body produces antibodies that attach and destroy the body's own cells. The ANA test measures the pattern and amount of these antibodies.

- Test results can be affected by:
  - Medication for high blood pressure, heart disease, and tuberculosis (TB).
- Normal range is:
  - 1:40 or less than 40.
- Abnormally high values are not used to diagnose a condition.

10.2.16 CD4+ count

Three types of leukocytes (WBC) important to fighting infection are T lymphocytes, T cells, and T-helper cells. The CD4+ count test measures the level of these leukocytes to assess the patient's immune system. Patients who have a low CD4+ count are at risk for opportunistic infections.

- Test results can be affected by:
  - Time when the CD4+ blood sample is taken, because CD4+ cells are normally lower in the morning.
  - The blood sample was not refrigerated.
  - Influenza, pneumonia, or herpes simplex, which can affect the test results.
  - Taking corticosteroids or undergoing chemotherapy.

- Normal CD4+ cell count range is:
  - 600 to 1200 cells/μl: not infected with human immunodeficiency virus (HIV).
  - Greater than 350 cells/μl: low risk for opportunistic infection.
- 200 to 350 cells/μl count may indicate:
  - Weak immune system.
  - Risk of opportunistic infection.
  - Start antiretroviral treatment.
- Under 200 cells/μl may indicate:
  - High risk for opportunistic infection.
  - Acquired immunodeficiency syndrome (AIDS).

10.2.17 Viral load measurement

HIV in a patient's blood is determined by the presence of HIV RNA. The amount of HIV RNA indicates whether the infection is decreasing, stabilized, or increasing. The viral load measurement test determines the amount of HIV RNA in the patient's blood. A viral load measurement test is administered when the patient is diagnosed with HIV and the result becomes the baseline. Results of subsequent viral load measurement tests are compared to the baseline to determine the infection's progress. A patient diagnosed with HIV who has a negative viral load measurement test result can infect another person. The viral load measurement test result is compared to the baseline test result and to previous tests results to determine the trend of the infection. There are three types of viral load measurement tests:

- Branched DNA (bDNA) test.
- Nucleic acid sequence-based amplification (NASBA) test.
- Reverse-transcriptase polymerase chain reaction (RT-PCR) test.
- Test results can be affected by:
  - Recent immunizations.
- Normal viral load measurement test result is (negative).
- Abnormal viral load measurement test result HIV RNA is found and is reported as copies per milliliter, where a copy is an HIV RNA.

10.2.18 Rheumatoid factor (RF)

The rheumatoid factor (RF) is an autoantibody that destroys the patient's own tissues, resulting in stiffness, joint pain, and inflammation. The RF test measures the amount of the RF in the blood sample and is used to differentiate rheumatoid arthritis from other forms of arthritis. There are two types of RF tests: the agglutination test and the nephelometry test.

- Test results can be affected by:
  - Age: Patients older than 65 years of age normally have a higher RF level.
- Normal test results: 1:20 to 1:40 or less.
- Higher levels may indicate:
  - Rheumatoid arthritis.
  - SLE.

10.3 Hematologic and Immune Medication

Commonly used medications for hematologic and immune disorders are anticoagulant medication, hematinic medication, heparin antagonist medication, blood derivatives, hemostatic medication, immune serums, and medication to treat HIV.

10.3.1 Anticoagulants

Anticoagulant medication is ordered to decrease the blood's ability to coagulate and is commonly prescribed for patients diagnosed with deep vein thrombosis (DVT).

- Medications:
  - Heparin.
  - Enoxaparin sodium (Lovenox).
  - Warfarin (Coumadin).
- Use: Reduce blood coagulation.
- Considerations:
  - Monitor platelet count.
  - PTT should be 1.5 to 2 times the normal value (heparin).
  - PT should be 1.5 to 3 times the normal value (warfarin).
  - Patient needs to avoid activities that may result in injury.
  - Heparin is administered intravenously or subcutaneously, not intramuscularly.
  - Lovenox is administered subcutaneously, not intramuscularly.
  - Warfarin is administered orally.
- Adverse effects:
  - Hemorrhage.
  - Fever.
  - Anorexia.
  - Decreased platelets (thrombocytopenia).

10.3.2 Hematinics medication

Hematinic medication is administered to reduce iron requirements of the body.

- Medications:
  - Ferrous sulfate.
- Use: Iron deficiency.
- Considerations:
  - Administer medication between meals to prevent upset stomach.
  - Give medication in orange juice, not with milk.
  - Avoid antacids when administering medication.
  - Use straw to administer medication to prevent staining teeth.

- Adverse effects:
  - Black stools.
  - Nausea/vomiting.
  - Epigastric pain.

10.3.3 Heparin antagonist

Heparin antagonist medication is administered to reverse the anticoagulation effect of heparin and is administered for a heparin overdose.

- Medications:
  - Protamine.
- Use: Reverse effects of heparin.
- Consideration:
  - Administer slowly.
  - Monitor for bleeding.
- Adverse effects:
  - Circulatory collapse.
  - Acute pulmonary hypertension.
  - Bradycardia.
  - Nausea.
  - Vomiting.

10.3.4 Blood derivatives

Blood derivative medication is administered to replace blood volume.

- Medications:
  - Plasma protein fractions.
  - Normal serum albumin 5% or 25%.
- Use: Hypoproteinemia, hypovolemic shock.
- Considerations:
  - No more than 250 g within 48 hours.
  - Monitor for vascular overload:
    - Pulmonary edema.
    - Heart failure.
  - Monitor input/output
  - Medication should appear clear, not cloudy.
- Adverse effects:
  - Fever.
  - Headache.
  - Vascular overload.

- Hypotension.
- Back pain.
- Difficulty breathing.

10.3.5 Hemostatics medication

Hemostatic medication is administered to reduce excessive bleeding caused by the use of anticlotting medication.

- Medications:
  - Aminocaproic acid (Amicar).
- Use: Excessive bleeding caused by anticlotting medication.
- Considerations:
  - Dilute medication with normal saline or lactated Ringer's solution.
  - Monitor PT, PTT, and INR for coagulation.
- Adverse effects:
  - Cramps.
  - Nausea/vomiting.
  - Circulatory collapse.
  - Pulmonary hypertension.
  - Bradycardia.

10.3.6 Immune serums

Immune serums are administered for exposure to hepatitis B.

- Medications:
  - Hepatitis B immune globulin (H-BIG).
  - Immune globulin.
- Use: Exposure to hepatitis B.
- Considerations:
  - Inject into the deltoid muscle or anterolateral thigh.
  - Administer with hepatitis B vaccine.
  - Risk of anaphylactic reaction.
- Adverse effects:
  - Hives.
  - Anaphylactic reaction.
  - Swelling.
  - Headache.
  - Muscle stiffness.
  - Chest tightness.

10.3.7 Protease inhibitors

Protease inhibitors are administered to treat HIV.

- Medications:
  - Indinavir (Crixivan).
  - Ritonavir (Norvir).
  - Saquinavir (Invirase).
- Use: Treatment of HIV.
- Considerations:
  - Patient must drink six glasses of water daily.
  - Administer on empty stomach (indinavir [Crixivan]).
  - Administer with food (ritonavir [Norvir]).
  - Monitor:
    - Liver functions.
    - Glucose.
- Adverse effects:
  - Seizure.
  - Nausea/vomiting.
  - Acute renal failure.
  - Portal hypertension.
  - Hyperglycemia.
  - Pain.
  - Rash.
  - Dizziness.

10.3.8 Immunosuppressant

Immunosuppressant medication is administered to reduce organ rejection after organ transplantation.

- Medications:
  - Cyclosporine.
- Use: Reduce organ rejection.
- Considerations:
  - Administer medication with fruit juice or milk.
  - Give medication in glass container.
  - Administer medication in the morning.
- Adverse effects:
  - Headache.
  - Increased risk of infection.
  - Seizures.
  - Kidney toxicity.

    - Hypertension.
    - Anaphylaxis.
    - Confusion.
    - Tremors.

10.3.9 Nucleoside analogs

Nucleoside analog medication is administered to treat HIV.

- Medications:
    - Zalcitabine (Hivid).
    - Lamivudine (Epivir).
    - Zidovudine (AZT, Retrovir).
    - Stavudine (Zerit).
- Use: Treatment of HIV.
- Considerations:
    - Monitor:
        - Liver function.
        - Pancreatic function.
        - Peripheral neuropathy.
    - Administer with other antiviral medication.
- Adverse effects:
    - Peripheral neuropathy.
    - Nausea/vomiting.
    - Headache.
    - Liver toxicity.
    - Fatigue.
    - Decreased platelets.
    - Seizures.
    - Anemia.
    - Fever.

10.3.10 Non-nucleoside reverse transcriptase inhibitors

Non-nucleoside reverse transcriptase inhibitors are administered to treat HIV.

- Medications:
    - Delavirdine (Rescriptor).
    - Nevirapine (Viramune).
- Use: Treatment of HIV.
- Considerations:
    - Administer with other antiviral medication.

- Adverse effects:
    - Rash.
    - Nausea/vomiting.
    - Pain.
    - Headache.
    - Anxiety.
    - Liver toxicity.
    - Fever.

10.4 Anemia

Anemia is a low hemoglobin or RBC count, which results in decreased oxygen-carrying capability of the blood. This may be due to blood loss, damage to the RBCs due to altered hemoglobin or destruction (hemolysis), nutritional deficiency (iron, vitamin B12, folic acid), lack of RBC production, or bone marrow failure. Some patients have a family history of anemia due to genetic transmission, such as thalassemia or sickle cell.

10.4.1 Signs and symptoms

- Fatigue due to hypoxia from less oxygen being available to the tissues of the body.
- Weakness due to hypoxia.
- Pallor due to less oxygen being available to the surface tissues.
- Tachycardia, as the body attempts to compensate for less available oxygen by beating more rapidly to increase blood supply.
- Systolic murmur due to increased turbulence of blood flow.
- Dyspnea or shortness of breath due to hypoxia as the body attempts to get more oxygen.
- Angina as the myocardium is not getting enough oxygen.
- Headache due to hypoxia.
- Lightheadedness due to hypoxia.
- Bone pain due to increased erythropoiesis as the body attempts to correct anemia.
- Jaundice in hemolytic anemia due to increased levels of bilirubin as RBCs break down.

10.4.2 Medical tests

- Hgb level is low.
- Hct level is low.
- RBC count is low.
- MCV shows size of cell: normal (normocytic), microcytic (low), or macrocytic (high).
- MCH shows color of cell: normal (normochromic), hypochromic (low).

- RDW (red cell distribution width) elevated; shows the variation of the cell sizes. The variation in cell size is greater when the body is attempting to compensate for anemia.
- Reticulocyte count elevated when RBC cell production is increased to compensate for the anemia.

10.4.3 Treatment

- Correction of the underlying cause is necessary. Treatment may include dietary modifications and supplementations.

10.4.4 Intervention

- Check vital signs for changes.
- Monitor CBC.
- Plan nursing care based on patient tolerance of activity.
- Monitor for angina.

10.5 Aplastic Anemia (Pancytopenia)

The bone marrow stops producing a sufficient amount of RBCs, WBCs, and platelets, increasing the risk of infection and hemorrhage. The red cells remaining in circulation are normal in size and color. This may be due to chemical exposure or high-dose radiation exposure, or exposure to toxins. Cancer treatments such as radiation therapy and chemotherapeutic agents may suppress bone marrow function, which will result in anemia (low RBC), thrombocytopenia (low platelets), and leukopenia (low WBC). The cause may also be unknown or idiopathic. The bone marrow dysfunction may be slow onset or sudden. The lifespan of the RBC is longer than the platelets and WBC, so the anemia may show up later than the effects of losing the other cells. Some exposures to toxic agents or medications are severe and potentially fatal in susceptible individuals.

10.5.1 Signs and symptoms

- Fatigue due to hypoxemia.
- Weakness due to tissue hypoxia.
- Pallor due to lack of oxygen reaching superficial tissues.
- Infections due to low WBC production, causing decreased ability to fight infection.
- Bruising (ecchymosis) and tiny under-skin hemorrhages (petechiae) due to decrease in platelets, altering clotting ability.
- Bleeding from mucous membranes (GI tract, mouth, nosebleeds, vaginal).

10.5.2 Medical tests

- Decreased:
  - Hgb.
  - Hct.

    - RBC count.
    - Platelet count (thrombocytopenia).
    - WBC (leukopenia).
    - Reticulocyte count
- Positive fecal occult blood test.
- Decreased cell counts in bone marrow biopsy as body stops producing RBCs, WBCs, and platelets

10.5.3 Treatment

- Administer:
    - Hematopoietic growth factor to correct anemia in patients with low erythropoietin levels.
    - Erythropoietin:
        - Epoetin alfa.
    - Human granulocyte colony-stimulating factor (G-CSF) to correct low WBC levels:
        - Filgrastim.
    - Granulocyte-macrophage colony stimulating factor (GM-CSF) sargramostim.
    - Packed RBC transfusions when anemia is symptomatic.
    - Platelet transfusion for severe bleeding.
    - Bone marrow transplant replaces functioning stem cells.
    - Immunosuppressive drugs:
        - Antithymocyte globulin.
        - Corticosteroids.
    - Splenectomy when spleen is enlarged and destroying RBCs.

10.5.4 Intervention

- Monitor vital signs for changes.
- Record intake and output of fluids.
- Protect patient from falls.
- Avoid intramuscular (IM) injections due to altered clotting ability.
- Instruct the patient:
    - No aspirin due to effect on platelet aggregation (clotting ability).
    - Plan to take rest periods during activities due to fatigue.
    - Only use an electric razor to decrease risk of bleeding due to decreased platelet count.
    - Call physician if there are signs of bleeding or bruising.

10.6 Iron Deficiency Anemia

In iron deficiency anemia, a lower than normal amount of iron in blood serum results in decreased formation of Hgb and a decreased ability for the blood to carry oxygen. Iron stores are typically depleted first, followed by serum iron levels. Iron deficiency may be due to blood loss, dietary deficiency, or increased demand due to pregnancy or lactation. As RBCs age, the body breaks them down and the iron is released. This iron is reused for the production of new blood cells. A small amount of iron is lost daily through the gastrointestinal tract, necessitating dietary replacement. When RBCs are produced without a sufficient amount of iron, the cells are smaller and paler than usual. Iron deficiency anemia is a common type of anemia. Typically, patients respond to oral supplementation of iron. Occasionally a patient will have problems absorbing iron from the intestinal tract. These patients will need parenteral supplementation. Once iron stores are replaced, the anemia should correct and Hgb levels return to normal. Some patients may need lifelong supplementation, depending on the cause of the deficiency.

10.6.1 Signs and symptoms

- Weakness due to anemia and tissue hypoxia.
- Pallor due to decreased amount of oxygen getting to surface tissues.
- Fatigue due to anemia and hypoxemia.
- Thin, concave-shaped nails raised at edges, also called spoon nails (koilonychia sign).
- Tachycardia and tachypnea on exertion due to increased demand for oxygen.

10.6.2 Medical tests

- Decreased:
  - Serum Hgb.
  - Serum ferritin.
  - Transferrin saturation.
- Normal then low:
  - MCV (microcytic anemia).
  - MCH (hypochromic anemia).
- Increased:
  - Serum iron-binding capacity.
  - Platelet count .
- Peripheral blood smear shows RBCs of different shapes (poikilocytosis).

10.6.3 Treatment

- Iron replacement therapy (3 to 6 months after the anemia has been corrected).
- Administer:
  - Iron:
    - Ferrous sulfate.
    - Ferrous gluconate.
    - Ferrous fumarate.
- Increase dietary intake of iron.

10.6.4 Intervention

- Monitor:
  - Intake and output.

- Vital signs for tachycardia or tachypnea.
- Reactions to parenteral iron therapy.
- Instruct the patient:
  - Check for bleeding.
  - Increase iron in diet.
  - Teach dietary sources of iron.

10.7 Pernicious Anemia

In pernicious anemia, the body is unable to absorb vitamin B12, which is needed to make RBCs, resulting in a decrease in RBC count. More common in people of northern European descent, the anemia typically develops in adulthood. Intrinsic factor is normally secreted by the parietal cells of the gastric mucosa, and it is necessary to allow intestinal absorption of vitamin B12. Destruction of the gastric mucosa due to an autoimmune response results in loss of parietal cells within the stomach. The ability of vitamin B12 to bind with intrinsic factor is lost, decreasing the amount that is absorbed. Typical onset is between the ages of 40 and 60. Ongoing replacement of vitamin B12 is necessary to correct the deficit and alleviate symptoms that may have developed. Without treatment, the neurologic effects will continue, ultimately leading to dementia.

10.7.1 Signs and symptoms

- Pallor due to anemia.
- Weakness and fatigue due to anemia.
- Tingling in hands and feet (feeling like stocking or glove on hands/feet) due to bilateral demyelination of dorsal and lateral columns of spinal cord nerves.
- Diminished vibratory and position sense.
- Poor balance due to effect on cerebral function.
- Dementia appears later in the disease.
- Beefy red tongue (atrophic glossitis).
- Nausea may lead to anorexia weight loss.
- Premature graying of hair.

10.7.2 Medical tests

- Decreased:
  - Hgb.
  - Hydrochloric acid (hypochlorhydria).
- Increased:
  - MCV (macrocytic anemia).
- Positive:
  - Schilling test due to decrease in intrinsic factor.
  - Romberg test due to ataxia and neurologic changes.

10.7.3 Treatment

- No oral B12 supplementation because patients cannot absorb vitamin B12 due to insufficient intrinsic factor.
- Vitamin B12 by IM injection.
- Transfusion of packed RBCs if anemia is severe.

10.7.4 Intervention

- Prevent injuries.
- Instruct the patient:
  - Use soft toothbrush due to oral changes.
  - Avoid activities that could lead to injury due to paresthesias or changes in balance.
  - Inspect feet each day for injury due to paresthesia.

10.8 Disseminated Intravascular Coagulation (DIC)

Blood coagulates through the entire body within the vascular compartment, depleting platelets and the blood's ability to coagulate. This results in bleeding in other areas. It occurs as a complication of some other condition. The coagulation sequence is activated in the body, which causes microthrombi to develop because levels of all the major anticoagulants are reduced. The clots that form are the result of coagulation proteins and platelets, resulting in severe hemorrhage. It is often due to obstetric complications, post trauma, sepsis, cancer, or shock.

10.8.1 Signs and symptoms

- Unexpected bleeding.
- Petechiae as clotting factors are lost.
- Purpura as clotting factors are lost.
- Severe hemorrhage as clotting factors are lost.
- Uncontrolled postpartum bleeding.
- Tissue hypoxia from microemboli.
- Hemolytic anemia as cells are destroyed trying to pass through partially blocked vessels.

10.8.2 Medical tests

- Decreased:
  - Platelet count: thrombocytopenia.
- Increased:
  - Fibrin degradation.
  - D-dimer.
  - PT.
  - PTT.

10.8.3 Treatment

- Administer:
  - Transfusion:
    - Packed RBCs to replace what has been lost due to bleeding:
      - Fresh frozen plasma: replaces coagulation factor deficiency.
      - Platelets.
      - Cryoprecipitate replaces fibrinogen.
  - Anticoagulant:
    - Heparin.
- Bed rest.

10.8.4 Intervention

- Monitor for bleeding.
- Avoid cleaning blood clots.
- Instruct the patient:
  - Avoid situations that might cause bleeding.
  - Use electric razor.
  - Use soft toothbrush.
  - Do not floss.

10.9 Hemophilia

The patient is missing a coagulation factor that is essential for normal blood clotting and as a result, the blood does not clot when the patient bleeds. It is an X-linked recessive inherited disorder, passed on so that it presents symptoms in males and rarely in females. Hemophilia A is the result of missing clotting factor VIII. Hemophilia B is the result of missing clotting factor IX and is also known as Christmas disease. The most common sites of bleeding are into the joints, muscles, or from the gastrointestinal tract. Mild forms of the disease will only cause bleeding after surgery or trauma, whereas severe forms of the disease will cause bleeding without any prior cause.

10.9.1 Signs and symptoms

- Tender joints due to bleeding.
- Swelling of knees, ankles, hips, and elbows due to bleeding.
- Blood in stool (tarry stool) due to gastrointestinal blood loss.
- Blood in the urine (hematuria).

10.9.2 Medical tests

- Increased:
  - PTT prolonged.

- Decreased:
  - Clotting factor VIII found in blood serum (hemophilia A).
  - Clotting factor IX found in blood serum (hemophilia B).

10.9.3 Treatment

- Avoid aspirin.
- Administer:
  - Factor VIII concentrates (hemophilia A).
  - Factor IX concentrates (hemophilia B).
  - Cryoprecipitate.
  - Desmopressin (DDAVP) (mild deficiency).

10.9.4 Intervention

- No IM injections.
- No aspirin.
- To stop bleeding:
  - Elevate site.
  - Apply direct pressure to the site.
- Instruct the patient:
  - Wear a medical alert identification.
  - Contact physician for any injury.
  - Avoid situations that injury might occur.

10.10 Leukemia

Leukemia is the replacement of bone marrow by abnormal cells, resulting in unregulated proliferation of immature WBCs entering the circulatory system. These leukemic cells may also enter the liver, spleen, or lymph nodes, causing these areas to enlarge. Leukemia is classified as acute/chronic and by:

- Lymphocytic leukemias involve immature lymphoctes originating in the bone marrow and typically infiltrate the spleen, lymph nodes, or central nervous system.
- Myelogenous or myelocytic leukemia involves the myeloid stem cells in the bone marrow and interfere with the maturation of all blood cell types (granulocytes, erythrocytes, thrombocytes).

10.10.1 Signs and symptoms

- Acute patients:
  - Fatigue and weakness due to anemia.

  - Fever due to increased susceptibility to infection.
  - Bleeding:
    - Petechiae.
    - Bruising (ecchymosis).
    - Nosebleed (epistaxis).
    - Gum bleeding (gingival).
- Bone pain due to bone infiltration and marrow expansion.
- Lymph nodes (lymphadenopathy) enlarged as leukemic cells invade nodes.
- Liver (hepatomegaly) and spleen (splenomegaly) enlarged as leukemic cells invade.
- Headache.
- Nausea.
- Vomiting.
- Weight loss.
- Chronic patients:
  - Fatigue due to anemia.
  - Weight loss due to chronic disease process and loss of appetite.
  - Poor appetite.
  - Enlarged lymph nodes (lymphadenopathy) due to infiltration of lymph nodes.
  - Enlarged spleen (splenomegaly) due to involvement of the spleen.

10.10.2 Medical tests

- Decreased:
  - RBC count.
  - Hgb levels.
  - Platelet count.
- Increased:
  - WBC count.
  - Immature WBCs shown in bone marrow biopsy.

10.10.3 Treatment

- Acute myelogenous leukemia:
  - Administer:
    - Anthracycline (idarubicin or daunorubicin) plus cytarabine.
    - Combination: Daunorubicin, vincristine, prednisone, asparaginase.
    - Platelet transfusions.
    - Filgrastim for neutropenia.
    - Antibiotics for infections.
    - Bone marrow transplant.
    - Immunosuppression to avoid transplant rejection.

- Chronic myelogenous leukemia:
  - Administer:
    - Signal transduction inhibitor:
      - Imatinib.
      - Interferon-α.
      - Busulfan.
      - Hydroxyurea.
- Chronic lymphocytic leukemia:
  - Administer:
    - Alkylating agents:
      - Cyclophosphamide.
      - Chlorambucil.
    - Antienoplastics:
      - Vincristine.
      - Prednisone.
      - Doxorubicin.
    - Monoclonal antibody targeted therapy:
      - Alemtuzumab.
      - Combination of fludarabine and rituxumab
      - Transfusion if hemolytic anemia or bleeding.
      - Packed RBCs.
      - Whole blood.
      - Platelets.
- Bone marrow transplant and immunosuppression.
- High-protein diet.

10.10.4 Intervention

- Monitor:
  - Bleeding.
  - Infection.
  - Pain control.
- Instruct the patient:
  - Avoid others with infection.
  - Report signs of infection.
  - Eat small, frequent meals.
  - Use an electric razor.
  - Use soft toothbrush.
  - Watch for bleeding, bruising.

10.11 Multiple Myeloma

In multiple myeloma, a malignancy of the plasma cells causes an excessive amount of plasma cells in the bone marrow. Masses within the bone marrow cause destructive lesions in the bone. Normal bone marrow function is reduced as the abnormal plasma cells continue to grow. Immune function is diminished and the patient develops anemia. The disease typically affects older adults.

10.11.1 Signs and symptoms

- Severe bone pain due to involvement of back or ribs.
- Anemia due to invasion of the bone marrow.
- Skeletal fractures due to loss of normal bone structure (osteoporosis).
- Increased risk of infection due to bone marrow failure to produce WBCs.
- Spinal cord compression as mass enlarges.
- Renal failure due to protein effect in renal tubules.

10.11.2 Medical tests

- Presence of the Bence Jones protein in urine.
- Serum protein electrophoresis shows a monoclonal protein spike.
- CBC shows anemia.
- Rouleau formation on peripheral smear: a group of RBCs clump together in a stack, like a stack of coins.
- Abnormal plasma cells in bone marrow biopsy.
- X-rays of bone show lytic lesions.
- Elevated calcium in blood (hypercalcemia).
- Protein in urine (proteinuria).
- Elevated erythrocyte sedimentation rate.

10.11.3 Treatment

- Pain management.
- Alkylating agent (melphalan) and prednisone:
  - Thalidomide and dexamethasone.
- Nonalkylating combination (vincristine, doxorubicin, and dexamethasone).
- Proteosome inhibitor (bortezomib) and thalidomide derivative (lenalidomide).
- Diet high in:
  - Protein.
  - Carbohydrate.
  - Vitamins.
  - Minerals.

- Small, frequent meals.
- Transfusion of packed RBCs if anemia severe.
- Bone marrow transplantation.

10.11.4 Intervention

- Protect the patient from falling.
- Monitor input and output due to renal function changes.
- Perform muscle-strengthening exercises.
- Instruct the patient:
  - No lifting.
  - Be alert for fractures.

10.12 Polycythemia Vera

Polycythemia vera is a myeloproliferative disorder that results in an overproduction of blood cells and a thickening of blood. The excess of cells present in the blood causes problems with the flow of blood through vessels, especially the smaller ones. There will be an increase in peripheral vascular resistance, increasing pressure, and vascular stasis in the smaller vessels, potentially causing thrombosis or tissue hypoxia. Organ damage may result because of these changes.

10.12.1 Signs and symptoms

- Facial skin and mucous membranes dark and flushed (plethora).
- Hypertension due to increased peripheral vascular resistance and thickening of the blood.
- Itching worse after warm shower due to histamine release.
- Headache.
- Difficulty concentrating.
- Vision blurred.
- Ringing in ears (tinnitus).
- Thrombosis due to vascular stasis.
- Spleen enlargement (splenomegaly).
- Tissue hypoxia.

10.12.2 Medical tests

- Increased:
  - RBC count.
  - Hgb.
  - Hct level.

  - WBC count.
  - Basophils.
  - Eosinophils.
  - Platelet count.
  - Uric acid level.
  - Potassium.
  - Vitamin B12 level.
- Bone marrow panhyperplasia.

10.12.3 Treatment

- Adequate hydration.
- Anticoagulants such as aspirin.
- Administer:
  - Myelosuppressive medication:
    - Hydroxyurea.
    - Anagrelide.
    - Radioactive phosphorus 32.
  - Medication to lower uric acid level, if necessary:
    - Allopurinol.
    - Alkylating agents.
    - Melphalan.
    - Busulfan.
  - Antihistamine for pruritis.
- Radiation therapy.

10.12.4 Intervention

- Monitor:
  - Vital signs.
  - For bleeding.
  - For signs of infections.
- Keep the patient mobilized to decrease chance of blood clot formation.
- Increase fluid intake.
- Instruct the patient:
  - Maintain activity.
  - Use electric razor.
  - Use soft toothbrush.
  - Avoid flossing to decrease chances of bleeding.
  - Avoid activities that could cause injury.

10.13 Sickle Cell Anemia

Sickle cell anemia is an autosomal recessive disorder in which an abnormal gene causes damage to the RBC membrane. The abnormal Hgb within the RBC is called hemoglobin S. Dehydration or drying of the RBC makes it more vulnerable to sickling (forming a crescent-like shape), as do hypoxemia and acidosis. Hemolytic anemia results as RBCs are destroyed due to damage to the outer membrane. The sickled cells can also clump together, causing difficulty getting through the smaller vessels.

10.13.1 Signs and symptoms

- Acute pain (especially back, chest, and long bones) from vascular occlusion of the small vessels as the sickled cells clump.
- Fever as the body responds to acute sickling episode and accompanying provoking event.
- Painful, swollen joints due to vaso-occlusive process.
- Fatigue due to chronic anemia.
- Stroke (cerebrovascular accident) due to vaso-occlusive process.
- Enlarged liver (heptaomegaly).
- Enlarged heart and systolic murmur.

10.13.2 Medical tests

- Decreased:
  - RBC count due to chronic hemolytic anemia; the RBCs have a shorter lifespan.
- Increased:
  - WBCs.
  - Reticulocytes.
  - Indirect bilirubin.
- Presence of Howell-Jolly bodies and target cells.
- Sickle cells appear in blood smear.
- Hgb electrophoresis shows majority Hgb S (80% to 98%).

10.13.3 Treatment

- Narcotic pain control necessary when pain is severe.
- Warm compresses on joint.
- Blood transfusion of packed RBCs when anemia indicates.
- Supplemental oxygen if hypoxic.
- Adequate hydration, using intravenous (IV) fluids.
- Administer:
  - Supplemental O_2 to increase available oxygen.

10.13.4 Intervention

- Increase fluid intake.
- Monitor IV fluids.
- Monitor pain control.
- Record fluid intake and output to monitor renal function.
- Instruct the patient:
  - Avoid the cold.
  - No cold compresses.
  - Plan for rest periods during the day.

10.14 Deep Vein Thrombosis (DVT)

Thrombophlebitis, or the formation of a clot within the vein, commonly occurs within the deep veins in the leg, but may also occur in the arm. Initially, platelets and white cells clump together, sticking to the inside of the vessel wall. As blood flows over the area, other cells may deposit onto the area, making the thrombus larger. Compression of blood flow, which will increase the venous pressure, or sluggishness of blood flow can increase the risk of clot formation. Immobility, obesity, or hormonal changes, such as pregnancy, all can contribute to increased risk.

10.14.1 Signs and symptoms

- Asymptomatic.
- Unilateral leg (or arm) pain or tenderness (calf, thigh, groin, upper or lower arm) depending on location of thrombosis.
- Unilateral swelling of leg (or arm) due to vascular occlusion.
- Positive Homan's sign (pain on dorsiflexion of foot) seen in minority of patients with DVT.
- Warmth over the site.

10.14.2 Medical tests

- Doppler flow studies.
- Venous duplex ultrasound.
- MRI direct thrombus imaging useful for inferior vena cava and pelvic vein locations.
- D-dimer to test for hypercoagulable state.

10.14.3 Treatment

- Bed rest with elevation of extremity.
- Warm, moist soaks of the area.

- Monitor:
  - PT.
  - PTT.
  - INR.
- Administer:
  - Weight-dosed heparin IV.
  - Low-molecular-weight heparin.
  - Warfarin.
  - Thrombolytic therapy to dissolve clot with drugs such as recombinant t-PA:
    - Activator (t-PA).
- Umbrella filter inserted into the inferior vena cava for patients with recurrent thrombophlebitis.
- Thrombectomy is the surgical removal of the thrombus.

10.14.4 Interventions

- Monitor:
  - Vital signs for changes.
  - For signs of bleeding or bruising.
  - For signs of pulmonary embolism:
    - Shortness of breath.
    - Chest pain.
    - Rapid heart rate.
    - Rapid respirations.
    - Sweating.
- Avoid massaging the area to lessen the possibility of dislodging the clot.
- Intermittent warm, moist soaks.
- Instruct the patient:
  - Avoid injury.
  - Use electric razor.
  - Soft toothbrush.
  - Avoid flossing between teeth.
  - Report signs of bleeding or bruising.

10.15 Idiopathic Thrombocytopenic Purpura (ITP)

ITP is an autoimmune disorder in which antibodies are developed to the patient's own platelets. The antibodies attach to the platelets and macrophages within the spleen recognize the antibodies. The body destroys the platelets within the spleen. The disease is typically more common in women and usually a chronic disease in adults with an onset in early to mid-adulthood.

10.15.1 Signs and symptoms

- Bleeding in mucous membranes or skin due to low platelet count.
- Nose bleeds (epistaxis).
- Oral bleeding.
- Heavy menstrual bleeding (menorrhagia).
- Purpura.
- Petechiae.

10.15.2 Medical tests

- Decreased:
  - Platelet count (thrombocytopenia).
- Mild anemia secondary to bleeding.

10.15.3 Treatment

- Administer:
  - Prednisone.
  - Immunoglobulin:
    - Danazol.
  - Immunosuppressive therapy:
    - Vincristine, azathioprine, cyclosporine, cyclophosphamide, and Rituximab.
- Stem cell transplantation.
- Splenectomy.

10.15.4 Interventions

- Monitor:
  - Vital signs for changes.
  - For signs of bleeding or bruising.
- Instruct the patient:
  - Avoid injury.
  - Use electric razor.
  - Soft toothbrush.
  - Avoid flossing between teeth.
  - Report signs of bleeding or bruising.

10.16 Acquired Immunodeficiency Syndrome (AIDS)

In AIDS, the human immunodeficiency virus (HIV) causes malfunction of T-cells to protect the body from invading microorganisms. When it enters a cell, HIV replicates, causing the cell to reproduce more infected cells, and frequently, cell death. The CD4 lymphocyte is most often affected, followed by B lymphocytes and macrophages.

10.16.1 Signs and symptoms

- Anorexia.
- Fatigue.
- Night sweats.
- Malnutrition.

10.16.2 Medical tests

- CD4 Less than 200 T cells per microliter.
- Positive HIV antibody titer 95% positive 6 weeks after contact.
- Positive Western blot.

10.16.3 Treatment

- Diet high in calories and protein.
- Administer:
  - Antibiotics to combat opportunistic infections:
    - Trimethoprim/sulfamethoxzole.
  - Antiviral medications:
    - Nucleoside analogs, have antiviral activity.
    - Didanosine.
    - Zidovudine.
    - Stavudine.
    - Zalcitabine.
    - Nucleotide analog.
    - Tenofovir.
  - Protease inhibitors, suppress HIV replication:
    - Fortovase.
    - Ritonavir.
    - Indinavir.
    - Nelfinavir.
  - Nonnucleoside reverse transcriptase inhibitors, stop reverse transcriptase at a different site.
    - Nevirapine.
    - Delavirdine.
    - Efavirenz.

  - Antiemetic to combat nausea:
    - Prochlorperazine.
  - Antifungal medication to combat fungal infections.
  - Fluconazole.

10.16.4 Intervention

- Maintain activity as tolerated and schedule rest periods to maintain physical functioning.
- Avoid exposure to blood to prevent the spread of the virus.
- Instruct the patient:
  - To use condoms to prevent the spread of the virus.

10.17 Anaphylaxis

An allergen, usually food or medication, enters the body, causing the release of histamines, which result in capillaries dilating and smooth muscle contracting. This results in edema, respiratory distress, hypotension, and skin changes, leading to an allergic reaction. Lesser degrees of extreme allergy are urticarial, which is hives, and angioedema, which is swelling caused by exudation.

10.17.1 Signs and symptoms

- Shortness of breath due to swelling of the larynx.
- Hypotension and shock due to generalized vasodilation.
- Sneezing.
- Anxiety secondary to difficulty in breathing.
- Rales (crackles) heard in the lungs due to fluid in the lungs.
- Wheezing (rhonchi) due to bronchospasm.

10.17.2 Medical tests

- Increased:
  - Tryptase levels are from mast cells.

10.17.3 Treatment

- Administer:
  - Emergency medications:
    - Epinephrine to open airways and reduce bronchospasm.
    - Corticosteroids to reduce symptoms.

        - Antihistamines to mitigate symptoms.
        - Circulatory volume expanders to treat hypotension†caused by vasodilation:
            - Saline.
            - Plasma.
            - IV fluids.
        - Vasopressors to counteract vasodilation and increase blood pressure:
            - Norepinephrine.
            - Dopamine.
    - Oxygen therapy to support breathing.
- Insert endotracheal tube to maintain airways.

10.17.4 Intervention

- Maintain airway to facilitate breathing.
- Monitor for hoarseness and difficulty breathing.
- Instruct the patient:
    - Avoid exposure to allergens to prevent further occurrences.
    - Seek medical help immediately if exposed to allergens to prevent anaphylaxis.

10.18 Kaposi's Sarcoma (KS)

With KS, overgrowth of blood vessels leads to malignant tumors and cancer of lymphatic tissue and skin. It is commonly found in patients with AIDS and usually seen in cases of advanced AIDS.

10.18.1 Signs and symptoms

- Red, brown, and purple lesions on the buccal mucosa, lips, gums, tongue, and palate because it is a malignancy affecting the skin and mucosa.
- Difficulty breathing (dyspnea) if the malignancy invades the pulmonary system.

10.18.2 Medical tests

- Biopsy to look for the HIV virus and B lymphocytes.
- CT scan to determine metastasis to the lesion to ascertain the severity of the disease.

10.18.3 Treatment

- Radiation in the affected tissue to shrink and treat tumors.
- Laser surgery may be used to remove some lesions.

- Administer:
  - Antiemetic medication to counter effects of chemotherapy and radiation:
    - Trimethobenzamide,
  - Chemotherapy medication to slow or halt the disease:
    - Doxorubicin.
    - Etoposide.
    - Vinblastine.
    - Vincristine.

10.18.4 Intervention

- Monitor skin for lesions to determine new lesions and/or metastasis.
- Daily weighing to determine changes in weight from baseline.
- Instruct the patient:
  - About the need for a high-protein, high-calorie diet.
  - To conserve energy.
  - About hospice care.

10.19 Lymphoma

In lymphoma, functionless and damaged cells of the lymphatic system undergo overgrowth, decreasing the effectiveness of the lymphatic system. There are two main types of lymphoma, characterized by painless lymph node swelling:

- Hodgkin's disease is a malignant lymphoma characterized by presence of Reed-Sternberg cells. There are four stages of Hodgkin's disease:
  - Stage I: Reed-Sternberg cells appear in one lymph node region.
  - Stage II: Reed-Sternberg cells appear in multiple lymph node regions on the same side of the diaphragm.
  - Stage III: Reed-Sternberg cells appear in multiple lymph node regions on both sides of the diaphragm
  - Stage IV: Reed-Sternberg cells appear throughout the body.
- Non-Hodgkin's lymphoma (NHL): Cancer of the B lymphocytes and are characterized by the absence of Reed-Sternberg cells.

10.19.1 Signs and symptoms

- Night sweats are characteristic of the disease.
- Anorexia due to effects of chemotherapy and the large lymph nodes.
- Enlarged painless, lymph nodes in cervical region, mesentery, abdomen, and pelvis.

10.19.2 Medical tests

- Lymph node biopsy contains Reed-Sternberg cells (Hodgkin's disease), which typify Hodgkin's disease.
- Bone marrow biopsy contains follicular type cells (NHL).

10.19.3 Treatment

- Radiation in the affected tissue to shrink the nodes.
- Administer:
  - Hodgkin's disease medication:
    - Vincristine.
    - Doxorubicin.
    - Bleomycin.
    - Dacarbazine.
  - NHL medication:
    - Cyclophosphamide.
    - Vincristine.
    - Doxorubicin.
    - Ritaximab.
    - Prednisone.
    - Radiation.

10.19.4 Intervention

- Monitor:
  - Vital signs to determine variations from baseline.
  - For complications such as new palpable lymph nodes and fever.
- Increase fluid intake
- Increase calories, protein, iron, calcium, and vitamins and minerals to counteract weight loss.
- Instruct the patient:
  - Consult with physician before using over-the counter medication.

10.20 Scleroderma

With scleroderma, antibodies attack connective tissues in an autoimmune response resulting in scar tissue (fibrosis) forming on skin, organs, gastrointestinal tract, blood vessels, and muscles, causing systemic sclerosis. It is a chronic disease of unknown etiology, usually seen in 30 to 50 year olds.

10.20.1 Signs and symptoms

- Stiffness and pain due to the fibrosis.
- Skin thickens.
- Edema.
- Malaise.
- Fever.

10.20.2 Medical tests

- Positive antinuclear antibody.
- Dermis appears thickened in skin biopsy.

10.20.3 Treatment

- No known medications are able to stop the disease.
- Medications may be used to treat the symptoms of the affected organs caused by scleroderma.
- Physical therapy to maintain joint mobility.

10.20.4 Intervention

- Monitor for increasing blood pressure, which is the leading cause of death of scleroderma patients, due to the renal effects of the disease.
- Instruct the patient:
  - There is no cure for scleroderma, but it may go into remission and then relapse.
  - Schedule rest periods during activities.
  - Avoid the cold.

10.21 Septic Shock

Septic shock starts with bacteremia, usually gram negative bacteria infecting the blood. The sources are usually the genitourinary system, gastrointestinal tract, and the lungs. The infection may be underlying for some time before shock develops. Once the cascade from bacteremia to septic shock starts, it may be difficult to halt the process. Shock may occur more quickly in patients who are elderly, immune compromised, or with other comorbidities.

10.21.1 Signs and symptoms

- Nausea and vomiting from the source of the infection.
- Temperature over 101°F due to infection.

- Hypotension due to fluid displacement, vasodilation.
- Tachycardia from fever and infection.
- Tachypnea from fever and infection.
- Lactic acidosis results from poor oxygenation.

10.21.2 Medical tests

- WBC 15,000 to 30,000 indicates infection.
- Decreased platelet count blood coagulopathies are common in shock.
- Abnormal PT and PTT blood coagulopathies.

10.21.3 Treatment

- Administer:
    - Antibiotics.

10.21.4 Intervention

- Monitor:
    - Vital signs, especially fever.
    - Fluid intake and output to assess for fluid overload and hydration status.
    - Coagulation factors.

Solved Problems

10.1 What test would you expect a prescriber to order if the patient is taking heparin?

PTT.

10.2 Why would a prescriber order a C-reactive protein test?

C-reactive protein is produced as part of the inflammatory process and attaches to the invading microorganism or damaged cells, enhancing phagocytosis in the destruction of the microorganism or damaged cell. The C-reactive protein test measures the C-reactive protein level in the blood. A high level indicates inflammation.

10.3 What might a low WBC indicate?

- Alcoholism.
- Lupus.
- Cushing's syndrome.
- Aplastic anemia.
- Enlarged spleen.
- Viral infection.

10.4 What might cause an abnormal false positive on a blood culture?

Contaminated sample or improper processing results in bacteria or fungi found in the blood sample but not in the patient's blood.

10.5 What CD4+ test result indicates that a patient is at risk for opportunistic infection?

Low CD4+ test results.

10.6 Would you expect a prescriber to order if a patient received a high dose of heparin?

Protamine.

10.7 What is pancytopenia?

Aplastic anemia in which bone marrow stops producing a sufficient amount of RBCs, WBCs, and platelets.

10.8 What is the underlying cause of pernicious anemia?

The body is unable to absorb vitamin B12, which is needed to make RBCs.

10.9 Why would a patient diagnosed with DIC bleed easily?

Blood coagulates through the entire body within the vascular compartment, depleting platelets and the body's ability to coagulate. This results in bleeding in other areas.

10.10 What would you expect the prescriber to order if a patient has a positive Homan's sign?

Doppler flow studies to rule out DVT.

10.11 What are the sources of septic shock?

Septic shock starts with bacteremia, usually gram-negative bacteria infecting the blood. The sources are usually the genitourinary system, gastrointestinal tract, and the lungs.

10.12 What is the purpose of performing a sedimentation rate test?

An increase in fibrinogen in blood during the inflammatory process causes erythrocytes (RBCs) to adhere to each other, forming a stack called rouleaux. The sedimentation rate test measures how many millimeters per hour of erythrocytes settle to the bottom of a test tube. Rouleaux settles quicker than erythrocytes. Therefore, an increased sedimentation rate indicates that the patient has inflammation.

10.13 Why would a prescriber order corticosteroids?

Corticosteroids are hormones that suppress the immune system.

10.14 What is the effect of interferon?

Interferon is a hormone produced by many cells when a virus is detected. Interferon causes cells to produce a protein that prevents the virus from replicating in other cells.

10.15 What begins the inflammation response?

Damage to cells.

10.16 What is prothrombin and what is the effect of prothrombin time?

There are 12 factors that must be present to coagulate (clot) blood. Prothrombin is clotting factor II synthesized by the liver with the assistance of vitamin K. When a blood vessel is injured, prothrombin is converted to thrombin, a protein, which forms a blood clot with other proteins to stop the bleeding. The prothrombin time (PT) test determines the time necessary for plasma to clot. The healthcare provider orders the prothrombin time test to assess the patient's risk for bleeding and to assess the therapeutic effect of anticoagulation medication.

10.17 What might a long PT indicate?

- Cirrhosis.
- Risk of bleeding.
- Vitamin K deficiency.
- Disseminated intravascular coagulation (DIC).
- Too much Coumadin or heparin.

10.18 What are immunoglobulins?

Immunoglobulins are antibodies made by the immune system in response to microorganisms that enter the body, an allergen, and abnormal cells such as cancer cells. An antibody is specific to an antigen. The immunoglobulin test measures the level of an immunoglobulin in the patient's blood. A low level of a specific immunoglobulin increases the risk of repeated infections from an antigen.

10.19 Why is the antinuclear antibody test ordered?

In autoimmune diseases, the body produces antibodies that attach to and destroy the body's own cells. The antinuclear antibody (ANA) test measures the pattern and amount of these antibodies.

10.20 Why would a prescriber order a viral load test?

The human immunodeficiency virus (HIV) in a patient's blood is determined by the presence of HIV RNA. The amount of HIV RNA indicates whether the infection is decreasing, stabilized, or increasing. The viral load measurement test determines the amount of HIV RNA in the patient's blood. A viral load measurement test is administered when the patient is diagnosed with HIV and becomes the baseline. Results of subsequent viral load measurement tests are compared to the baseline to determine the infection's progress. A patient diagnosed with HIV who has a negative viral load measurement test result can infect another person. The viral load measurement test result is compared to the baseline test result and to previous tests results to determine the trend of the infection.

10.21 What can affect the results of a viral load test?

Recently received immunizations.

10.22 What is the purpose of ordering an RF test?

The rheumatoid factor (RF) is an autoantibody that destroys the patient's own tissues, resulting in stiffness, joint pain, and inflammation. The rheumatoid factor test measures the amount of the rheumatoid factor in the blood sample and is used to differentiate rheumatoid arthritis from other forms of arthritis.

10.23 Why would a prescriber order cyclosporine?

Cyclosporine is an immunosuppressant used to reduce organ rejection following an organ transplant.

10.24 Why would a patient with anemia feel fatigue?

The patient has a decreased amount of red blood cells and therefore has a reduced amount of oxygen being carried to cells resulting in fatigue.

10.25 What would you say if a patient who is receiving warfarin asks to shave?

Use only an electric razor.

INDEX

AACN. *See* American Association of Critical Care Nurses
Abbreviated Mental Test Scores (AMTS), 289
Abdomen. *See also* Gastrointestinal system
  computed tomography scan of, 171–172
  pain in, 170
  quadrants of, 167
  rigidity of, 170, 205
  sounds of, 170
  trauma of, 201–202
  x-ray of, 171
Abdominal reflex, 292
Abducens nerve, 291
ABG. *See* Arterial blood gas
Abscess, of brain, 300–301
Absence seizures, 312
Accessory nerve, 292
ACE. *See* Angiotensin-converting enzyme inhibitors
Acid-base
  balance, kidneys and, 209, 236
  blood gas test results, 37
  values, 270
Acknowledgement, of stressors, 10, 11
ACLS. *See* Advanced cardiac life support
Acoustic nerve, 291
Acquired immunodeficiency syndrome (AIDS), 365–366
ACS. *See* Acute coronary syndrome
ACTH. *See* Adrenocorticotropic hormone
Activated charcoal, 274
Active listening, stress and, 11
Acute coronary syndrome (ACS), 107–108, 115
Acute glomerulonephritis, 223
Acute inflammation, 30, 42
Acute Physiology and Chronic Health Evaluation (APACHE), 3
Acute renal failure, 227
Acute respiratory distress syndrome (ARDS), 134–135, 161
Acute respiratory failure, 150–151
Acute stroke, 105–107, 115
Acute tubular necrosis, 232
Adaptation, stages of, 12
Addison's disease, 252–253, 266
ADH. *See* Antidiuretic hormone
Adrenal gland, 240
Adrenaline. *See* Epinephrine
Adrenergic blocking, 70–71
Adrenergic medications, 69–70, 220
Adrenocorticotropic hormone (ACTH), 38
Advanced cardiac life support (ACLS), 100–101
Advocate, patient, 16
Aerosol therapy, 154–155
Afterload, 45
Aging, physiologic reserve and, 2, 17
AIDS. *See* Acquired immunodeficiency syndrome
Albumin, 28, 42
Aldosterone hormone, 209
Alkalinizing agent, 222–223
Alpha-adrenergic blocking medications, 70
Alteplase, 297, 323
Altered mental status (AMS), 287
Aluminum hydroxide, 175, 206
American Association of Critical Care Nurses (AACN)
  responsibilities of critical care nurse defined by, 15
  standards for critical care nursing, 15
  standards of practice of critical care nurse defined by, 15
Ammonia detoxicant, 177
AMS. *See* Altered mental status
AMTS. *See* Abbreviated Mental Test Scores
ANA. *See* Antinuclear antibodies
Analgesics, 273
Anaphylaxis, 366–367
Anemia, 348–349, 374
  aplastic, 349–350, 372
  iron deficiency, 350–352
  pernicious, 352–353, 372
  sickle cell, 361–362
Aneurysm
  aortic, 73–74
  cerebral, 303–304, 323, 324
Angina pectoris, 75–76, 115, 116
  chest pain and, 50
Angiotensin II receptor blocker (ARB), 64–65
Angiotensin-converting enzyme inhibitors (ACE), 64
Antacids, 175, 206

Anti-angina, 61–63
Antiarrhythmics, 58–61
Antibiotics, 273
Anticholinergics, 131, 160
Anticoagulants, 66–68, 296, 343, 373
  oral, 68
Anticonvulsants, 296
Antidiuretic hormone (ADH), 177–178, 206, 209, 239
Antiemetic medications, 175–176, 206
Antihypertensive medications, 63–65
Anti-inflammatory medications, 131–132
Antilipemics, 71–73
Antinuclear antibodies (ANA), 341, 373
Antiplatelets, 67–68, 296, 323
Antithyroid medication, 247
Aortic aneurysm, 73–74
  dissecting, chest pain and, 50
Aortic valve, 44
APACHE. *See* Acute Physiology and Chronic Health Evaluation
Aplastic anemia, 349–350, 372
Appendicitis, 178–179
Appropriate action, failure to take, 16
ARB. *See* Angiotensin II receptor blocker
ARDS. *See* Acute respiratory distress syndrome
Arterial blood gas (ABG)
  environmental critical care and, 269–270, 285
  respiratory system and, 125–126
Arterial blood pressure, monitoring of, 56
Arteries
  circumflex, 44
  left coronary, 44
  right coronary, 44
Artery, carotid, edema and, 46
Ascending Guillain-Barré, 306
Asthma, 135–137, 161
Astrocytoma, 302
Asystole, 92–94
Atelectasis, 137–138, 161
Atonic seizures, 312
Atopic asthma, 135
Atrial fibrillation, 91–92, 115
Atrioventricular valves (AV), 44
Atrophic gastritis, 189
Auscultation
  in cardiovascular system assessment, 47–49
  in endocrine system assessment, 242
  in environmental critical care assessment, 268
  in gastrointestinal system assessment, 167–168
  in renal system assessment, 211, 236
  in respiratory system assessment, 121–122
Autonomic nervous system, 39
Autonomy, 19
  loss of, 10
AV. *See* Atrioventricular valves

Bacteria, 29
Bacterial meningitis, 307
Balloon catheterization, 112
Balloon inflation lumen, 56
Barbiturates, 296
Barrett's esophagus, 187
Basic life support, 99–100
Basilar skull fracture, 317
Basophils, 326
Bell's palsy, 300
Beneficence, 13
Benzodiazepines, 132–133, 161, 296
Beta-adrenergic blockers, 62
Beta-adrenergic blocking medications, 70–71
Bile-sequestering medication, 71–72
Biot's respiration, 119
Bladder, cancer of, 229–230
Bleeding
  gastrointestinal system and, 188–189, 206
  platelets and, 28, 42, 272, 285
Blood, 26
  carbon dioxide and, 24
  creatinine level, 209, 236
  culture, 339, 372
  in diarrhea, with pus, 199, 207
  oxygen and, 24
  pH value, 125, 160
  plasma, 28
  red blood cells, 27
  Rh group, 28–29
  in stool, 170, 205
  type of, 28, 330
  in vomit, 170, 205
  white blood cells, 27–28
Blood chemistry, for environmental critical care, 271
Blood derivatives, 344–345
Blood flow, heart and, 43
Blood gas test results, 37. *See also* Arterial blood gas
Blood glucose, 24
Blood pressure
  kidneys and, 41, 209
  liver disease and, 41
  monitoring of, 55–56
    arterial, 56
    central venous, 56
    pulmonary arterial, 56, 114
Blood supply, to heart, 44
Blood tests
  for endocrine system, 244–246
  for renal system, 215–217
Blood transfusion capability chart, 330
Blood urea nitrogen (BUN), 215
Blunt abdominal trauma, 201
Body hair, on legs, 46, 114
Body surface area (BSA), 278, 279
Bone marrow, 27, 325, 327
Boredom, stress and, 10
Bradycardia, 101, 104
Brain, computed tomography scan of, 293–294, 323
Brain abscess, 300–301
Brain tumor, 302–303
Breach, 16

Breath sounds
  abnormal, 121
  misplaced, 122
  normal, 121
  voice, 122
Bronchiectasis, 138, 161
Bronchitis, 139–141
Bronchodilators, 130–131
Bronchophony, 122
Bronchoscopy
  for environmental critical care, 269, 285
  for respiratory system, 126–127
BSA. *See* Body surface area
BUN. *See* Blood urea nitrogen
Burns, 278–282
  fluid replacement for, 281, 286
  voice changes and, 286

CABG. *See* Coronary artery bypass graft
Calcitonin, 240
Calcitrol, 31
Calcium, serum, assessment of, 244, 264
Calcium channel blockers, 62–63, 297, 323
Calcium gluconate, 266
Calculi basketing, 233, 238
Cancer
  of bladder, 229–230
  of kidneys, 231
Carbon dioxide (CO_2), blood and, 24
Cardiac arrest, 98–99
  advanced cardiac life support, 100–101
  basic life support, 99–100
  bradycardia treatment, 101, 104
Cardiac catheterization, 52–54
Cardiac contusion, 108–109
Cardiac glycosides, 57
Cardiac impulses, 45
Cardiac index, 54
Cardiac markers, 50–51, 114
Cardiac output, 45
  maintenance of, 25
  monitoring of, 54–55, 114
Cardiac rub, 49, 114
Cardiac tamponade, 78–79, 115
Cardiogenic shock, 79–80
Cardiovascular system, 24–25, 40–41
  acute coronary syndrome, 107–108, 115
  acute stroke, 105–107, 115
  angina, 75–76, 115, 116
  aortic aneurysm, 73–74
  assessment of
    auscultation, 47–49
    chest pain and, 49–50
    inspection, 46
    palpation, 46–47
    percussion, 47
  asystole, 92–94
  atrial fibrillation, 91–92, 115
  balloon catheterization, 112
  cardiac arrest, 98–99
    advanced cardiac life support, 100–101
    basic life support, 99–100
    bradycardia treatment, 101, 104
  cardiac contusion, 108–109
  cardiac output maintenance, 25
  cardiac tamponade, 78–79, 115
  cardiogenic shock, 79–80
  conduction system, 26
  congestive heart failure, 81–83
  coronary artery bypass graft, 109–110
  coronary circulation, 26, 40
  critical care definitions, 43
  endocarditis, 80–81
  fibrinolytic therapy, 104–105
  heart chambers, 26
  hypertension, 83–85, 115
  hypertensive crisis, 83–85, 115
  hypovolemic shock, 85–86, 115
  medications for
    adrenergic blocking, 70–71
    adrenergics, 69–70
    anti-angina, 61–63
    antiarrhythmics, 58–61
    anticoagulants, 66–68
    antihypertensive, 63–65
    antilipemics, 71–73
    cardiac glycosides, 57
    diuretics, 65–66
    phosphodiesterase inhibitors, 57–58
    thrombolytics, 68–69
  murmurs, 48–49, 114
  myocardial infarction, 76–78
  myocarditis, 86–87
  pacemaker, 113
  pericarditis, 87–89
  physiologic reserve of, 7
    measurement in, 2
  pulmonary edema, 89–90, 115
  synchronized cardioversion, 112–113
  tests for
    blood pressure monitoring, 55–56
    cardiac catheterization, 52–54
    cardiac function measurements, 55–56
    cardiac markers, 50–51, 114
    cardiac output monitoring, 54–55, 114
    echocardiogram, 52, 114
    electrocardiogram, 51–52
  thrombophlebitis, 90–91
  valve surgery, 110–111
  vascular assist device, 112
  vascular surgery, 111
  ventricular fibrillation, 94–96
  ventricular tachycardia, 96–98
Carotid artery, edema and, 46
Catecholamines, 69
  serum, assessment of, 244, 264
CBC. *See* Complete blood count
CD4+ count, 341–342, 372

Cells
  cytotoxic T, 28, 41, 327
  function of, 21–22, 40
  glucose and, 24
  helper T, 28, 41, 327
  lymphokine-producing, 327
  memory T, 28, 41, 327
  suppressor T, 28, 41, 327
  T, 41
Central nervous system (CNS), 39
  magnetic resonance imaging of, 294
Central venous blood pressure, monitoring of, 56
Cerebellum, 39
Cerebral aneurysm, 303–304, 323, 324
Cerebral angiograph, 295, 322
Cerebral cortex, 39
Cerebral edema, 298
Cerebral hemorrhage, 298–299, 322
Cerebrospinal fluid, 39
Cerebrovascular accident (CVA), 105, 310–311, 321
Chemical burns, irrigation of, 286
Chest
  pain in, 49–50
  x-ray of, 127–128, 160
Chest tube, 158–159, 162
Cheyne-Stokes, 119–120
CHF. *See* Congestive heart failure
Cholecystitis, 179–180
Cholesterol absorption inhibitors, 72
Chronic inflammation, 30, 42
Chronic obstructive pulmonary disease (COPD), 139
Chronic renal failure, 227
Chvostek's sign, 242
Cincinnati Prehospital Stroke Scale (CPSS), 106
Circumflex artery, 44
Cirrhosis of liver, 180–183, 206
CK-MB. *See* Creatinine kinase-MB
Clonic seizures, 312
Closed pneumothorax, 146
CNS. *See* Central nervous system
CO_2. *See* Carbon dioxide
Coagulation, physiologic reserve of, 7
Coffee ground emesis, 170, 205
Cold agglutinins, 336
Comminuted skull fracture, 317
Communication, stress and, 10, 11
Complement system, 30, 327
Complete blood count (CBC), 333–336
Complex partial seizures, 312
Compound skull fracture, 317
Computed tomography (CT) scan
  of abdomen, 171–172
  of brain, 293–294, 323
  for endocrine system, 243
  of renal system, 212–213, 236
  of spine, 293–294
  thoracic, 128
Concussion, 298, 313–314, 322–323
Conduction system, 26
Congestive heart failure (CHF), 81–83
Conn's syndrome. *See* Primary aldosteronism
Consortium, loss of, 16
Continuous positive airway pressure therapy (CPAP), 155, 161
Contractility, 45
Contrecoup injury, 298
Contusion, 298, 314–315, 322, 323
COPD. *See* Chronic obstructive pulmonary disease
Cope sign. *See* Obturator sign
Coping skills, lack of, 10, 11
Cor pulmonale, 141–142, 161
Coronary artery bypass graft (CABG), 109–110
Coronary circulation, 26, 40
Corpus callosum, 39
Corticosteroids, 248, 265, 266, 273, 297, 327, 372
Corticotropin, 239
Cortisol, 240
  serum, assessment of, 244, 265
  urine analysis and, 246
Cough, 118
Coup injury, 298, 314, 322
CPAP. *See* Continuous positive airway pressure therapy
CPSS. *See* Cincinnati Prehospital Stroke Scale
Crackles, 121
Cranial nerves, function of, 290–292
C-reactive protein (CRP), 332–333, 371
Creatinine blood level, 209, 236
Creatinine clearance, 208, 216, 237
Creatinine kinase-MB (CK-MB), 51, 114
Critical care. *See also* Multisystem critical care
  cost of, 14
  documentation, 12
  emergency medicine compared to, 1, 17
  ethical challenges of, 12–13
    ethical dilemma, 14, 19–20
    ethical principles, 13–14
  family and, 11–12, 19
  legal issues, 15–16
  patient risk factor measurement, 3
  physiological compensation in
    multiorgan dysfunction syndrome, 2–3, 17
    physiologic reserve measurement, 2
  standards, 15, 20
Critical care assessment, 4
  critical factors of, 8–9
Critical care patient, 1, 16–17
Critical care stressors, 9–10
  nurse role to reduce, 10, 18–19
Critical care thinking, 3–4
  critical care assessment, 4
  Glasgow Coma Scale, 5, 6
  physical assessment, 4–5
Critical care unit, 1
  rules of, 12
  staff of, goal of, 17
Crohn's disease, 183–184
CRP. *See* C-reactive protein
CT. *See* Computed tomography scan

Cullen's sign, 195, 207
Cushing's syndrome, 254–255, 265
CVA. *See* Cerebrovascular accident
Cytotoxic T cells, 28, 41, 327

Damages, 16
Death, fear of, 9, 11
Deep vein thrombosis, 362–363
Deep-partial thickness burn, 278
Defamation, 16
Depressed skull fracture, 317
Descending Guillain-Barré, 306
Detoxification, in renal system, 208–209
Developing awareness, in adaptation, 12
Diabetes mellitus, 260–263
  gestational, 260
Diagnose, failure to, 16
Dialysis, for environmental critical care, 272, 285
Diaphragmatic hernia. *See* Hiatal hernia
Diarrhea, 170
  blood in, with pus, 199, 207
Diastatic skull fracture, 317
Diastole, 45
DIC. *See* Disseminated intravascular coagulation
Diffuse axonal injury, 316–317
Digestion, 22–23. *See also* Gastrointestinal system
  gallbladder and, 164
  liver and, 24, 41, 164
  pancreas and, 164
Dignity, loss of, 10
Digoxin, 57, 114
Dilantin, seizures and, 324
Dilated pupils, 290
Disbelief, in adaptation, 12
Discomfort, stress and, 10
Disruption, minimum, stress and, 10
Disseminated intravascular coagulation (DIC), 353–354, 372
Distal lumen, 56
Diuretics, 297
  loop, 65, 220–221
  potassium-sparing, 66, 221–222
  thiazide, 65, 221
Diverticulitis, 184–185
Document, failure to, 16
Documentation, critical care, 12
Duodenal ulcer, 197
Duty, 16, 20
Dye dilution test, 54
Dysmetabolic syndrome. *See* Metabolic syndrome
Dyspnea. *See* Shortness of breath

Early diastolic murmur, 48
EBV. *See* Epstein-Barr virus antibody test
Echocardiogram, 52, 114
Edema, 46, 113
  cerebral, 298
Education, stress and
  of family, 11
  of patient, 10
Egophony, 122
Electrocardiogram
  for cardiovascular system, 51–52
  for environmental critical care, 271
Electrolytes, 31–32
  balance of, 209
  critical thinking, 34–36
  tests for, 32–33
  treatment for, 33–34
Emergency medicine, critical care compared to, 1, 17
Emphysema, 142–144
Encephalitis, 304–305, 322, 323
Endocarditis, 80–81
Endocrine system, 38
  Addison's disease, 252–253, 266
  assessment of, 241–242
    auscultation, 242
    inspection, 241–242
    palpation, 242
    signs and symptoms, 242–243
  critical care definitions, 239
  Cushing's syndrome, 254–255, 265
  cycle, 239–241
  diabetes insipidus, 255–256, 265
  diabetes mellitus, 260–263
  hyperparathyroidism, 258–260
  hyperthyroidism, 251–252, 265, 266
  hypothyroidism, 250–251, 264, 265, 266
  medication for, 246–250
    antithyroid, 247
    corticosteroids, 248, 265
    insulin, 248–249
    oral antidiabetic, 249–250
    thyroid hormone replacement, 246–247, 266
  metabolic syndrome, 263–264
  pheochromocytoma, 257–258, 265
  primary aldosteronism, 256–257
  syndrome of inappropriate antidiuretic hormone
      secretion, 253–254, 265
  tests for, 243–246
    blood, 244–246
    computed tomography scan, 243
    radionuclide thyroid imaging, 243–244, 264, 266
    urine analysis, 246
Endoscopy
  lower gastrointestinal, 173
  upper gastrointestinal, 172–173
Endotracheal rapid sequence intubation, 155–157
Endotracheal suctioning, 159, 162
End-tidal carbon dioxide monitor, 126, 160
Environmental critical care
  assessment of, 267–269
    auscultation, 268
    inspection, 268
    signs and symptoms, 268, 284–285
  burns, 278–282, 286
  definitions, 267
  hyperthermia, 274–276, 285, 286
  hypothermia, 276–278, 286

Environmental critical care (*Cont.*)
medications in
activated charcoal, 274
analgesics, 273
antibiotics, 273
corticosteroids, 273
nonsteroidal anti-inflammatory drugs, 273
sorbitol, 274, 285
poisoning, 282–284, 286
procedures for, 269–272
bronchoscopy, 269, 285
dialysis, 272, 285
gastric lavage, 272
tests for
arterial blood gas, 269–270, 285
blood chemistry, 271
electrocardiograph, 271
hematologic studies, 272
treatment goals, 267, 284
Eosinophils, 326
Epidural hematoma, 298
Epinephrine, 240
EPO. *See* Erythropoietin
Epstein-Barr virus (EBV) antibody test, 339
Erosive gastritis, 189
Erythrocytes. *See* Red blood cells
Erythropoietin (EPO), 31, 42
Esophageal varices, 170, 205
Estrogen, 241
ESWL. *See* Extracorporeal shock wave lithotripsy
Ethical challenges, of critical care, 12–13, 19
ethical dilemma, 13, 14, 19–20
ethical principles, 13–14
Expectations, setting of, stress and, 12
Expiration, stridor on, 121, 122, 160
Extracorporeal shock wave lithotripsy (ESWL), 233–234, 238
Extrinsic asthma. *See* Atopic asthma

Facial nerve, 291
Factor Xa inhibitor, 66–67
Family
critical care and, 11–12, 19
education of, stress and, 11
Fe. *See* Iron
Fecal test, 174–175
Feeling exploration, stress and, 11
Fibric acid derivative medication, 72
Fibrinogen, 28, 42
Fibrinolytic therapy, 104–105
Fidelity, 13–14
First degree burn, 278
Flick Method, 54
Fluid volume excess, 35–36
Fluid volume loss, 34–35
Fluids, 31–32
balance of, 209
replacement of, for burns, 281, 286
Follicle-stimulating hormone (FSH), 38, 239
Fracture, of skull, 317–319
Frustration, stress and, 10, 11
FSH. *See* Follicle-stimulating hormone
Full thickness burn, 278

Gallbladder. *See also* Cholecystitis
digestion and, 164
Gastric lavage
for environmental critical care, 272
for gastrointestinal system, 203
Gastric ulcer, 197
Gastritis, 189–190
Gastroenteritis, 185–186, 206
Gastroesophageal reflux disease (GERD), 187–188
Gastrointestinal system
abdominal trauma, 201–202
appendicitis, 178–179
assessment of, 164–170
auscultation, 167–168
inspection, 166–167
palpation, 168–169
percussion, 168
signs and symptoms, 169–170
bleeding in, 188–189, 206
cholecystitis, 179–180
cirrhosis of liver, 180–183, 206
critical care definitions, 163
Crohn's disease, 183–184
cycle, 163–164
diverticulitis, 184–185
gastritis, 189–190
gastroenteritis, 185–186, 206
gastroesophageal reflux disease, 187–188
hepatitis, 190–192
hiatal hernia, 192–193
intestinal obstruction, 193–194, 207
medications for
ammonia detoxicant, 177
antacids, 175, 206
antidiuretic hormone, 177–178, 206
antiemetics, 175–176, 206
histamine-2 receptor antagonists, 176, 206
proton pump inhibitors, 177
pancreatitis, 193–194, 207
paralytic ileus, 193–194, 207
peptic ulcer disease, 197–199, 205
peritonitis, 196–197, 205
procedures of
gastric lavage, 203
nasogastric decompression, 203–204, 207
nasogastric intubation, 202–203, 207
paracentesis, 204–205, 207
tests for
abdominal computed tomography scan, 171–172
abdominal x-ray, 171
fecal, 174–175
liver function, 174
lower endoscopy, 173
magnetic resonance imaging, 172

spleen-liver scan, 173–174
upper endoscopy, 172–173
ulcerative colitis, 199–200, 207
GCS. *See* Glasgow Coma Scale
GERD. *See* Gastroesophageal reflux disease
Gestational diabetes, 260
GFR. *See* Glomerular filtration rate
GH. *See* Growth hormone
Glasgow Coma Scale (GCS), 5, 6
Glioblastoma, 302
Gliomas, 302
Glomerular filtration rate (GFR), 209
Glossopharyngeal nerve, 291
Glucagon, 240
Glucose
blood, 24
cells and, 24
Glucose tolerance test, 244, 264
Gonads, 240–241
Graves' disease. *See* Hyperthyroidism
Greasy stools, 175, 206
Growth hormone (GH), 239
Grunting, rapid respirations and, 122, 160
Guillain-Barré syndrome, 305–307, 323

Headaches, migraine, 297, 324
Heart. *See also* Cardiovascular system
blood flow and, 43
blood supply to, 44
chambers of, 26
cycle of
cardiac output, 45
diastole, 45
stroke volume, 45, 55
systole, 44–45
impulses of, 45
sounds
abnormal, 47–48
normal, 47
valves of, 44
Heart failure, left sided, edema and, 46
Heat stroke. *See* Hyperthermia
Helicobacter pylori, 340
Helper T cells, 28, 41, 327
Hematinics, 343–344
Hematologic studies, for environmental critical care, 272
Hematologic system
acquired immunodeficiency syndrome, 365–366
anaphylaxis, 366–367
anemia, 348–349, 374
aplastic anemia, 349–350, 372
assessment of, 328–329
inspection, 329
palpation, 329
signs and symptoms, 329
critical care definitions, 325
cycle, 325–326
deep vein thrombosis, 362–363
disseminated intravascular coagulation, 353–354, 372
hemophilia, 354–355
idiopathic thrombocytopenic purpura, 363–364
iron deficiency anemia, 350–352
Kaposi's sarcoma, 367–368
leukemia, 355–357
lymphoma, 368–369
medications for
anticoagulants, 343, 373
blood derivatives, 344–345
hematinics, 343–344
hemostatics, 345
heparin antagonist, 344, 372
immune serums, 345
immunosuppressants, 346–347, 374
non-nucleoside reverse transcriptase inhibitors, 347–348
nucleoside analogs, 347
protease inhibitors, 346
multiple myeloma, 358–359
pernicious anemia, 352–353, 372
polycythemia vera, 359–360
scleroderma, 369–370
septic shock, 370–371
sickle cell anemia, 361–362
tests for
antinuclear antibodies, 341, 373
blood culture, 339, 372
blood type, 330
CD4+ count, 341–342, 372
cold agglutinins, 336
complete blood count, 333–336
C-reactive protein, 332–333, 371
Helicobacter pylori, 340
immunoglobulins, 340–341, 373
iron, 338
mononucleosis, 339–340
partial thromboplastin time, 331, 371
prothrombin time, 336–337, 373
reticulocyte count, 337
rheumatoid factor, 342, 373
sedimentation count, 337–338, 372
total serum protein, 331–332
viral load measurement, 342, 373
Hematoma
epidural, 298
intracerebral, 319–320, 322
subdural, 298, 315–316
Hematopoietic system, physiologic reserve measurement in, 2
Hemodialysis, 234–235
Hemophilia, 354–355
Hemorrhage
cerebral, 298–299, 322
intracerebral, 298
subarachnoid, 298, 320–321
Hemorrhagic stroke, 310
Hemorrhoids, 170, 205
Hemostatics, 345
Heparin antagonist, 344, 372
Heparins, 67

Hepatitis, 190–192
Hernia
  hiatal, 192–193
  rolling hiatal, 192
  sliding hiatal, 192, 193
Hiatal hernia, 192–193
Histamine-2 receptor antagonists, 176, 206
Histamines, 42
HIV. *See* Human immunodeficiency virus
Hodgkin's disease, 368
Holosystolic murmur, 48
Homan's sign, 372
Hormonal mechanism, 38
Hormones, 266
  aldosterone, 209
  antidiuretic, 177–178, 206, 239
  corticosteroids, 327, 372
  follicle-stimulating, 239
  growth, 239
  interferon, 327, 372
  interleukin, 327
  luteinizing, 240
  thyrotropic, 38
  tumor necrosis factor, 327
  tymosin, 327
Human immunodeficiency virus (HIV), 342, 347–348, 365, 373
Humoral mechanism, 38
17- Hydroxycorticosteroid test, 246
Hyperparathyroidism, 258–260
Hypertension, 83–85, 115
Hypertensive crisis, 83–85, 115
Hyperthermia, 274–276, 285, 286
Hyperthyroidism, 251–252, 265, 266
Hypertrophic pyloric stenosis, 205
Hypocalcemia, 266
Hypoglossal nerve, 292
Hypoparathyroidism, 264
Hypothalamus, 39
Hypothermia, 276–278, 286
Hypothyroidism, 250–251, 264, 265, 266
Hypovolemia, 227
Hypovolemic shock, 85–86, 115

IDDM. *See* Insulin-dependent diabetes mellitus
Identifying change, in adaptation, 12
Idiopathic thrombocytopenic purpura (ITP), 363–364
Iliopsoas sign, 169–170
IMA. *See* Ischemia modified albumin
Immune serums, 345
Immune system, 29–30
  acquired immunodeficiency syndrome, 365–366
  anaphylaxis, 366–367
  anemia, 348–349, 374
  aplastic anemia, 349–350, 372
  assessment of, 328–329
    inspection, 329
    palpation, 329
    signs and symptoms, 329
  critical care definitions, 325
  cycle, 326–328
  deep vein thrombosis, 362–363
  disseminated intravascular coagulation, 353–354, 372
  hemophilia, 354–355
  idiopathic thrombocytopenic purpura, 363–364
  infection, 30–31, 42
  inflammation, 30–31, 42
  iron deficiency anemia, 350–352
  Kaposi's sarcoma, 367–368
  leukemia, 355–357
  lymphoma, 368–369
  medications for
    anticoagulants, 343, 373
    blood derivatives, 344–345
    hematinics, 343–344
    hemostatics, 345
    heparin antagonist, 344, 372
    immune serums, 345
    immunosuppressants, 346–347, 374
    non-nucleoside reverse transcriptase inhibitors, 347–348
    nucleoside analogs, 347
    protease inhibitors, 346
  multiple myeloma, 358–359
  pernicious anemia, 352–353, 372
  physiologic reserve and, 2, 17
  polycythemia vera, 359–360
  scleroderma, 369–370
  septic shock, 370–371
  sickle cell anemia, 361–362
  tests for
    antinuclear antibodies, 341, 373
    blood culture, 339, 372
    blood type, 330
    CD4+ count, 341–342, 372
    cold agglutinins, 336
    complete blood count, 333–336
    C-reactive protein, 332–333, 371
    Helicobacter pylori, 340
    immunoglobulins, 340–341, 373
    iron, 338
    mononucleosis, 339–340
    partial thromboplastin time, 331, 371
    prothrombin time, 336–337, 373
    reticulocyte count, 337
    rheumatoid factor, 342, 373
    sedimentation count, 337–338, 372
    total serum protein, 331–332
    viral load measurement, 342, 373
Immunoglobulins, 340–341, 373
Immunosuppressants, 346–347, 374
Inderal. *See* Propranolol
Infection, 30–31, 327–328
  chain of, 31, 42, 328
  corticosteroids and, 248, 266
  urinary tract, 229, 238
Inflammation, 30–31, 327–328, 372
  acute, 30, 42
  chronic, 30, 42

Injury
contrecoup, 298
coup, 298, 314, 322
diffuse axonal, 316–317
to spinal cord, 308–310, 322, 324
Inspection
in cardiovascular system assessment, 46
in endocrine system assessment, 241–242
in environmental critical care assessment, 268
in gastrointestinal system assessment, 166–167
in hematologic system assessment, 329
in immune system assessment, 329
in renal system assessment, 211
in respiratory system assessment, 119–120
Insulin, 24, 240, 248–249
guide, 261
Insulin-dependent diabetes mellitus (IDDM), 260
Interferon, 327, 372
Interleukin, 327
Intestines
large, 23, 164
obstruction in, 193–194, 207
small, 23, 164
Intracerebral hematoma, 319–320, 322
Intracerebral hemorrhage, 298
Intravenous pyelogram (IVP), 214–215, 237
Intrinsic asthma. *See* Nonatopic asthma
Iron (Fe), 338
Iron deficiency anemia, 350–352
Ischemia modified albumin (IMA), 51
Ischemic stroke, 310
ITP. *See* Idiopathic thrombocytopenic purpura
IVP. *See* Intravenous pyelogram

Jaundice, 170
Jugular vein distention, edema and, 46
Justice, 14

Kaposi's sarcoma, 367–368
Kayexalate. *See* Sodium polystyrene sulfonate
17- Ketosteroid test, 246
Kidney stones, 225–226, 238
Kidneys, 31. *See also* Renal system
acid-base balance and, 209, 236
blood pressure and, 41, 209
cancer of, 231
red blood cell production and, 209, 236
trauma of, 224–225
Koilonychia sign, 351
KUB radiography, 213, 237

Lactulose, 177, 206
LAPSS. *See* Los Angeles Prehospital Stroke Scale
Large intestine, 23, 164
Laryngeal edema, after thyroid surgery, 266
Left coronary artery, 44
Left sided heart failure, edema and, 46
Legs, body hair on, 46, 114
Leukemia, 355–357
Leukocytes. *See* White blood cells
Level of conscience (LOC), 287
LH. *See* Luteinizing hormone
Linear skull fracture, 317
Liver
cirrhosis of, 180–183, 206
digestion and, 24, 41, 164
disease of, blood pressure and, 41
physiologic reserve of, 7
Liver function tests, 174
LOC. *See* Level of conscience
Loop diuretics, 65, 220–221
Los Angeles Prehospital Stroke Scale (LAPSS), 106
Loss of consortium, 16
Lower gastrointestinal endoscopy, 173
Lumbar puncture, 295
Lund and Browder Classification, 278
Luteinizing hormone (LH), 38, 240
Lymph system, 327
Lymphocytes, 326
Lymphocytic leukemia, 355
Lymphokine-producing cells, 327
Lymphoma, 368–369

Magnetic resonance imaging (MRI)
of central nervous system, 294
of gastrointestinal system, 172
of renal system, 213
thoracic, 128
Malpractice, 15
Mannitol, 282, 286
McBurney's Point, 169, 206
Mechanical ventilation, 157–158
Medically futile, 18
Medulla, 39
Melatonin, 240
Memory T cells, 28, 41, 327
Meningiomas, 302, 323
Meningitis, 307–308, 322
Metabolic acidosis, 125, 270
Metabolic alkalosis, 125, 270
Metabolic syndrome, 263–264
MI. *See* Myocardial infarction
Mid-diastolic murmur, 48
Midsystolic murmur, 48
Migraine headaches, 297, 324
Milestones, stress and
provide family with, 11
provide patient with, 10
Mitral valve, 44
MOF. *See* Multiple organ failure
Monocytes, 326
Mononucleosis, 339–340
Monospot test, 339
Mortality Probability Model (MPM), 3
Motor function, 292
MPM. *See* Mortality Probability Model
MRI. *See* Magnetic resonance imaging
Mucus, in stools, 175, 206

Multiorgan dysfunction syndrome, 2–3, 17
Multiple myeloma, 358–359
Multiple organ failure (MOF), 3
Multisystem critical care
  acid-base, blood gas test results, 37
  blood, 26
    plasma, 28
    platelets, 28, 42
    red blood cells, 27
    Rh group, 28–29
    type of, 28
    white blood cells, 27–28
  cardiovascular system, 24–25, 40–41
    cardiac output maintenance, 25
    conduction system, 26
    coronary circulation, 26, 40
    heart chambers, 26
  cells
    function of, 21–22, 40
    glucose and, 24
  digestion and, 22–23
    liver and, 24, 41
  electrolytes, 31–32
    critical thinking, 34–36
    tests for, 32–33
    treatment for, 33–34
  endocrine system, 38
  fluids, 31–32
  immune system, 29–30
    infection, 30–31, 42
    inflammation, 30–31, 42
  kidneys, 31, 41
  neurologic system, 39
Murmurs, 48–49, 114
Myelogenous leukemia, 355
Myocardial infarction (MI), 76–78
  chest pain and, 50
Myocarditis, 86–87
Myoclonic seizures, 312
Myoglobin, 51
Myxedema. *See* Hypothyroidism

Nasogastric (NG)
  decompression, 203–204, 207
  intubation, 202–203, 207
Negligence, 15
Nerves
  abducens, 291
  accessory, 292
  acoustic, 291
  cranial, function of, 290–292
  facial, 291
  glossopharyngeal, 291
  hypoglossal, 292
  olfactory, 291
  optic, 291
  trigeminal, 291
  trochlear, 291
  vagus, 291
Neurologic system, 39
  assessment of, 288–292
    cranial nerve function, 290–292
    motor function, 292
    pupil changes, 290
    reflexes, 292
    signs and symptoms of, 290–292
  Bell's palsy, 300
  brain abscess, 300–301
  brain tumor, 302–303
  cerebral aneurysm, 303–304, 323, 324
  cerebral hemorrhage, 298–299, 322
  cerebrovascular accident, 310–311, 321
  concussion, 313–314, 322–323
  contusion, 314–315, 322, 323
  critical care definitions, 287
  critical condition treatment goals, 287
  diffuse axonal injury, 316–317
  encephalitis, 304–305, 322, 323
  Guillain-Barré syndrome, 305–307, 323
  intracerebral hematoma, 319–320, 322
  medications for
    anticoagulants, 296
    anticonvulsants, 296
    antiplatelets, 296, 323
    barbiturates, 296
    benzodiazepines, 296
    calcium channel blockers, 297, 323
    corticosteroids, 297
    diuretics, 297
    opioid analgesics, 297, 323
    serotonin inhibitors, 297
    thrombolytics, 297, 323
  meningitis, 307–308, 322
  procedures for
    cerebral angiograph, 293–295, 322
    lumbar puncture, 295
  seizure disorder, 311–313, 323
  skull fracture, 317–319
  spinal cord injury, 308–310, 322, 324
  subarachnoid hemorrhage, 320–321
  subdural hematoma, 315–316
  tests for
    brain computed tomography scan, 293–294, 323
    central nervous system magnetic resonance imaging, 294
    cerebral angiograph, 295, 322
    spinal computed tomography scan, 293–294
    spinal x-ray, 293
Neuromuscular blocking medications, 133–134, 161
Neutrophils, 326
NG. *See* Nasogastric
NHL. *See* Non-Hodgkin's lymphoma
NIDDM. *See* Non-insulin dependent diabetes mellitus
Nitrates, 61–62
Nonatopic asthma, 135
Noncatecholamines, 69–70
Non-Hodgkin's lymphoma (NHL), 368
Non-insulin dependent diabetes mellitus (NIDDM), 260

Nonmaleficence, 13
Non-nucleoside reverse transcriptase inhibitors, 347–348
Nonsteroidal anti-inflammatory drugs (NSAIDs), 273
Norepinephrine, 240
Normal mechanism, 38
NSAIDs. *See* Nonsteroidal anti-inflammatory drugs
Nucleoside analogs, 347
Nurse, role of, in critical care stressor reduction, 10, 18–19

O_2. *See* Oxygen
Obturator sign, 169
OGTT. *See* Oral glucose tolerance test
Olfactory nerve, 291
Oligodendroglioma, 302
Open pneumothorax, 146
Opioid analgesics, 297, 323
Optic nerve, 291
Oral antidiabetic, 249–250
Oral glucose tolerance test (OGTT), 261
Oral hypoglycemic agents, 261
Oropharyngeal suctioning, 159
Oxygen (O_2), 40
  blood and, 24
Oxygen saturation, 124, 160
Oxygen therapy, 154
Oxytocin, 38, 239

P wave, 51, 271
Pacemaker, 113
Pacemaker lumen, 56
Pain
  in abdomen, 170
  in chest, 49–50
Palpation
  in cardiovascular system assessment, 46–47
  in endocrine system assessment, 242
  in gastrointestinal system assessment, 168–169
  in hematologic system assessment, 329
  in immune system assessment, 329
  in renal system assessment, 211–212, 236
  in respiratory system assessment, 120
Pancreas, 240
  digestion and, 164
Pancreatitis, 193–194, 207
Pancytopenia. *See* Aplastic anemia
Paracentesis, 204–205, 207
Paralytic ileus, 193–194, 207
Parathyroid gland, 240
Parathyroid hormone (PTH), 240
Parkland formula, 281, 286
Partial thromboplastin time (PTT), 331, 371
Patient advocate, failure to be, 16
Patient education, stress and, 10
Patient interaction, stress and, 10
Patient privacy, failure to maintain, 16
Pattern recognition receptors (PRR), 30, 42
Pediatrics
  burns and, 278, 279
  respiratory system assessment in, 123
Penetrating abdominal trauma, 201
Pepsin, 23
Peptic ulcer disease (PUD), 197–199, 205
Percussion
  in cardiovascular system assessment, 47
  in gastrointestinal system assessment, 168
  in renal system assessment, 211
  in respiratory system assessment, 120–121
Pericarditis, 87–89
  chest pain and, 50
Peripheral nervous system, 39
Peritoneal dialysis, 235–236
Peritonitis, 196–197, 205
Permanent disability, fear of, 10, 11
Pernicious anemia, 352–353, 372
pH blood value, 125, 160
Pheochromocytoma, 257–258, 265
Phosphodiesterase inhibitors, 57–58
Physiologic reserve, measurement of, 2, 17
  hematopoietic system, 2
  pulmonary system, 2
  renal system, 2
Pineal, 240
Pinpoint pupils, 290
Pituitary gland, 39, 239
Plantar reflex, 292
Plasma, 28
Plasma expander, for spinal cord injury, 324
Platelets, 28, 42, 326
  bleeding and, 272, 285
Pleural effusion, 144–145, 161
Pleural friction rub, 121
Pneumonia, 145–146
Pneumothorax, 146–147
Poisoning, 282–284, 286
Polycythemia vera, 359–360
Postrenal failure, 227
Potassium-sparing diuretics, 66, 221–222
PR interval (PRI), 51, 271
Preload, 45
Prerenal failure, 227
PRI. *See* PR interval
Primary aldosteronism, 256–257
Prinzmetal's angina, 74
Privacy
  failure to maintain, 16
  lack of, 10
Progesterone, 241
Projectile vomiting, 170, 205
Prolactin, 38
Propranolol (Inderal), 59–60, 114
Protease inhibitors, 346
Prothrombin time (PT), 336–337, 373
Proton pump inhibitors, 177
Proximal lumen, 56
PRR. *See* Pattern recognition receptors
Psoas sign. *See* Iliopsoas sign
PT. *See* Prothrombin time
PTH. *See* Parathyroid hormone

PTT. *See* Partial thromboplastin time
PUD. *See* Peptic ulcer disease
Pulmonary angiography, 129–130, 160
Pulmonary arterial blood pressure, monitoring of, 56, 114
Pulmonary edema, 89–90, 115
Pulmonary embolism, 151–153, 161
  chest pain and, 50
Pulmonary system, physiologic reserve measurement in, 2
Pulmonary vascular resistance, 55–56
Pulmonic valve, 44
Pulse oximetry, 124
Pulses, 46–47
Pupils, changes in, 290
Pyelonephritis, 226–227, 238

QRS complex, 52, 271
QT interval (QTI), 52, 271

Radionuclide thyroid imaging, 243–244, 264, 266
Rapid respirations, grunting and, 122, 160
RBC. *See* Red blood cells
Rebound tenderness, 169
Red blood cells (RBC), 27, 325
  production, kidneys and, 209, 236
Reed-Sternberg cells, 368
Reflexes, 292
Renal angiograph, 215, 237
Renal calculi. *See* Kidney stones
Renal failure, 227–228
Renal scan, 214, 237
Renal system
  acute glomerulonephritis, 223
  acute tubular necrosis, 232
  assessment of, 209–212
    auscultation, 211, 236
    inspection, 211
    palpation, 211–212, 236
    percussion, 211
    signs and symptoms, 212
  bladder cancer, 229–230
  critical care definitions, 208
  cycle, 208–209
  detoxification in, 208–209
  kidney cancer, 231
  kidney stones, 225–226, 238
  kidney trauma, 224–225
  medications for
    adrenergics, 220
    alkalinizing agent, 222–223
    diuretics, 220–222
    sulfonate cation-exchange resin, 222
  physiologic reserve of, 7
    measurement in, 2
  procedures for
    calculi basketing, 233, 238
    extracorporeal shock wave lithotripsy, 233–234, 238
    hemodialysis, 234–235
    peritoneal dialysis, 235–236
  pyelonephritis, 226–227, 238
  renal failure, 227–228
  tests for
    intravenous pyelogram, 214–215, 237
    KUB radiography, 213, 237
    renal angiograph, 215, 237
    renal blood tests, 215–217
    renal scan, 214, 237
    urinary computed tomography scan, 212–213, 236
    urinary magnetic resonance imaging, 213
    urinary ultrasound, 214
    urine analysis, 217–219, 236, 237, 238
  urinary tract infection, 229, 238
Renin, 3
Reorganization, in adaptation, 12
Resolution, in adaptation, 12
Respiratory acidosis, 125, 147–148, 270
Respiratory alkalosis, 125, 270
Respiratory arrest, 153
Respiratory system
  acute respiratory distress syndrome, 134–135, 161
  acute respiratory failure, 150–151
  assessment of, 118–122
    auscultation, 121–122
    inspection, 119–120
    palpation, 120
    in pediatrics, 123
    percussion, 120–121
    signs and symptoms, 122–123
  asthma, 135–137, 161
  atelectasis, 137–138, 161
  bronchiectasis, 138, 161
  bronchitis, 139–141
  cor pulmonale, 141–142, 161
  critical care definitions, 117
  cycle, 117
  emphysema, 142–144
  medication for
    anticholinergics, 131, 160
    anti-inflammatory, 131–132
    bronchodilators, 130–131
    neuromuscular blocking, 133–134, 161
    sedatives, 132–133, 161
  pleural effusion, 144–145, 161
  pneumonia, 145–146
  pneumothorax, 146–147
  procedures for
    aerosol therapy, 154–155
    chest tube, 158–159, 162
    continuous positive airway pressure therapy, 155, 161
    endotracheal rapid sequence intubation, 155–157
    endotracheal suctioning, 159, 162
    mechanical ventilation, 157–158
    oropharyngeal suctioning, 159
    oxygen therapy, 154
    tracheotomy, 158, 162
  pulmonary embolism, 151–153, 161
  respiratory acidosis, 147–148
  respiratory arrest, 153

tests for
arterial blood gas, 125–126
bronchoscopy, 126–127
chest x-ray, 127–128, 160
end-tidal carbon dioxide monitor, 126, 160
pulmonary angiography, 129–130, 160
pulse oximetry, 124
sputum analysis, 127, 160
thoracic computed tomography scan, 128
thoracic magnetic resonance imaging scan, 128
ventilation perfusion scan, 128–129, 160
tuberculosis, 148–149
Reticulocyte count, 337
RF. *See* Rheumatoid factor
Rh blood group, 28–29
Rheumatoid factor (RF), 342, 373
Rhonchi, 121
Right coronary artery, 44
Rolling hiatal hernia, 192
Rubs, 49
Rule of Nines, 278, 279

S3 heart sound, 47
S4 heart sound, 47–48
SAPS. *See* Simplified Acute Physiology Score
Scleroderma, 369–370
Second degree burn, 278
SED. *See* Sedimentation count
Sedatives, 132–133, 161
Sedimentation count (SED), 337–338, 372
Seizure disorder, 311–313, 323
Seizures, Dilantin and, 324
Self-determination, failure to adhere to, 16
Semilunar valves, 44
Separation, stress and, 10, 11
Septic shock, 370–371, 372
Sequential Organ Failure Assessment Score (SOFA), 3
Serotonin inhibitors, 297
Shock
cardiogenic, 79–80
hypovolemic, 85–86, 115
septic, 370–371, 372
warming, 278, 286
Shortness of breath, 118–119
SIADH. *See* Syndrome of inappropriate antidiuretic hormone secretion
Sickle cell anemia, 361–362
Simple partial seizures, 312
Simplified Acute Physiology Score (SAPS), 3
Skin, 326
bronzing of, 266
shiny, 46, 114
Skull fracture, 317–319
Sleep disruption, stress and, 10
Sliding hiatal hernia, 192, 193
Small intestine, 23, 164
Sodium polystyrene sulfonate (Kayexalate), 222, 238
SOFA. *See* Sequential Organ Failure Assessment Score
Somatic nervous system, 39
Somatotropin, 38, 239
Sorbitol, 274, 285
Spinal cord injury, 308–310, 322
plasma expander for, 324
Spine
computed tomography scan of, 293–294
x-ray of, 293
Spleen, immune system and, 327
Spleen-liver scan, 173–174
Spontaneous pneumothorax, 146
Sputum analysis, 127, 160
ST segment, 52, 271
Stable angina, 74
Stools
blood in, 170, 205
greasy, 175, 206
mucus in, 175, 206
Stressors, critical care patient and, 9–11
nurse role in reduction of, 18–19
Stridor, on expiration, 121, 122, 160
Stroke
hemorrhagic, 310
ischemic, 310
Stroke volume, 45, 55
Subarachnoid hemorrhage, 298, 320–321
Subdural hematoma, 298, 315–316
Sulfonate cation-exchange resin, 222
Superficial burn, 278
Superficial partial-thickness burn, 278
Suppressor T cells, 28, 41, 327
Sympatholytic medications, 63
Synchronized cardioversion, 112–113
Syndrome of inappropriate antidiuretic hormone secretion (SIADH), 253–254, 265
Syndrome X. *See* Metabolic syndrome
Systemic vascular resistance, 55
Systole, 44–45

T cells, 41. *See also* Cells
T3. *See* Triiodothyronine
T4. *See* Thyroxine
Tactile stimulation, 292
TEE. *See* Transesophageal echocardiography
Temperature, body, measurement of, 286
Tension pneumothorax, 146
Testes, 241
Testosterone, 241
Thalamus, 39
Thermistor connector lumen, 56
Thermodilution, 54
Thiazide diuretics, 65, 221
Third degree burn, 278
Thoracic
computed tomography scan of, 128
magnetic resonance imaging scan of, 128
Thrombolytic agent (t-PA), 68–69, 297, 323, 324
Thrombophlebitis, 90–91
edema and, 46
Thymopoietin, 240

Thymosin, 240
Thymus, 327
Thyroid gland, 240
Thyroid hormone replacement, 246–247, 266
Thyroid releasing hormone (TRH), 21
Thyroid stimulating hormone (TSH), 38, 239, 245, 265
Thyrotropic hormone, 38
Thyroxine (T4), 240
TIA. *See* Transient ischemic attack
TIBC. *See* Total iron binding capacity test
TNF. *See* Tumor necrosis factor
Tonic seizures, 312
Tonic/clonic seizures, 312
Total iron binding capacity (TIBC) test, 338
Total serum protein, 331–332
Toxin, 29
t-PA. *See* Thrombolytic agent
Tracheotomy, 158, 162
Transesophageal echocardiography (TEE), 52
Transient ischemic attack (TIA), 105, 310
Trauma
  of abdomen, 201–202
  of kidneys, 224–225
TRH. *See* Thyroid releasing hormone
Tricuspid valve, 44
Trigeminal nerve, 291
Triiodothyronine (T3), 240
Trochlear nerve, 291
Troponin, 51
Trousseau's sign, 242
Trust, establishment of, 11
TSH. *See* Thyroid stimulating hormone
Tuberculosis, 148–149
Tumor, of brain, 302–303
Tumor necrosis factor (TNF), 327
Turner's sign, 195, 207
Tymosin, 327

Ulcer
  duodenal, 197
  gastric, 197
Ulcerative colitis, 199–200, 207
Ultrasound, of renal system, 214
Unstable angina, 74
Upper gastrointestinal endoscopy, 172–173
Urinary tract infection, 229, 238
Urine
  analysis of
    for endocrine system, 246
    for renal system, 217–219, 236, 237, 238
  cloudy, 218, 238

Vagus nerve, 291
Valves
  of heart, 44
  surgery for, 110–111
Varicosities, edema and, 46
Vascular assist device, 112
Vascular surgery, 111
Vasodilating medications, 63–64
Vasopressin, 38
Vasospastic angina, 74
Venous insufficiency, edema and, 46
Ventilation perfusion scan, 128–129, 160
Ventricular fibrillation, 94–96
Ventricular tachycardia, 96–98
Veracity, 13
Viral load measurement, 342, 373
Viral meningitis, 307
Virus, 29
Voice, changes in, burns and, 286
Vomit. *See also* Coffee ground emesis
  blood in, 170, 205
  projectile, 170, 205

Warming shock, 278, 286
WBC. *See* White blood cells
Wheezes, 121
Whispered pectoriloquy, 122
White blood cells (WBC), 27–28, 325–326, 371
Wrongful death, 16

X-ray
  of abdomen, 171
  of chest, 127–128, 160
  of spine, 293